HIV/AIDS

ISSN 2332-3841

HIV/AIDS

Barbara Wexler

INFORMATION PLUS® REFERENCE SERIES
Formerly Published by Information Plus, Wylie, Texas

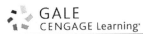
GALE
CENGAGE Learning·

Farmington Hills, Mich • San Francisco • New York • Waterville, Maine
Meriden, Conn • Mason, Ohio • Chicago

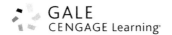

HIV/AIDS

Barbara Wexler

Kepos Media, Inc.: Steven Long and Janice Jorgensen, Series Editors

Project Editors: Laura Avery, Tracie Moy

Rights Acquisition and Management: Ashley Maynard, Carissa Poweleit

Composition: Evi Abou-El-Seoud, Mary Beth Trimper

Manufacturing: Rita Wimberley

For product information and technology assistance, contact us at
Gale Customer Support, 1-800-877-4253.
For permission to use material from this text or product,
submit all requests online at **www.cengage.com/permissions.**
Further permissions questions can be e-mailed to
permissionrequest@cengage.com

Cover photograph: © Susan Walsh/AP Photo.

While every effort has been made to ensure the reliability of the information presented in this publication, Gale, a part of Cengage Learning, does not guarantee the accuracy of the data contained herein. Gale accepts no payment for listing; and inclusion in the publication of any organization, agency, institution, publication, service, or individual does not imply endorsement of the editors or publisher. Errors brought to the attention of the publisher and verified to the satisfaction of the publisher will be corrected in future editions.

Gale
27500 Drake Rd.
Farmington Hills, MI 48331-3535

ISBN-13: 978-0-7876-5103-9 (set)
ISBN-13: 978-1-5730-2665-9

ISSN 2332-3841

This title is also available as an e-book.
ISBN-13: 978-1-5730-2709-0 (set)
Contact your Gale sales representative for ordering information.

Printed in the United States of America
1 2 3 4 5   20 19 18 17 16

TABLE OF CONTENTS

HIV/AIDS, knowledge and tolerance, and the persistence of misinformation about HIV/AIDS. Efforts to heighten public awareness, such as the AIDS Memorial Quilt, AIDS activist organizations, and celebrity activists, are also highlighted.

PREFACE

HIV/AIDS is part of the *Information Plus Reference Series*. The purpose of each volume of the series is to present the latest facts on a topic of pressing concern in modern American life. These topics include the most controversial and studied social issues of the 21st century: abortion, capital punishment, care of older adults, crime, the environment, health care, immigration, national security, sports, women, youth, and many more. Although this series is written especially for high school and undergraduate students, it is an excellent resource for anyone in need of factual information on current affairs.

By presenting the facts, it is the intention of Gale, Cengage Learning, to provide its readers with everything they need to reach an informed opinion on current issues. To that end, there is a particular emphasis in this series on the presentation of scientific studies, surveys, and statistics. These data are generally presented in the form of tables, charts, and other graphics placed within the text of each book. Every graphic is directly referred to and carefully explained in the text. The source of each graphic is presented within the graphic itself. The data used in these graphics are drawn from the most reputable and reliable sources, such as the various branches of the U.S. government and private organizations and associations. Every effort has been made to secure the most recent information available. Readers should bear in mind that many major studies take years to conduct and that additional years often pass before the data from these studies are made available to the public. Therefore, in many cases the most recent information available in 2016 is dated from 2013 or 2014. Older statistics are sometimes presented as well if they are landmark studies or of particular interest and no more-recent information exists.

Although statistics are a major focus of the *Information Plus Reference Series*, they are by no means its only content. Each book also presents the widely held positions and important ideas that shape how the book's subject is discussed in the United States. These positions are explained in detail and, where possible, in the words of their proponents. Some of the other material to be found in these books includes historical background, descriptions of major events related to the subject, relevant laws and court cases, and examples of how these issues play out in American life. Some books also feature primary documents or have pro and con debate sections that provide the words and opinions of prominent Americans on both sides of a controversial topic. All material is presented in an evenhanded and unbiased manner; readers will never be encouraged to accept one view of an issue over another.

HOW TO USE THIS BOOK

The spread of the acquired immunodeficiency syndrome (AIDS) has become a global epidemic. As of 2014, an estimated 37 million people worldwide were living with the human immunodeficiency virus (HIV), according to the Joint United Nations Programme on HIV/AIDS. That same year there were 2 million new HIV cases diagnosed and 1.2 million HIV-related deaths. This book includes information on the nature of HIV/AIDS and the HIV/AIDS epidemic; symptoms and transmittal; patterns and trends in surveillance; populations at risk; children, adolescents, costs, and treatment; people living with HIV/AIDS; testing, prevention, and education; HIV/AIDS worldwide; and knowledge, awareness, behavior, and opinion of those affected by HIV/AIDS.

HIV/AIDS consists of 10 chapters and three appendixes. Each chapter is devoted to a particular aspect of HIV/AIDS. For a summary of the information that is covered in each chapter, please see the synopses that are provided in the Table of Contents. Chapters generally begin with an overview of the basic facts and background information on the chapter's topic, then proceed to examine subtopics of particular interest. For example,

Chapter 4: Populations at Risk begins with a description of the prevalence rates of HIV infection—that is, the total number of people with HIV/AIDS in a population at a specified time. The chapter then describes rates of HIV infection and AIDS in various populations, noting changes such as a decreasing percentage of infections attributable to male-to-male sexual contact and an increasing proportion of cases among heterosexuals. The chapter describes the epidemiology of HIV/AIDS in terms of specific populations by examining differences based on age, race, geography, sex, and transmission category. It also discusses HIV/AIDS among hemophiliacs, prisoners, and sex workers. Readers can find their way through a chapter by looking for the section and subsection headings, which are clearly set off from the text. They can also refer to the book's extensive Index if they already know what they are looking for.

Statistical Information

The tables and figures featured throughout *HIV/AIDS* will be of particular use to readers in learning about this issue. These tables and figures represent an extensive collection of the most recent and important statistics on HIV/AIDS and related issues—for example, graphics cover the number of people living with HIV infection, pediatric AIDS cases, the number of annual AIDS deaths, an HIV replication cycle, home HIV tests, and recommended laboratory tests for HIV. Gale, Cengage Learning, believes that making this information available to readers is the most important way to fulfill the goal of this book: to help readers understand the issues and controversies surrounding HIV/AIDS in the United States and to reach their own conclusions.

Each table or figure has a unique identifier appearing above it, for ease of identification and reference. Titles for the tables and figures explain their purpose. At the end of each table or figure, the original source of the data is provided.

To help readers understand these often complicated statistics, all tables and figures are explained in the text. References in the text direct readers to the relevant statistics. Furthermore, the contents of all tables and figures are fully indexed. Please see the opening section of the Index at the back of this volume for a description of how to find tables and figures within it.

Appendixes

Besides the main body text and images, *HIV/AIDS* has three appendixes. The first is the Important Names and Addresses directory. Here, readers will find contact information for a number of government and private organizations that can provide further information on HIV/AIDS. The second appendix is the Resources section, which can also assist readers in conducting their own research. In this section, the author and editors of *HIV/AIDS* describe some of the sources that were most useful during the compilation of this book. The final appendix is the detailed Index. It has been greatly expanded from previous editions and should make it even easier to find specific topics in this book.

COMMENTS AND SUGGESTIONS

The editors of the *Information Plus Reference Series* welcome your feedback on *HIV/AIDS*. Please direct all correspondence to:

Editors
Information Plus Reference Series
27500 Drake Rd.
Farmington Hills, MI 48331-3535

CHAPTER 1
THE NATURE OF HIV/AIDS

Acquired immunodeficiency syndrome (AIDS) is the late stage of an infection caused by the human immuno-deficiency virus (HIV). HIV is a retrovirus that destroys certain white blood cells. The targeted destruction weakens the body's immune system and makes the infected person susceptible to infections and diseases that ordinarily would not be life threatening. AIDS is a blood-borne, sexually transmitted disease because HIV is spread through contact with blood, semen, or vaginal fluids from an infected person.

In 1981 the Centers for Disease Control and Prevention (CDC) reported that five previously healthy young men in California had been diagnosed with an unusual pattern of infections indicative of compromised immune systems. The cause of their conditions was not known at the time. The CDC's report attracted the attention of doctors around the country who had patients with similar symptoms, and by the end of the year 270 cases of severe immune deficiency had been reported. In 1982 the CDC established a case definition for the disease, which it termed AIDS. In 1983 a research team at the Pasteur Institute in Paris, France, led by Luc Montagnier (1932–), Françoise Barré-Sinoussi (1947–), and Harald zur Hausen (1936–) first isolated HIV and identified it as the cause of AIDS. Montagnier, Barré-Sinoussi, and zur Hausen were awarded the Nobel Prize in Physiology or Medicine for this discovery in 2008.

Over time, awareness grew as the annual number of diagnosed cases and deaths steadily increased. In "First 500,000 AIDS Cases—United States, 1995" (*Morbidity and Mortality Weekly Report*, vol. 44, no. 46, November 24, 1995), the CDC stated that the number of U.S. AIDS cases reported since 1981 reached the half-million mark in 1995. It also indicated that HIV infection was the leading cause of death among Americans aged 25 to 44 years.

By 1998, however, HIV/AIDS deaths among this age group had fallen dramatically. That year HIV infection was the fifth most-common cause of death among people in the United States aged 25 to 44 years. By 2013 HIV as a cause of death had dropped to eighth place among people aged 25 to 34 years, with the disease claiming 631 lives, and to ninth place among those aged 35 to 44 years, claiming 1,246 lives. (See Table 1.1.)

Overall, HIV mortality (death) rates plateaued in 1995 and began to decline in 1996, even before the widespread use of effective drug treatments such as protease inhibitors. In 1997 HIV infection was the 14th leading cause of death overall in the United States. By 1999 HIV infection no longer ranked among the 15 leading causes of death in the United States. Figure 1.1 shows that after a sharp decline in deaths from HIV/AIDS in the mid-1990s the annual number of deaths has been slowly declining.

Although the overall decline in HIV/AIDS deaths between 1995 and 2012 was a positive trend for people infected with HIV and those suffering from AIDS, the reality is that the total number of people living with HIV/AIDS increased during this period. In other words, even though not as many people were dying from HIV/AIDS, more people were living with the disease due to successful therapies.

The observed decline in HIV/AIDS deaths is small reassurance at best to the many thousands of people who are diagnosed with an HIV infection each year in the United States. The CDC indicates in *HIV Surveillance Report: Diagnoses of HIV Infection in the United States and Dependent Areas, 2013* (February 2015, http://www.cdc.gov/hiv/pdf/g-l/hiv_surveillance_report_vol_25.pdf#Page=5) that in 2013 there were an estimated 47,352 new cases of HIV infection in adults, adolescents, and children. In "Basic Statistics" (May 11, 2015, http://www.cdc.gov/hiv/statistics/basics.html), the CDC reports that an estimated 1.2 million people were living with HIV infection in 2013. About 13% of these people were unaware of their infection.

TABLE 1.1

Deaths and death rates for the 15 leading causes of death among persons aged 25–44, 2013

Rank*	Cause of death	Number	Percent of total deaths	Rate
All races, both sexes, 25–34 years				
...	All causes	45,463	100.0	106.1
1	Accidents (unintentional injuries)	16,209	35.7	37.8
2	Intentional self-harm (suicide)	6,348	14.0	14.8
3	Assault (homicide)	4,236	9.3	9.9
4	Malignant neoplasms	3,673	8.1	8.6
5	Diseases of heart	3,258	7.2	7.6
6	Diabetes mellitus	684	1.5	1.6
7	Chronic liver disease and cirrhosis	676	1.5	1.6
8	Human immunodeficiency virus (HIV) disease	631	1.4	1.5
9	Cerebrovascular diseases	508	1.1	1.2
10	Influenza and pneumonia	449	1.0	1.0
11	Pregnancy, childbirth and the puerperium	441	1.0	1.0
12	Congenital malformations, deformations and chromosomal abnormalities	423	0.9	1.0
13	Septicemia	333	0.7	0.8
14	Chronic lower respiratory diseases	291	0.6	0.7
15	Nephritis, nephrotic syndrome and nephrosis	266	0.6	0.6
...	All other causes (residual)	7,037	15.5	16.4
All races, both sexes, 35–44 years				
...	All causes	69,573	100.0	172.0
1	Accidents (unintentional injuries)	15,354	22.1	38.0
2	Malignant neoplasms	11,349	16.3	28.1
3	Diseases of heart	10,341	14.9	25.6
4	Intentional self-harm (suicide)	6,551	9.4	16.2
5	Assault (homicide)	2,581	3.7	6.4
6	Chronic liver disease and cirrhosis	2,491	3.6	6.2
7	Diabetes mellitus	1,952	2.8	4.8
8	Cerebrovascular diseases	1,687	2.4	4.2
9	Human immunodeficiency virus (HIV) disease	1,246	1.8	3.1
10	Influenza and pneumonia	881	1.3	2.2
11	Septicemia	820	1.2	2.0
12	Chronic lower respiratory diseases	760	1.1	1.9
13	Nephritis, nephrotic syndrome and nephrosis	627	0.9	1.5
14	Congenital malformations, deformations and chromosomal abnormalities	441	0.6	1.1
15	Essential hypertension and hypertensive renal disease	409	0.6	1.0
...	All other causes (residual)	12,083	17.4	29.9

*Rank based on number of deaths.

SOURCE: Adapted from "LCWK2. Deaths, Percent of Total Deaths, and Death Rates for the 15 Leading Causes of Death in 10-year Age Groups, by Race and Sex: United States, 2013," in *National Vital Statistics System: Mortality Tables*, Centers for Disease Control and Prevention/National Center for Health Statistics, December 31, 2014, http://www.cdc.gov/nchs/data/dvs/LCWK2_2013.pdf (accessed July 9, 2015)

The American Foundation for AIDS Research notes in "Thirty Years of HIV/AIDS: Snapshots of an Epidemic" (2015, http://www.amfar.org/thirty-years-of-hiv/aids-snapshots-of-an-epidemic) that between 1996 and 1997 the number of AIDS deaths declined 42%. This dramatic decrease was due to the introduction and use of effective antiretroviral drugs that slow the progression of HIV infection. This decline continued in the following years, but at a slower pace, with deaths dropping 21% between 1997 and 1998, and 5% between 1998 and 1999. This may be due to a combination of several factors, including complicated drug treatment regimens that were difficult for patients to maintain and a lack of access to prompt testing or treatment. In "Basic Statistics," the CDC notes that as of 2012 an estimated 658,507 people diagnosed with AIDS in the United States had died, including 13,712 people that year alone.

The AIDS epidemic is not restricted to the United States. According to the CDC, in 2013 approximately 2.1 million new cases of HIV occurred worldwide, and an estimated 35 million people were living with HIV/AIDS that year. As of 2013 a total of about 39 million people around the world had died of AIDS, including roughly 1.5 million deaths that year. Although the countries of sub-Saharan Africa continue to have the world's highest annual rates of HIV infection and death, the epidemic has also taken a toll on Southeast Asia, Central Asia, Eastern Europe, and Latin America.

THE HUMAN IMMUNODEFICIENCY VIRUS

A virus is a tiny infectious agent composed of genes that are surrounded by a protective coating. Until a virus contacts a host cell, it is essentially an inert bag of genetic material. Viruses are parasites. They must invade other cells and commandeer the host cell's replication machinery to reproduce. A frequent outcome of viral infection is the destruction of the host cell, as the newly made virus particles burst out of the cell. This host cell's destruction can harm the organism that the host cell is a part of (in the case of HIV, a human).

HIV belongs to a group of viruses called retroviruses. The name arises from the presence of a special enzyme—reverse transcriptase—that reverses the usual pattern of translating the genetic message. (See Figure 1.2.) In animals, genes consist of deoxyribonucleic acid (DNA). DNA is the blueprint from which another type of genetic material called ribonucleic acid (RNA) is made, in a process called transcription. In turn, the RNA serves as the blueprint for the proteins used in the organism. In contrast to animals, retroviruses store their genes in RNA. After HIV infects a human cell, the viral reverse transcriptase transcribes HIV RNA into DNA. The viral DNA then becomes part of the host DNA—a process called integration—and is replicated along with the host DNA to produce new HIV particles.

Before 1980 retroviruses had been found in some animals. As far back as 1911 Francis Peyton Rous (1879–1970) isolated an infectious and debilitating virus from a chicken. The Rous sarcoma virus was later shown to be a cancer-causing virus and the first known retrovirus. The first known human retroviruses, human T-cell leukemia virus (HTLV-I) and the closely related human T-cell lymphotropic virus (HTLV-II), were discovered in 1980 by Robert C. Gallo (1937–) and his colleagues at the National Cancer Institute (NCI). This breakthrough provided the groundwork for discovery of the virus that would eventually be known as HIV.

FIGURE 1.1

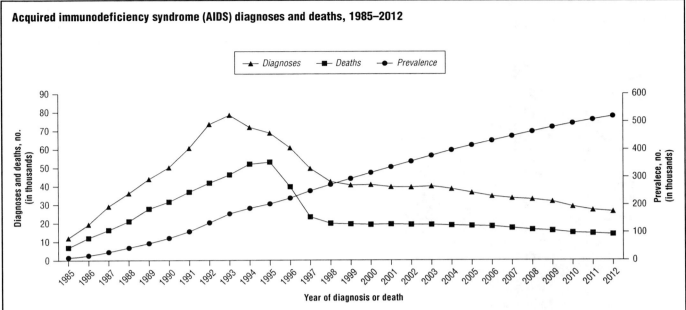

Acquired immunodeficiency syndrome (AIDS) diagnoses and deaths, 1985–2012

Note: All displayed data have been statistically adjusted to account for reporting delays, but not for incomplete reporting. Deaths of persons with HIV infection, stage 3 (AIDS) may be due to any cause.

SOURCE: "Stage 3 (AIDS) Classifications and Deaths of Persons with HIV Infection Ever Classified as Stage 3 (AIDS), among Adults and Adolescents, 1985–2012—United States and 6 Dependent Areas," in *Trends in HIV Infection, Stage 3 (AIDS)*, Centers for Disease Control and Prevention, June 5, 2015, http://www.cdc.gov/hiv/pdf/statistics_surveillance_aidstrends.pdf (accessed July 9, 2015)

Identifying the Virus

In September 1983 Montagnier and his colleagues at the Pasteur Institute took a sample from a lymph node biopsy of a patient and identified a retrovirus they named lymphadenopathy-associated virus (LAV). Eight months later Gallo's group at the NCI isolated the same virus in AIDS patients, which they called HTLV-III. LAV and HTLV-III were found to be identical and are now referred to as HIV. A conflict arose about which researcher should be credited with the discovery. In 1991, in an intense, politically charged atmosphere, Gallo dropped his claim to the discovery of HIV.

The original HIV is now known as HIV-1. This is due to the 1986 discovery by scientists at the Pasteur Institute of another AIDS-causing virus in West Africans, which was labeled HIV-2. Although the two forms of HIV have similar modes of transmission, the symptoms of HIV-2 were found to be milder than those of HIV-1. Furthermore, HIV-2 was shown to differ in molecular structure from HIV-1 in a way that ties it more closely to a virus that causes AIDS in macaque monkeys. Antoine Benard et al. indicate in "Immunovirological Response to Triple Nucleotide Reverse-Transcriptase Inhibitors and Ritonavir-Boosted Protease Inhibitors in Treatment-Naive HIV-2–Infected Patients: The ACHIEV2E Collaboration Study Group" (*Clinical Infectious Diseases*, vol. 52, no. 10, May 2011) that HIV-2 is generally diagnosed in western Africa, and small numbers of cases are diagnosed in Europe and North America each year. (Unless otherwise specified, the term *HIV* in the remainder of this edition refers to HIV-1.)

The Origins of the Virus

Montagnier and Gallo, along with other investigators, believed that HIV had been present in Central Africa and other regions for some time, and at some point the virus crossed the species barrier from primates to humans. The rural nature of these societies and limited access to the outside world by those infected with the virus may have confined the spread of HIV for decades. However, once the migration of tribal Central Africans to urban areas began, the more liberated sexual practices there promoted the spread of HIV. Within a comparatively short time, the once rare and remote disease was spread by globe-trotting HIV-infected people.

It was long speculated that HIV evolved from simian immunodeficiency virus (SIV), a retrovirus that infects monkeys. The theory was that HIV evolved from a human infection with a mutated form of SIV that was infectious to humans. Consistent with this theory was the finding that HIV is a part of the lentivirus family, which includes SIV.

In 1982 Isao Miyoshi (1932–) of Kochi University identified an HTLV-related virus in Japanese macaque monkeys. Genetically similar to HTLV, it was designated as the simian T-lymphotropic virus (STLV). Further studies identified STLV in both Asian and African monkeys and apes, with an infection rate ranging from 1% to 40%.

FIGURE 1.2

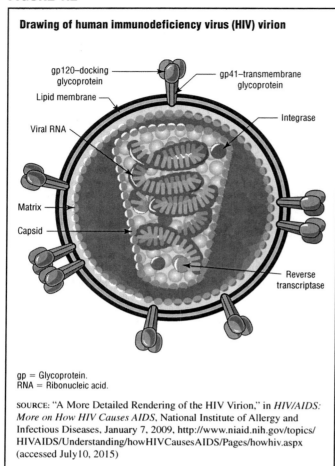

Drawing of human immunodeficiency virus (HIV) virion

gp120–docking glycoprotein

gp41–transmembrane glycoprotein

Lipid membrane

Integrase

Viral RNA

Matrix

Capsid

Reverse transcriptase

gp = Glycoprotein.
RNA = Ribonucleic acid.

SOURCE: "A More Detailed Rendering of the HIV Virion," in *HIV/AIDS: More on How HIV Causes AIDS*, National Institute of Allergy and Infectious Diseases, January 7, 2009, http://www.niaid.nih.gov/topics/HIVAIDS/Understanding/howHIVCausesAIDS/Pages/howhiv.aspx (accessed July 10, 2015)

In 1988 Max Essex (1939–) and Phyllis Jean Kanki (1956–) of the Harvard School of Public Health discovered that the simian virus found in African chimpanzees and African green monkeys was more homologous (related in primitive origin) to the human virus than to the simian virus in Asian macaques. This discovery provided strong support for an evolved version of African STLV as being the origin of human HTLV.

In 1999 an international team of researchers at the University of Alabama announced that the genetic sequence of a simian virus isolated from a tissue sample obtained from a chimpanzee was virtually identical to the HIV discovered by Montagnier. Interestingly, chimpanzees are only rarely infected with SIV. This implies that chimpanzee may be temporary carriers of the virus, which normally resides in some other, as yet unidentified, primate species. A common chimpanzee subspecies, *Pan troglodytes troglodytes*, which along with the bonobo is the closest living species to humans, naturally harbors HIV-1, and there have been documented occurrences of cross-species transmission from them to humans. Because these chimpanzees are still poached for bushmeat, humans may be at risk for continued exposure. A complete understanding of the mechanisms of cross-species transmission

and the ability of these chimpanzees to resist infection may help researchers develop strategies to protect humans from HIV as well as from other viruses that originate in animals, such as H1N1, SARS coronavirus, hantaviruses, and the Ebola and Marburg viruses.

In October 2014 Nuno Faria et al. reconstructed and described the genetic history and spread of HIV in humans in "The Early Spread and Epidemic Ignition of HIV-1 in Human Populations" (*Science*, vol. 346, no. 6205). The researchers assert that HIV likely emerged in Kinshasa, the capital and largest city of the Democratic Republic of the Congo, around 1920. It subsequently spread from Africa to Haiti, and then to the United States, from where it spread worldwide. Faria et al. explain that although various strains of HIV jumped from primates to humans at least 13 times, just one of these transmissions led to the HIV pandemic (global epidemic).

ATTACKING THE IMMUNE SYSTEM

As with other infections, HIV must evade the immune system, which functions to detect and destroy invaders. To learn how HIV first attacks healthy cells while evading attack by the immune system, it is important to understand the complex structure of HIV and how normal white blood cells work.

Healthy White Blood Cells at Work

White blood cells are major components of the coordinated system of organs and cells that make up the human immune system. These organs and cells work to prevent invasion by foreign substances. There are five types of white blood cells: macrophages (scavenger cells of the immune system), T4 or helper T cells, T8 or killer T cells, plasma B cells, and memory B cells. T and B white blood cells are also called lymphocytes. Lymphocytes bear the major responsibility for carrying out immune system activities.

Each type of white blood cell has a specific function. Macrophages, which begin as smaller monocytes (single cells), ready the T4 cells to respond to particular invaders such as viruses. During a viral attack, macrophages, which are sometimes referred to as the vacuum cleaner of the immune system, swallow viral cells, but leave a portion displayed so that the T4 cells can make contact. Macrophages also stimulate the production of thousands of T4 cells, which are programmed to battle the invader. Figure 1.3 shows how the virus attaches to an immune cell and reproduces.

When T4 lymphocytes attack an invading virus, they also send out chemical messages that cause the multiplication of B cells and T8 killer cells. These cells, along with the help of some T4 cells, destroy the infected cell. Other T4 cells, which are not actively involved in destroying the infected cells, send chemical messages to

FIGURE 1.3

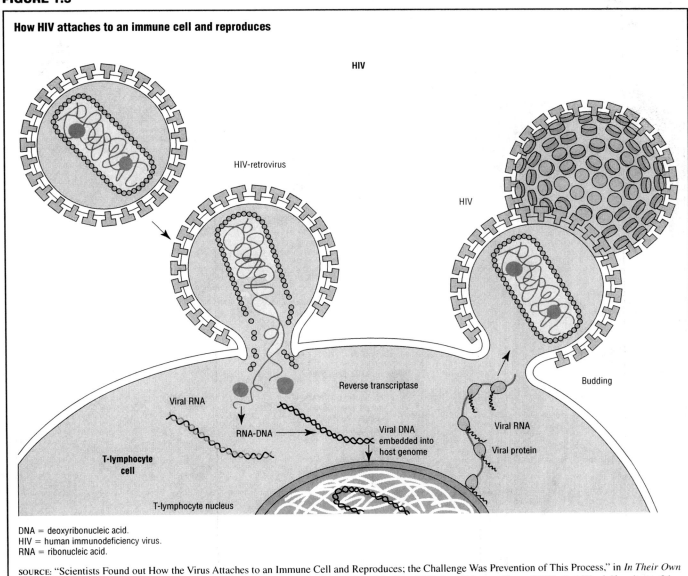

How HIV attaches to an immune cell and reproduces

DNA = deoxyribonucleic acid.
HIV = human immunodeficiency virus.
RNA = ribonucleic acid.

SOURCE: "Scientists Found out How the Virus Attaches to an Immune Cell and Reproduces; the Challenge Was Prevention of This Process," in *In Their Own Words...NIH Researchers Recall the Early Years of AIDS*, National Institutes of Health, June 2001, http://history.nih.gov/NIHInOwnWords/docs/page_04 .html (accessed July 10, 2015)

B cells, causing them to reproduce and divide into groups of either plasma cells or memory cells. Plasma cells make antibodies that cripple the invading virus, whereas memory cells increase the immune response if the invader ever attacks again.

HIV's Molecular Structure

HIV has nine genes. Three of these—designated env, gag, and pol code—form the structural components of the virus that surround the genetic material and the outer surface of the virus particle. The remaining genes—tat, nef, rev, vpr, vpu, and vif—are involved in regulating the genetic activities that are necessary to create copies of the infecting virus.

HIV's complement of nine genes is minuscule compared with the 30,000 genes in human DNA. Nevertheless,

HIV is more complex than most other retroviruses, which have only three or four genes. Scientists believe these genes direct the production of proteins that make up parts of the virus and regulate its reproduction. The HIV core contains genes that are protected by a protein shell, and the virus is surrounded and protected by a fatty membrane dotted with glycoproteins (proteins with sugar units attached). (See Figure 1.2.) Figure 1.4 shows the steps in the replication cycle of HIV.

Once HIV enters the human body, its primary target is a subset of immune cells that contain a molecule called CD4. In particular, the virus attaches itself to CD4+ T cells and, to a lesser extent, to macrophages. Figure 1.5 shows the cell-to-cell spread of HIV through the CD4-mediated fusion of an infected cell with an uninfected cell.

FIGURE 1.4

HIV replication cycle

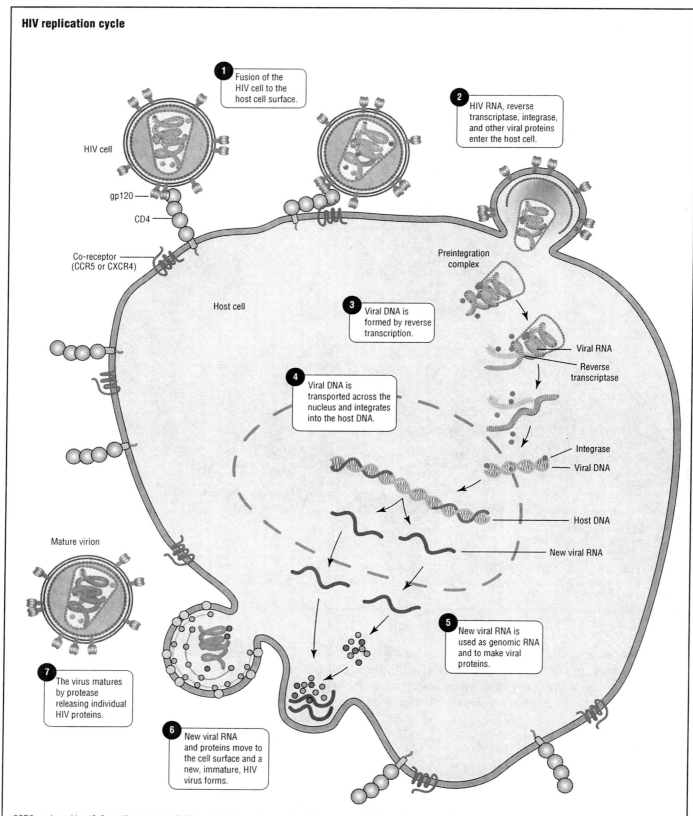

CCR5 = chemokine (C-C motif) receptor 5. CXCR4 = CXC chemokine receptor. CD4 = cluster of differentiation 4. gp120 = glycoprotein.

SOURCE: M. Wayengera, "Figure 1. Schematics of the Retroviral Replication Cycle," in "On the General Theory of the Origins of Retroviruses," *Theoretical Biology and Medical Modelling*, vol. 7, no. 5, February 16, 2010, OpenI, U.S. National Library of Medicine, Lister Hill National Center for Biomedical Communications, http://openi.nlm.nih.gov/detailedresult.php?img=2830970_1742-4682-7-5-1&req=4 (accessed July 10, 2015)

FIGURE 1.5

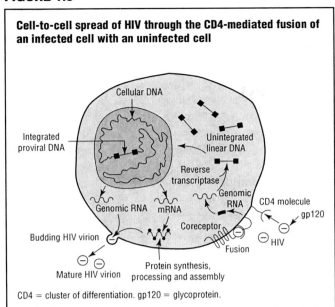

Cell-to-cell spread of HIV through the CD4-mediated fusion of an infected cell with an uninfected cell

CD4 = cluster of differentiation. gp120 = glycoprotein.

SOURCE: "Cell-to-Cell Spread of HIV Also Can Occur through the CD4-Mediated Fusion of an Infected Cell with an Uninfected Cell," in *HIV/AIDS: More on How HIV Causes AIDS*, National Institute of Allergy and Infectious Diseases, May 12, 2009, http://www.niaid.nih.gov/TOPICS/HIVAIDS/UNDERSTANDING/HOWHIVCAUSESAIDS/Pages/howhiv.aspx (accessed July 10, 2015)

Degrading the Immune System

In November 1995 Ute-Christiane Meier et al. proposed in "Cytotoxic T Lymphocyte Lysis Inhibited by Viable HIV Mutants" (*Science*, vol. 270, no. 5240) that HIV defuses the killer cells that are supposed to destroy virus-stricken cells. The researchers isolated HIV from AIDS patients and demonstrated that the virus had undergone a mutation, or change, in its genetic structure. When killer T cells approached cells infected with the mutated virus, the T cells failed to kill the stricken cells, perhaps because they no longer recognized them. In fact, the T cells were unable to kill even cells infected with the original, un-mutated virus. The mutations not only allowed the altered strains to multiply but also allowed unaltered strains to flourish.

Not all researchers agree that the alteration of killer T cells is the underlying basis for the establishment of an HIV infection. Some believe that other cells in the immune system attack and kill CD4-containing cells. The CD4-containing cells that have not been invaded by the virus, but that display fragments of it, become targets for other cells—besides the killer cells—which see the infected cells as a camouflaged virus and kill them. In addition, HIV-infected cells may send out protein signals that weaken or destroy other healthy cells in the immune system.

It is, however, agreed that HIV subsequently exhibits various behaviors, depending on the kind of cell it has invaded and how the cell behaves. The virus can remain dormant in T cells for two to 20 years, hidden from the immune system. When the cells are stimulated, however, the viral genes that have been incorporated into the DNA of the T4 cells can be replicated and the gene products assembled into new virus particles that then break free of the T4 cells and attack other cells. Once a T4 cell has been infected, it cannot respond adequately and may reproduce to form as few as 10 cells. An uninfected T4 cell usually reproduces 1,000 or more times to form the army needed to fight the HIV invader. When these crippled T4 cells do encounter the invader, the virus inside them reproduces and the cells are destroyed. Worse still, HIV reproduces itself at a rate far greater than any other known virus. The T4 cells become factories for the invading enemy soldiers, ultimately producing them in overwhelming numbers.

The Attack

The immune system is unable to produce sufficient antibodies to fight off the complex HIV. The battle between HIV and the immune system begins when the virus slips into the bloodstream via a CD4 receptor enzyme on a T4 cell, to which it preferentially attaches itself. A CD4 receptor alone, however, is not enough to cause infection, and for years scientists searched for some other protein on the cell surface that HIV exploits to gain entry.

This protein was discovered in May 1996 by a team of scientists at the National Institute of Allergy and Infectious Diseases (NIAID). The scientists named the protein fusin because it helps the virus fuse with a healthy cell membrane and inject genetic material into the cell. The CD4-containing cell signals to killer T cells that it is infected by displaying fragments of HIV proteins on its surface. This triggers the killer cells to spring into action by multiplying and seeking out the infected CD4-containing cells to pierce them open and destroy them.

CONFIRMING A HIDING PLACE

Typically, an HIV infection begins with a sudden, flu-like illness. Shortly after this first episode, the virus virtually disappears and symptoms may not materialize for as long as 20 years. Over time, the immune system eventually collapses and the virus appears in ever-increasing amounts of CD4-containing cells floating free in the patient's blood. Although previous studies focused on the presence of the virus in the blood, two independently conducted studies in 1993—Janet Embretson et al.'s "Massive Covert Infection of Helper T Lymphocytes and Macrophages by HIV during the Incubation Period of AIDS" (*Nature*, vol. 362, no. 6418, March 25, 1993) and Anthony S. Fauci et al.'s "Multifactorial Nature of Human Immunodeficiency Virus Disease: Implications for Therapy" (*Science*, vol. 262, no. 5136, November 12, 1993)—confirmed that HIV hides in a patient's lymph nodes and similar tissue during the first or early stage of infection.

Searching for an Active Virus

Research by Fauci et al. focused on the search for the virus in the blood and lymphoid tissue (the lymph nodes, spleen, tonsils, and adenoids) of 12 HIV-infected patients whose infections had progressed to varying severities. Initially, the virus is concentrated almost entirely in the lymphoid tissues. Fauci et al. believe the virus infiltrates the lymph nodes within weeks of the initial infection. Particles of the virus coated with antibodies adhere to the follicular dendritic cells, a group of filtering cells that trap foreign material. Nearby CD4-containing cells "see" the trapped material and are stimulated to attack the invaders. The stronger virus counterattacks and reproduces itself on some of these CD4-containing cells.

After this infiltration, performance of the immune system declines. This decline, which ultimately is dramatically debilitating, occurs over an extended period—up to 20 years in some people. During this decline the follicular dendritic cells also begin to deteriorate, and the quantity of HIV in the CD4-containing cells floating free in the blood increases significantly. In the final stage of the disease, there is an almost complete dissolution of the follicular dendritic cell network. At this point the amount of HIV in the blood and in the CD4-containing cells has grown to equal the amount in the lymph nodes.

NOT JUST THE IMMUNE SYSTEM

For some time scientists believed HIV attacked and affected only the immune system. Many early AIDS cases that provided evidence of the involvement of other regions of the body were not counted due to the narrower definitions of AIDS that existed before 1993. However, after 1993 clear evidence showed that the free virus (not attached to any other cells) could appear in the fluid surrounding the brain and spinal cord and in the bloodstream. HIV can be found not only in T4 lymphocytes but also in other immune system cells, as well as in cells in the nervous system, intestine, and bone marrow.

CDC researchers proposed another reason HIV infections are so difficult to eliminate and why the immune system is so susceptible to them. HIV can infect and grow in immature bone marrow cells, offering no clues about what the mature HIV-infected cells will become. The virus reproduces without revealing itself to the immune system, which under normal circumstances would destroy it. By developing in immature bone marrow cells, a great quantity of the virus can be produced before the body ever attempts to resist it.

As they mature, the cells change, becoming infected monocytes and macrophages that may not only fail to fight infections but may also spread the virus to other immune system cells. Infected marrow cells can seed the virus into other parts of the body, including the brain.

SEARCHING FOR ANSWERS

Researchers have long been puzzled by the fact that AIDS is virtually always fatal, even though relatively small amounts of the virus are found in patients, compared with other lethal viral infections. How the virus kills cells has been hotly debated. Certainly, it is inconsistent with other retroviruses, which do not kill all the infected host cells. Although HIV is considered to be a slow virus (one that exerts its effect over a long period), some AIDS activity occurs quickly and may be associated with the coincidental presence of infectious mycoplasma (bacteria that lack a cell wall).

Restoring Immune Response

In December 1993 the NCI reported that the immune function had been restored to HIV-infected cells grown in a laboratory through the addition of interleukin-12 (IL-12). IL-12 is a member of a group of natural blood proteins called cytokines that were discovered in 1991 by scientists at the Wistar Institute and Hoffmann-La Roche Inc. Despite this promising result, the U.S. Food and Drug Administration (FDA) halted human testing of IL-12 in June 1995, after two patients died. After testing the protein on animals, researchers concluded that the problem was not in IL-12 itself, but in the timing of the doses. Consequently, human testing resumed in November 1995.

In December 1995 a new class of drugs called protease inhibitors received FDA approval. These drugs block the ability of HIV to mature and to infect new cells by suppressing the protein-degrading activity of a viral enzyme. Enzymes with this activity are classified as proteases, hence the designation of the enzyme blocker as a protease inhibitor. If protease inhibitors block the spread of HIV in the immune system, then AIDS will not develop. Although patients may be HIV positive the rest of their life, they may never die from HIV infection.

Theories of HIV/AIDS Progression

Even after three decades of research, there is no consensus among HIV experts about the origination and development of AIDS. There is, however, agreement that the latent period between the establishment of an HIV infection and the appearance of the symptoms of AIDS averages from two to 11 years, although some people remain symptom free for as long as 20 years. Furthermore, as many as 20% of all HIV-infected people do not develop AIDS. Called long-term nonprogressors, these individuals are believed to have genetic and immune response characteristics that slow or halt the course of disease progression. Much research centers on these people, because an understanding of the physiological characteristics that allow them to suppress the infection could be invaluable for treating the disease in other patients.

After HIV infection is established, the immune system regenerates cells only up to a certain point, which would explain a gradual progression to AIDS. The early regulatory functions of the immune system limit viral replication until a certain threshold is reached. When the number of different viral mutants becomes too large, the regulatory system is overwhelmed and shuts down, opening the door to opportunistic infections.

When the total CD4+ T-cell count falls from the normal 500 to 1,600 per cubic millimeter of blood to 200 per cubic millimeter, the rate of immune decline accelerates and the HIV-positive person becomes prone to the opportunistic infections and other illnesses that are characteristic of AIDS.

SOME INCONSISTENCIES WITH CURRENT THEORIES. Most scientists agree that there are still gaps and inconsistencies in the knowledge of how HIV causes AIDS. One inconsistency concerns the infection and killing of the helper T cells. Initially, researchers thought that the main tactic of HIV was to infect and destroy the T cells. As these cells died, the numerical strength of the helper T-cell force was depleted, thus causing the immune deficiency associated with AIDS patients.

Other scientists, however, consider this theory too simplistic because so few T cells—no more than one infected cell in 500—are infected. Rather, two studies published in 2001 in the *Journal of Experimental Medicine*—Hiroshi Mohri et al.'s "Increased Turnover of T Lymphocytes in HIV-1 Infection and Its Reduction by Antiretroviral Therapy" (vol. 194, no. 9, November 5, 2001) and Joseph A. Kovacs et al.'s "Identification of Dynamically Distinct Subpopulations of T Lymphocytes That Are Differentially Affected by HIV" (vol. 194, no. 12, December 17, 2001)—support the idea that HIV does not block the production of T cells but instead accelerates the division of existing T cells. This causes the existing T cells to die off more quickly than normal.

Another inconsistency involves the observation that the rapid decline in the number of T cells comes relatively late in the infection, even though there are clear indications that the immune system has been impaired much earlier.

OPPORTUNISTIC INFECTIONS

Once HIV has destroyed the immune system, the body can no longer protect itself against bacterial, fungal, protozoal, and other viral agents that take advantage of the compromised condition and cause infections. These sorts of infections, which would not otherwise occur but for an impaired immune system, are known as opportunistic infections (OIs). In the non-AIDS community, OIs occur in hospitals, where ill, newborn, or older patients may also have less than adequately functioning immune systems. Because

patients are considered to have AIDS if at least one OI appears, OIs are also referred to as "AIDS-defining events," even though OIs are not the only AIDS-defining events.

By 1997 the leading OI for Americans suffering from HIV/AIDS was *Pneumocystis carinii* pneumonia (PCP), a lung disease caused by a fungus. Before the discovery of HIV/AIDS, PCP was found almost exclusively in cancer and transplant patients with weakened immune systems. During the 1980s PCP was the AIDS-defining illness for two-thirds of people diagnosed with AIDS in the United States, and it was estimated that 75% of HIV-infected people would develop PCP during their lifetime. According to Laurence Huang et al., in "An Official ATS Workshop Summary: Recent Advances and Future Directions in Pneumocystis Pneumonia (PCP)" (*Proceedings of the American Thoracic Society*, vol. 3, no. 8, November 2006), the incidence of PCP decreased 3.4% per year between 1992 and 1995 and then declined 21.5% annually between 1996 and 1998, when powerful combinations of antiretroviral therapy (ART) were beginning to be used. NAM, a U.K.-based charitable organization that produces and distributes information about HIV/AIDS, explains in "PCP" (June 6, 2012, http://www.aidsmap .com/PCP/page/1044747) that effective HIV treatment and improved treatment for PCP, including the use of antibiotics to prevent its occurrence, have made PCP infection uncommon among people with HIV in the United States. PCP, however, remains the most frequently occurring serious OI among HIV-infected people in developing countries.

Although prescription drugs such as trimethoprim-sulfamethoxazole were found to be effective at preventing PCP during the late 1980s, and their widespread use along with the addition of ART a decade later markedly reduced the cases of PCP, researchers find that people who do not adhere to treatment remain at risk of developing the disease.

In "Primary Relationships, HIV Treatment Adherence, and Virologic Control" (*AIDS and Behavior*, vol. 16, no. 6, August 2012), Mallory O. Johnson et al. find that patients' positive appraisals of their relationships and positive beliefs about the effectiveness of treatment are associated with greater adherence, whereas concerns about partners and medication are associated with less adherence. In addition, HIV-positive people who smoke are three times more likely to develop PCP than non-smokers. In "Doctor-Patient Relationship: Active Patient Involvement (DPR:API) Is Related to Long Survival Status and Predicts Adherence Change in HIV" (*Journal of AIDS & Clinical Research*, vol. 6, no. 2, February 20, 2015), Gail Ironson, Aurelie Lucette, and Roger C. McIntosh find that patients who are actively involved in their care are more likely to adhere to treatment and have better health outcomes and long-term survival.

Esophageal candidiasis, an infection of the esophagus, and extrapulmonary cryptococcosis, a systemic fungus that enters the body through the lungs and may invade any organ, are also OIs frequently diagnosed in AIDS patients.

Other illnesses such as Burkitt's lymphoma, cervical cancer, and primary brain lymphoma are also considered AIDS-defining events. Wasting syndrome (which is characterized by drastic weight loss and lethargy) is another illness that may be considered an AIDS-defining event. Other examples of AIDS-defining events include diagnosis of *Mycobacterium avium* complex, a serious bacterial infection that may occur in the liver, bone marrow, and spleen or spread throughout the body; cytomegalovirus disease, a member of the herpesvirus group; Kaposi's sarcoma, a once-rare cancer of the blood vessel walls that causes purple lesions on the skin; and toxoplasmic encephalitis, an inflammation of the brain. Patients may experience more than one OI or AIDS-defining event.

In 2006 NIAID researchers identified a critical human cell surface molecule—protein xCT—as the receptor that can make cells vulnerable to infection with Kaposi's sarcoma herpesvirus (KSHV). Although Kaposi's sarcoma was less common in the United States in 2013 than it had been during the early years of the AIDS pandemic; it was the second most-common cancer associated with HIV infection. Figure 1.6 shows how KSHV fuses to and enters a human cell after binding to the protein xCT.

HIV and Tuberculosis

Tuberculosis (TB) is a communicable infection caused by the bacterium *Mycobacterium tuberculosis*. TB was a widespread pandemic in North America during the late 19th and early 20th centuries, and then it faded from prominence. TB, however, regained a foothold during the 1990s, with the number of cases increasing in the United States. Part of this increase is the parallel increase in the occurrence of the infection in HIV-positive individuals. HIV infection has become one of the strongest known risk factors for the progression of TB from infection to disease.

TB is spread from person to person through the inhalation of airborne particles containing *M. tuberculosis*. The particles, called droplet nuclei, are produced when a person with infectious TB forcefully exhales, such as when coughing, sneezing, speaking, or singing. These infectious particles remain suspended in the air and may be inhaled by someone sharing the same air. The risk of transmission is increased when ventilation is poor and when susceptible people share air for prolonged periods with a person who has untreated TB.

Approximately 85% of TB infections occur in the lungs. This infection is called pulmonary TB. Nevertheless, TB may occur at any site of the body, such as the larynx, lymph nodes, brain, kidneys, or bones. These cases

are called extrapulmonary TB. Except for laryngeal TB, people with extrapulmonary TB are usually not considered infectious.

According to the CDC, in "Tuberculosis" (September 24, 2015, http://www.cdc.gov/tb/statistics/default.htm), the number of TB cases in the United States declined 1.5% between 2013 and 2014; however, TB remains one of the leading causes of death of people who are HIV infected.

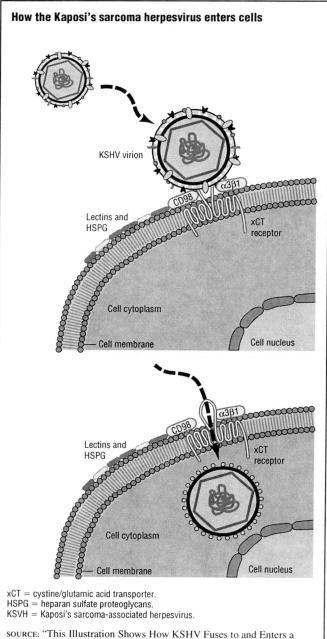

FIGURE 1.6

How the Kaposi's sarcoma herpesvirus enters cells

xCT = cystine/glutamic acid transporter.
HSPG = heparan sulfate proteoglycans.
KSVH = Kaposi's sarcoma-associated herpesvirus.

SOURCE: "This Illustration Shows How KSHV Fuses to and Enters a Human Cell after Binding to the Protein xCT," in *Landmark Discovery of a Kaposi's Sarcoma-Associated Herpesvirus Receptor Provides New Perspectives on Disease Associated with HIV/AIDS*, National Institute of Allergy and Infectious Disease, April 2006, http://www.nih.gov/news/pr/apr2006/niaid-06.htm (accessed July 10, 2015)

This is because people who are not HIV infected can usually defend themselves successfully against TB infection. The risk that TB will develop in people infected only with *M. tuberculosis* is 10% within their lifetime. People with HIV, who have weakened immune systems, are less able to resist infection and are more likely to develop active TB. HIV-infected people with either latent TB infection or active TB disease can be effectively treated with prescription drugs that kill the bacteria.

Varieties of TB have developed that are resistant to drug therapy, posing a threat to public health initiatives aimed at reducing TB infections. Multidrug-resistant TB (MDR-TB) is a variety of the disease that does not respond to the two first-line anti-TB drugs—rifampicin and isoniazid. Extensively drug-resistant TB (XDR-TB) does not respond to any of the drugs conventionally used to combat the disease. In "Treatment Outcomes for Extensively Drug-Resistant Tuberculosis and HIV Co-infection" (*Emerging Infectious Diseases*, vol. 19, no. 3, March 2013), Max R. O'Donnell et al. report that even when treated, many MDR-TB and XDR-TB patients do not fare well. In a study of 6,127 patients with either MDR-TB or XDR-TB, the researchers find a high mortality rate (48%) and a low rate of successful treatment (22%). O'Donnell et al. call for more rapid HIV and TB testing to enable prompt treatment, ongoing drug susceptibility testing to ensure that patients are receiving effective medication, and the development of more potent anti-TB drugs.

HIV and Cancer

People with AIDS are susceptible to cancer. Some malignant tumors, such as Kaposi's sarcoma and cancers of the lymph system, have been common among AIDS patients since the disease was first discovered in 1981. More recently, however, physicians and researchers have found that certain forms of cancer are more prevalent among HIV/AIDS patients who are living longer.

Most AIDS-related cancers are believed to be caused by viruses. These cancers are more common among HIV-infected people because HIV suppresses the immune system, enabling cancer-causing viruses to attack more successfully. These cancers include non-Hodgkin's lymphoma (found in lymph tissues) and primary lymphoma of the brain. People infected with HIV are also at greater risk of anal, cervical, liver, lung, oral, and skin cancers as well as myeloma (malignant tumors of the bone marrow), brain tumors, testicular cancers, and leukemia (cancer of the blood cells).

Because anti-HIV-combination drug therapies, such as ART, have become widely used, researchers report a decline in Kaposi's sarcoma and primary lymphoma of the brain. One possible explanation for the decline may be that the combination drug therapies enable the body to recover partial immunity, which in turn helps prevent the development of cancer.

Lung cancer is the third most commonly diagnosed cancer among people with HIV, after non-Hodgkin's lymphoma and Kaposi's sarcoma. Allison A. Lambert, Christian A. Merlo, and Gregory D. Kirk of the Johns Hopkins School of Medicine observe in "Human Immunodeficiency Virus–Associated Lung Malignancies" (*Clinics in Chest Medicine*, vol. 34, no. 2, June 2013) that lung cancer in HIV-positive patients is diagnosed at younger ages than it is in the general population. Research has shown that HIV increases the lung cancer risk among smokers, but that it is also associated with increased risk of lung cancer in non-smokers. It is not known exactly how HIV influences the development of lung cancer; it may promote its development directly or increase susceptibility to it by compromising immune function.

In "Excess Cancers among HIV-Infected People in the United States" (*Journal of the National Cancer Institute*, vol. 107, no. 4, April 2015), Hilary A. Robbins et al. explain that since the introduction of ART, the incidence of AIDS-defining infections and cancers, including Kaposi's sarcoma, non-Hodgkin's lymphoma, and cervical cancer, have decreased significantly. Nevertheless, the incidence and numbers of deaths that are attributable to non-AIDS-related malignancies and other diseases have increased. This shift is the result of increased life expectancy and the reduction of competing causes of death.

TOWARD A VACCINE OR A CURE: THE HOPE AND THE REALITIES

The different routes of attack of HIV on the immune system and the ability of the virus to mutate has prompted some observers to opine that an effective vaccine will be difficult to achieve. This sentiment is contrary to the 1984 prediction made by Margaret M. Heckler (1931–), the U.S. secretary of health and human services, that the identification of HIV would lead to a vaccine within two years.

The intervening years have made many AIDS researchers realize that developing a vaccine to prevent AIDS (confer immunity on the person receiving the vaccine) is challenging. Testing the effectiveness of an AIDS vaccine is also difficult, because it would be unethical and illegal to deliberately expose people to HIV to check if the vaccine worked. As a consequence, studies often take the approach of offering potential vaccines to people who are at a high risk of exposure to HIV and then monitoring their health.

One example is the RV144 HIV vaccine study conducted in Thailand in 2009. This study offered vaccine trials in provinces where the rate of HIV infection was very high. The scientists conducting the study also warned their subjects that the vaccine might not work, advised the subjects to practice safe sex, and supplied condoms to help prevent infection. The Thai study involved the use of two vaccines. When these vaccines were combined, they reduced the risk of infection by 30%. The RV 144 HIV vaccine was found to confer protection in some study subjects but not in others.

In "HIV Vaccine Awareness Day" (May 18, 2015, http://www.niaid.nih.gov/news/newsreleases/2015/Pages/HVAD2015.aspx), the National Institutes of Health (NIH) reports that vaccine efforts continue. For example, the bulletin says that NIAID (one of the NIH institutes) formed the Pox-Protein Public-Private Partnership (P5), a diverse group of public and private organizations committed to building on the success of the RV144 HIV vaccine trial. In 2015 NIAID and P5 launched a trial of a vaccine that is based on RV144, called HVTN, in South Africa. Research was also underway on the possibility of administering antibodies directly in lieu of a vaccine. (Vaccines work by inducing people's immune systems to produce antibodies.)

Despite the challenges, clinical trials of HIV vaccines continue. In "HIV/AIDS Clinical Trials" (October 19, 2015, http://aidsinfo.nih.gov/clinical-trials), AIDSinfo, a service of the U.S. Department of Health and Human Services, notes that eight clinical trials of HIV vaccines were recruiting subjects as of October 2015.

Antiretroviral Therapy Is Effective

Although an effective vaccine remains elusive, great strides have been made in treating people infected with HIV. During the mid-1990s a "hit-hard-early" strategy gained favor. In this strategy a cocktail of anti-HIV drugs was given to patients shortly after they were diagnosed. The idea of ART is to suppress the reproduction of the virus as much as possible. Some of the drugs target the virus's reverse transcriptase. By inhibiting the enzyme's activity, the ability of HIV to reproduce is thwarted. However, ART has a downside. Although it is able to suppress the viral load, it is unable to eradicate it, and once ART is initiated, treatment must be ongoing. The therapy can be expensive and hard to maintain, and its long-term use is associated with a number of serious side effects. If patients do not adhere to the treatment, then they may not adequately suppress the virus.

In "The Clinical Role and Cost-Effectiveness of Long-Acting Antiretroviral Therapy" (*Clinical Infectious Diseases*, vol. 60, no. 7, April 1, 2015), Eric L. Ross et al. report that development of long-acting antiretroviral therapy is underway and could improve outcomes in people with poor adherence to daily ART.

ART INCREASES RISK FOR HEART DISEASE. Because ART has reduced AIDS-related deaths, people with HIV infections are living longer and suffering from many of the same diseases, such as heart disease, as their uninfected age peers. Furthermore, Lars G. Hemkens and Heiner C. Bucher aver in "HIV Infection and Cardiovascular Disease" (*European Heart Journal*, vol. 35, no. 21, June 1, 2014) that ART-induced metabolic changes, such as increases in cholesterol and triglycerides, lead to an elevated risk of heart disease.

Promise, Progress, and Setbacks

As of 2015, Timothy Ray Brown (1966–) is the only person believed to have been functionally cured of HIV. In "I Am the Berlin Patient: A Personal Reflection" (*AIDS Research and Human Retroviruses*, vol. 31, no. 1, January 2015), Brown, who was known as the "Berlin Patient" before going public, describes his story. He was diagnosed with HIV in 1995, and spent 11 years on ART to keep the infection under control. In 2006 he was diagnosed with life-threatening leukemia. To combat the leukemia Brown went through several rounds of chemotherapy and received two bone marrow stem-cell transplants.

Aware of Brown's HIV infection, Brown's doctors successfully sought out a bone marrow donor who had a rare genetic mutation that made that individual resistant to HIV infection. (Bone marrow is where much of the body's blood and immune system cells are generated.) The hope was that the combination of the chemotherapy and the new bone marrow would free Brown of his infection. To test this hypothesis, Brown stopped his ART before the transplants. In the years since he has remained off of ART and has been closely monitored, but no signs of an HIV infection have been found.

Brown's cure was exciting news, but unfortunately it did not hold out the prospect of an immediate treatment for other people with HIV. While Brown eventually recovered fully, the treatment he received was extremely debilitating and ran a substantial risk of killing him. It was attempted only because the leukemia was likely to kill Brown otherwise. Nevertheless, that even one person has been cured gives hope to those searching for more widely applicable treatments, as well as inspiring more research into the factors in Brown's case that might help others.

Unfortunately, other HIV-infected patients treated with chemotherapy and bone marrow cell transplants have not fared as well as Brown. In "Antiretroviral-Free HIV-1 Remission and Viral Rebound after Allogeneic Stem Cell Transplantation: Report of 2 Cases" (*Annals of Internal Medicine*, vol. 161, no. 5, September 2, 2014), Timothy J. Henrich et al. report that two people with HIV who were suffering from lymphoma underwent a treatment involving chemotherapy and bone marrow transplants. Both individuals discontinued ART after their transplants, and initially they had undetectable levels of HIV, resulting in hope that they had been cured. The virus, however, eventually reappeared, after 12 weeks in one patient and 32 weeks in the other, leading them to resume ART. Researchers theorize that HIV lurking within cells outside the blood may contribute to the persistence of HIV. In an editorial in the same issue of the journal, "Finding a Cure for HIV: Much Work to Do," Sharon R. Lewin observes that the relationship between HIV infectivity and human immune responses is complicated and "the amount of residual infectious virus left after ART and an effective immune response are both likely to be key in achieving long-term HIV remission." She concludes, "the most sobering lesson was that these cases . . . have raised the possibility that total elimination of every last virus or infected cell to achieve lifelong remission may not be possible."

Another case of an individual thought to be cured only to later show signs of infection is described by Deborah Persaud et al. in "Absence of Detectable HIV-1 Viremia after Treatment Cessation in an Infant" (*New England Journal of Medicine*, October 23, 2013). In this case, a baby born to an HIV-infected mother was treated with an aggressive regimen of antiretroviral drugs within 30 hours of birth, before it was even known if the baby was infected. While the virus was later detected, confirming an infection, by the time the baby was one month old, virus levels were undetectable. The baby's mother discontinued the drug treatment when the baby was about 18 months old. As a consequence, doctors expected to find high virus levels when the child was 24 months old; instead, they found very small amounts of viral genetic material but no virus that was able to replicate. After 30 months without treatment and with no detectable plasma HIV levels, the child was considered cured of HIV infection. However, in "Virus Detected in Baby 'Cured' of HIV" (CNN.com, July 11, 2014), Saundra Young and Jacque Wilson report that HIV was once again detected in the then four-year-old child in July 2014. The child was also found to have a low T-cell count, indicating a weakened immune system. More than two years after her ART had been stopped, the drug therapy was resumed.

CHAPTER 2
DEFINITION, SYMPTOMS, AND TRANSMITTAL

A DEFINITION OF AIDS

The Centers for Disease Control and Prevention (CDC) is the federal government's clearinghouse, research center, and monitoring agency for all infectious diseases, including HIV/AIDS. The CDC tracks the diseases in the United States and notifies health officials of their occurrence via *Morbidity and Mortality Weekly Report* notices and a website that is updated frequently.

The CDC defines AIDS as a disease caused by infection with HIV that weakens the immune system and increases the risk of certain infections and cancers. The CDC first outlined a surveillance (a constant observation of a process) case definition in 1982, and then revised it in 1983, 1985, 1987, 1993, 2000, 2008 and again in 2014 as knowledge about HIV infection increased and additional symptoms were included in the definitions. The 1993 definition emphasized the clinical importance of the CD4+ T-cell count and included the addition of three clinical conditions. CD4+ T-helper cells are white blood cells that also are called CD4 cells, T-helper cells, or T4 cells because one of their key functions is to send signals to other types of immune cells, including cells that kill viruses or other infectious agents.

THE 1993 AND 2008 CLASSIFICATION REVISIONS AND EXPANDED SURVEILLANCE CASE DEFINITIONS

The "1993 Revised Classification System for HIV Infection and Expanded Surveillance Case Definition for AIDS among Adolescents and Adults" (*Morbidity and Mortality Weekly Report*, vol. 41, no. RR-17, December 18, 1992), by Kenneth G. Castro et al. of the CDC, was revised in 2014 and published as "Revised Surveillance Case Definitions for HIV Infection—United States, 2014" (*Morbidity and Mortality Weekly Report*, vol. 63, no. 3, April 11, 2014), by Richard M. Selik et al. of the CDC. As of October 2015, it was the standard surveillance case definition.

The 1993 revision addressed the concerns of many women and physicians, who strongly advocated the inclusion of diseases such as pelvic inflammatory disease (inflammation of the female reproductive organs by microorganisms) and vaginal candidiasis (a fungal infection, commonly called a yeast infection or thrush) as conditions that could precede the development of AIDS, so that women infected with HIV would be included in the revised definition. Advocates cautioned that if the CDC omitted such inclusive criteria, many women would be denied access to treatment, education, and disability benefits.

Although reporting criteria include recommendations for diagnosing HIV infection, the primary purpose of the original and updated case definitions is public health surveillance as opposed to the diagnosis of individual patients.

The 2014 Revised Definition and Classification: Classifies Stages 1 to 3 Based on CD4+ Counts

The 2014 revision combined the adult and pediatric criteria for a confirmed case of HIV infection and specifies different criteria for staging HIV infection among three age groups (children less than age one, one to five years old, and age six or older). Table 2.1 shows HIV infection stage based on age-specific CD4+ T-lymphocyte counts. The 2014 revision also redefined the laboratory criteria for a confirmed case, in response to the development of new diagnostic testing algorithms (sets of rules for solving problems) that do not require confirmatory tests. People with laboratory tests presumed to be positive are still expected to have additional tests to confirm their diagnoses. However, they may be included in the surveillance database before those test results are available. Laboratory criteria for distinguishing between HIV-1 and HIV-2 infection and recognizing early HIV infection also are included in the new surveillance case definition.

Another important change is the addition of "stage 0"—test results indicative of early HIV infection, which

TABLE 2.1

Surveillance case definition for HIV infection among adults and adolescents, 2014

Stage	Age on date of CD4+ T-lymphocyte test					
	<1 yr		1–5 yrs		≥6 yrs	
	Cells/µL	%	Cells/µL	%	Cells/µL	%
1	≥1,500	≥34	≥1,000	≥30	≥500	≥26
2	750–1,499	26–33	500–999	22–29	200–499	14–25
3	<750	<26	<500	<22	<200	<14

Notes: The stage is based primarily on the CD4+ T-lymphocyte count; the CD4+ T-lymphocyte count takes precedence over the CD4 T-lymphocyte percentage, and the percentage is considered only if the count is missing. There are three situations in which the stage is not based on this table: (1) if the criteria for stage 0 are met, the stage is 0 regardless of criteria for other stages (CD4 T-lymphocyte test results and opportunistic illness diagnoses); (2) if the criteria for stage 0 are not met and a stage-3-defining opportunistic illness has been diagnosed, then the stage is 3 regardless of CD4 T-lymphocyte test results; or (3) if the criteria for stage 0 are not met and information on the above criteria for other stages is missing, then the stage is classified as unknown.

SOURCE: Richard M. Selik et al., "Table. HIV Infection Based on Age-Specific CD4+ T-Lymphocyte Count or CD4+ T-Lymphocyte Percentage of Total Lymphocytes," in "Revised Surveillance Case Definitions for HIV Infections—United States, 2014,"*MMWR*, vol. 63, no. 3, April 11, 2014, http://www.cdc.gov/mmwr/pdf/rr/rr6303.pdf (accessed July 16, 2015)

TABLE 2.2

Stage 3 defining opportunistic illnesses in HIV infection

- Bacterial infections, multiple or recurrent[a]
- Candidiasis of bronchi, trachea, or lungs
- Candidiasis of esophagus
- Cervical cancer, invasive[b]
- Coccidioidomycosis, disseminated or extrapulmonary
- Cryptococcosis, extrapulmonary
- Cryptosporidiosis, chronic intestinal (>1 month's duration)
- Cytomegalovirus disease (other than liver, spleen, or nodes), onset at age >1 month
- Cytomegalovirus retinitis (with loss of vision)
- Encephalopathy attributed to HIV
- Herpes simplex: chronic ulcers (>1 month's duration) or bronchitis, pneumonitis, or esophagitis (onset at age >1 month)
- Histoplasmosis, disseminated or extrapulmonary
- Isosporiasis, chronic intestinal (>1 month's duration)
- Kaposi sarcoma
- Lymphoma, Burkitt (or equivalent term)
- Lymphoma, immunoblastic (or equivalent term)
- Lymphoma, primary, of brain
- *Mycobacterium avium* complex or *Mycobacterium kansasii*, disseminated or extrapulmonary
- *Mycobacterium tuberculosis* of any site, pulmonary[b], disseminated, or extrapulmonary
- Mycobacterium, other species or unidentified species, disseminated or extrapulmonary
- *Pneumocystis jirovecii* (previously known as *"Pneumocystis carinii"*) pneumonia
- Pneumonia, recurrent[b]
- Progressive multifocal leukoencephalopathy
- *Salmonella* septicemia, recurrent
- Toxoplasmosis of brain, onset at age >1 month
- Wasting syndrome attributed to HIV

[a]Only among children aged <6 years.
[b]Only among adults, adolescents, and children aged ≥6 years.

SOURCE: Richard M. Selik et al., "Appendix: Stage-3-Defining Opportunistic Illnesses in HIV Infection," in "Revised Surveillance Case Definitions for HIV Infections—United States, 2014," *MMWR*, vol. 63, no. 3, April 11, 2014, http://www.cdc.gov/mmwr/pdf/rr/rr6303.pdf (accessed July 16, 2015)

occurs before the antibody response has fully developed. The addition of stage 0 allows for routine monitoring of the number of cases diagnosed within months of infection, which includes the most infectious period when viral loads and the potential for transmission are very high. The 2014 revision classifies stages 1 to 3 of HIV infection on the basis of the CD4+ T-lymphocyte count unless people have had a stage-3–defining opportunistic illness.

The 2014 revision also eliminates the requirement that evidence of HIV infection in a child's mother is necessary to define a case of HIV infection in a child less than 18 months old when laboratory testing confirms HIV infection. It uses CD4+ T-lymphocyte counts and percentages for determining the stage of HIV infection in children as well as adults and adolescents, and stages children ages six to 12 years the same way adults and adolescents are staged. In the 2008 case definition, only the presence or absence of opportunistic illnesses was used to stage cases in children younger than age 13. Table 2.2 lists stage 3–defining opportunistic illnesses in HIV infection.

The Impact of the 1993 Definition on Case Reporting

CDC data indicate that expansion of the AIDS surveillance criteria changed both the process of AIDS surveillance and the number of reported cases. In "Current Trends Update: Impact of the Expanded AIDS Surveillance Case Definition for Adolescents and Adults on Case Reporting—United States, 1993" (*Morbidity and Mortality Weekly Report*, vol. 43, no. 9, March 11, 1994), the CDC reports that in 1993, 103,500 AIDS cases were reported in the United States among adults and

adolescents aged 13 years and older. This number was just over twice the 49,016 cases reported in 1992 and likely represented a one-time effect of the 1993 expansion of the AIDS definition. The steep increase represented the reporting of people who were diagnosed with the newly added conditions before 1993. New reported AIDS cases declined again beginning in 1996 in response to antiretroviral therapy (ART), which slowed the progression from HIV infection to AIDS. Between 1998 and 1999 the decline in the incidence of AIDS began to level. (See Figure 2.1.) Between 1999 and 2012 the number of new diagnoses declined, and the number of AIDS-related deaths declined very slightly.

Table 2.3 shows the estimated numbers and rates of people living with HIV infection in 2009, 2010, 2011 and 2012. The number and rate of people living with diagnosed HIV infection increased each year during this period.

DIAGNOSIS AND SYMPTOMS OF HIV INFECTION AND AIDS

Only a qualified health professional can diagnose HIV infection and AIDS. There are three types of diagnostic tests, called immunoassays, for HIV—antibody

FIGURE 2.1

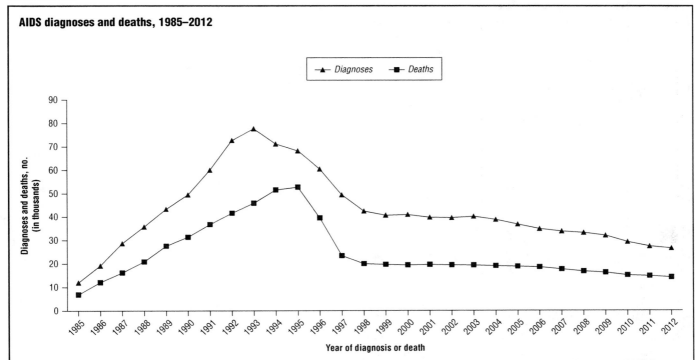

AIDS diagnoses and deaths, 1985–2012

Note: All displayed data have been statistically adjusted to account for reporting delays, but not for incomplete reporting. Deaths of persons with HIV infection, stage 3 (AIDS) may be due to any cause.

SOURCE: "Stage 3 (AIDS) Classifications and Deaths of Persons with HIV Infection Ever Classified as Stage 3 (AIDS), among Adults and Adolescents, 1985–2012—United States and 6 Dependent Areas," in *Epidemiology of HIV Infection through 2013*, Centers for Disease Control and Prevention, National Center for HIV/AIDS, Viral Hepatitis, Sexual Transmitted Diseases, and Tuberculosis Prevention, Division of HIV/AIDS Prevention, June 5, 2015, http://www.cdc.gov/hiv/pdf/g-l/cdc-hiv-genepislideseries-2013.pdf (accessed July 17, 2015)

tests, antigen/antibody tests, and nucleic acid (RNA) tests. Antibody tests detect proteins the body makes to combat HIV while antigen and RNA tests detect HIV itself. New tests with improved sensitivity can detect early HIV-1 infection, when the risk of transmitting the virus is much higher than the risk from people with established infection. Figure 2.2 shows how these immunoassays are used to detect HIV infection.

To evaluate a patient with a positive HIV test, the health care practitioner performs a complete physical examination and collects the patient's social and family history. Diagnostic laboratory tests are also performed. These tests typically include complete blood count and routine chemistry; CD4+ T-cell count; assays (analyses) that measure the amount of HIV-1 ribonucleic acid (RNA) in plasma; tuberculin skin tests to detect the presence of the bacterium that causes tuberculosis; and assays for the microbial agents that cause syphilis, toxoplasmosis, and hepatitis B and C. Females are screened for cervical cancer.

From HIV to AIDS

Through 2015, among people who were not treated with ART, the average time from initial HIV infection to the development of AIDS was about 10 years, according to the U.S. Department of Health and Human Services (HHS)

in "Stages of HIV Infection" (August 27, 2015, https://www.aids.gov/hiv-aids-basics/just-diagnosed-with-hiv-aids/hiv-in-your-body/stages-of-hiv). Advances in treatment, however, have significantly increased the life expectancy of AIDS patients.

Margaret T. May et al. indicate in "Impact on Life Expectancy of HIV-1 Positive Individuals of CD4+ Cell Count and Viral Load Response to Antiretroviral Therapy" (*AIDS*, vol. 28, no. 8, May 2014) that many people diagnosed with HIV infection in the 21st century will have normal life expectancies. Research finds that HIV-infected people, especially those who begin treatment with a low CD4+ count and maintain cell counts that are near normal, can anticipate a life span that is comparable to their uninfected peers.

THE EARLY STAGE. Although the timing and progression of HIV infection vary, the disease follows a basic pattern. In the beginning of the early stage, shortly after the virus has entered the bloodstream, the T4 cell count is normal (about 1,000 per cubic millimeter), and the virus is undetectable using assays that detect the presence of anti-HIV antibodies. Antibody assays can remain negative for up to six weeks. In unusual cases antibodies may remain undetectable for a year or more. Even after testing

TABLE 2.3

Number of people living with HIV infection by year and selected characteristics, 2009–12

	2009 No.	2009 Estimated[a] No.	2009 Estimated[a] Rate	2010 No.	2010 Estimated[a] No.	2010 Estimated[a] Rate	2011 No.	2011 Estimated[a] No.	2011 Estimated[a] Rate	2012 No.	2012 Estimated[a] No.	2012 Estimated[a] Rate
Age at end of year												
<13	539	543	1.0	448	452	0.8	366	370	0.7	305	309	0.6
13–14	472	475	5.7	325	328	3.9	253	255	3.1	192	194	2.3
15–19	2,700	2,721	12.4	2,555	2,582	11.6	2,297	2,330	10.6	1,972	2,009	9.3
20–24	7,023	7,114	32.6	7,616	7,753	35.3	8,106	8,297	37.0	8,292	8,539	37.3
25–29	15,664	15,856	72.1	16,008	16,273	76.0	16,344	16,693	77.5	16,683	17,138	79.2
30–34	27,900	28,165	139.5	28,164	28,551	140.2	28,402	28,857	138.9	28,661	29,227	138.1
35–39	49,572	49,901	239.5	45,668	46,064	226.4	42,917	43,397	218.5	41,315	41,881	212.1
40–44	83,602	83,972	394.5	79,380	79,831	377.0	74,569	75,096	352.5	70,161	70,739	332.2
45–49	105,662	105,943	458.1	107,429	107,765	470.3	106,738	107,139	477.5	103,599	103,979	473.5
50–54	83,229	83,337	378.2	89,688	89,826	397.1	95,328	95,479	418.2	100,925	100,976	442.1
55–59	53,868	53,878	280.2	59,189	59,189	295.3	65,398	65,362	318.7	71,829	71,662	340.9
60–64	27,404	27,400	170.7	31,910	31,880	185.1	36,310	36,225	200.7	40,936	40,707	225.6
≥65	20,971	20,926	52.1	24,082	23,999	58.5	27,759	27,614	65.8	32,441	32,138	73.4
Race/ethnicity												
American Indian/Alaska Native	1,352	1,356	—	1,412	1,417	—	1,477	1,483	—	1,539	1,544	—
Asian[b]	4,883	4,927	—	5,191	5,249	—	5,486	5,557	—	5,788	5,878	—
Black/African American	193,674	194,277	—	200,417	201,203	—	206,409	207,362	—	212,686	213,559	—
Hispanic/Latino[c]	109,361	109,872	—	112,762	113,380	—	115,839	116,570	—	119,029	119,846	—
Native Hawaiian/other Pacific Islander	381	384	—	415	419	—	439	444	—	468	474	—
White	152,027	152,391	—	154,964	155,376	—	157,505	157,956	—	159,883	160,187	—
Multiple races	16,928	17,024	—	17,301	17,406	—	17,632	17,743	—	17,918	18,010	—
Transmission category												
Male adult or adolescent												
Male-to-male sexual contact	203,865	227,712	—	211,110	236,842	—	217,903	245,335	—	224,666	253,865	—
Injection drug use	50,858	59,621	—	50,208	59,199	—	49,535	58,663	—	48,931	58,127	—
Male-to-male sexual contact and injection drug use	30,416	33,113	—	30,512	33,330	—	30,492	33,418	—	30,457	33,436	—
Heterosexual contact[d]	33,768	41,109	—	34,973	42,843	—	36,097	44,398	—	37,085	45,849	—
Perinatal	2,144	2,151	—	2,230	2,238	—	2,300	2,310	—	2,346	2,355	—
Other[e]	43,780	2,283	—	46,246	2,262	—	48,355	2,246	—	50,777	2,238	—
Subtotal	**364,831**	**365,989**	**291.2**	**375,279**	**376,714**	**297.4**	**384,682**	**386,369**	**302.2**	**394,262**	**395,870**	**306.7**
Female adult or adolescent												
Injection drug use	26,477	33,265	—	26,329	33,355	—	26,050	33,275	—	25,851	33,197	—
Heterosexual contact[d]	60,090	77,018	—	62,090	80,370	—	63,860	83,429	—	65,495	86,367	—
Perinatal	2,227	2,236	—	2,348	2,360	—	2,445	2,459	—	2,512	2,526	—
Other[e]	24,442	1,180	—	25,968	1,199	—	27,384	1,212	—	28,886	1,230	—
Subtotal	**113,236**	**113,699**	**86.7**	**116,735**	**117,283**	**88.1**	**119,739**	**120,375**	**89.7**	**122,744**	**123,320**	**91.1**
Child (<13 yrs at end of year)												
Perinatal	518	521	—	428	432	—	344	348	—	288	292	—
Other[e]	21	21	—	20	20	—	22	22	—	17	17	—
Subtotal	**539**	**543**	**1.0**	**448**	**452**	**0.8**	**366**	**370**	**0.7**	**305**	**309**	**0.6**
Region of residence												
Northeast	132,381	133,326	241.2	134,265	135,322	244.4	135,858	137,035	246.5	137,523	138,725	248.7
Midwest	50,643	50,793	76.0	52,479	52,664	78.6	54,268	54,486	81.1	56,098	56,295	83.6
South	189,674	189,829	167.5	196,909	197,202	171.7	203,565	203,980	175.8	210,291	210,539	179.6
West	95,226	95,875	134.0	98,015	98,784	137.0	100,207	101,083	138.8	102,357	103,285	140.5
U.S. dependent areas	10,682	10,408	236.9	10,794	10,477	254.5	10,889	10,531	258.1	11,042	10,655	263.5
Total[f]	**478,606**	**480,231**	**154.2**	**492,462**	**494,449**	**157.7**	**504,787**	**507,115**	**160.7**	**517,311**	**519,500**	**163.4**

[a]Estimated numbers resulted from statistical adjustment that accounted for reporting delays and missing transmission category, but not for incomplete reporting. Rates are per 100,000 population. Rates by race/ethnicity are not provided because U.S. census information for U.S. dependent areas is limited. Rates are not calculated by transmission category because of the lack of denominator data.
[b]Includes Asian/Pacific Islander legacy cases.
[c]Hispanics/Latinos can be of any race.
[d]Heterosexual contact with a person known to have, or to be at high risk for, HIV infection.
[e]Includes hemophilia, blood transfusion, and risk factor not reported or not identified.
[f]Because column totals for estimated numbers were calculated independently of the values for the subpopulations, the values in each column may not sum to the column total.

SOURCE: "Table 14b. Persons Living with Diagnosed HIV Infection, by Year and Selected Characteristics, 2009–2012—United States and 6 Dependent Areas," in *HIV Surveillance Report: Diagnoses of HIV Infection in the United States and Dependent Areas, 2013*, vol. 25, Centers for Disease Control and Prevention, National Center for HIV/AIDS, Viral Hepatitis, Sexual Transmitted Diseases, and Tuberculosis Prevention, Division of HIV/AIDS Prevention, February 2015, http://www.cdc.gov/hiv/pdf/g-l/hiv_surveillance_report_vol_25.pdf#Page=56f (accessed July 17, 2015)

positive for the virus or for the presence of the antiviral antibodies, many people remain asymptomatic for years.

During this period, which is known as the acute infection stage, the virus uses CD4 cells to make copies of itself

FIGURE 2.2

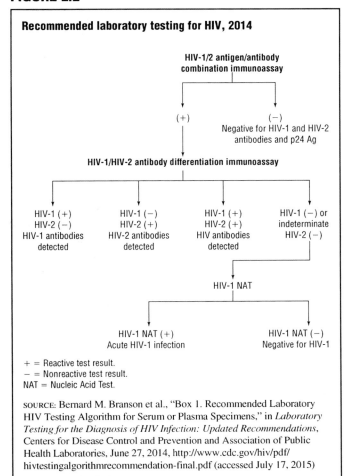

Recommended laboratory testing for HIV, 2014

HIV-1/2 antigen/antibody combination immunoassay

(+)

(−)
Negative for HIV-1 and HIV-2 antibodies and p24 Ag

HIV-1/HIV-2 antibody differentiation immunoassay

HIV-1 (+)
HIV-2 (−)
HIV-1 antibodies detected

HIV-1 (−)
HIV-2 (+)
HIV-2 antibodies detected

HIV-1 (+)
HIV-2 (+)
HIV antibodies detected

HIV-1 (−) or indeterminate
HIV-2 (−)

HIV-1 NAT

HIV-1 NAT (+)
Acute HIV-1 infection

HIV-1 NAT (−)
Negative for HIV-1

+ = Reactive test result.
− = Nonreactive test result.
NAT = Nucleic Acid Test.

SOURCE: Bernard M. Branson et al., "Box 1. Recommended Laboratory HIV Testing Algorithm for Serum or Plasma Specimens," in *Laboratory Testing for the Diagnosis of HIV Infection: Updated Recommendations*, Centers for Disease Control and Prevention and Association of Public Health Laboratories, June 27, 2014, http://www.cdc.gov/hiv/pdf/hivtestingalgorithmrecommendation-final.pdf (accessed July 17, 2015)

and destroys these cells in the process. Because of this, the CD4 count can fall quickly.

HIV is most readily transmitted during this stage because the amount of virus in the blood is very high. Over time, the immune response reduces the amount of virus in the body, and the CD4 count increases but generally does not return to pre-infection levels. Some people may develop symptoms like those of infectious mononucleosis—fatigue, fever, swollen glands, and a rash. Often, these symptoms disappear within weeks, and a connection with an HIV infection is not made. Throughout this stage, however, the virus is multiplying and destroying healthy cells. Most people continue to feel fine, although some may have chronically swollen lymph nodes. This stage lasts about five years.

THE MIDDLE STAGE. During a period known as clinical latency (because the virus is relatively inactive or dormant), HIV is still active but reproduces at very low levels and often produces no symptoms. Toward the end of this stage, the viral load rises, the CD4 cell count decreases, and the T4 cell count is reduced by half, to about 500 per cubic millimeter. Even with this physiological change, many people are still asymptomatic. As the infection advances,

skin tests will likely show that cell-mediated immunity, a form of immunological defense, is disintegrating. The deterioration of the immune system has begun.

People on ART may live in this phase for decades. For those who are not on ART, this stage can last up to a decade. Although ART greatly reduces the risk of transmitting HIV during this phase, it is still very possible for HIV to be transmitted. Symptoms of HIV infection—including weight loss; profound, unexplained fatigue; nausea; fever; night sweats; swollen lymph glands; a persistent, dry cough; easy bruising or unexplained bleeding; watery diarrhea; loss of memory; balance problems; mood changes; blurring or loss of vision; and oral lesions, such as thrush (a fungal infection caused by *Candida albicans*, which produces a white coating on the tongue and throat)—appear as the immune system weakens and is unable to defend against them.

ART involves taking a combination of three or more anti-HIV medications from at least two different drug classes daily. ART prevents HIV from reproducing, which helps people infected with HIV live longer, healthier lives and may reduce the risk of HIV transmission. The U.S. Food and Drug Administration (FDA) indicates in "Antiretroviral Drugs Used in the Treatment of HIV Infection" (October 8, 2015, http://www.fda.gov/forpatients/illness/hivaids/treatment/ucm118915.htm) that as of October 2015 there were 37 anti-HIV medications available, including nine combination drugs containing two or more anti-HIV medications. Because HIV mutates, it can become resistant to some of these drugs, necessitating a change of drug regimen.

THE FINAL STAGE. AIDS is the stage of infection that occurs when the immune system is so damaged that it cannot fend off infections and infection-related cancers. The third stage of HIV infection is reached when the CD4+ T-cell count drops to 200 per cubic millimeter or below. (Normal CD4 counts are between 500 and 1,600 cells per cubic millimeter.) The appearance of one or more opportunistic infections (OIs), regardless of the CD4 count, is also considered to be diagnostic for AIDS. Without treatment, people diagnosed with AIDS typically survive about three years.

Although many patients are still asymptomatic at the beginning of this stage, the functioning of the immune system is now markedly weakened. The body is far less able to defend itself from invasion. As a consequence, the risk of infection due to opportunistic bacteria, viruses, fungi, and parasites and the possibility of cancer increase dramatically. To prevent *Pneumocystis carinii* pneumonia, a lung disease that is caused by a fungus and one of the most common OIs, patients are often treated with antibiotics during this stage.

At the onset of this stage, patients may experience weight loss, diarrhea, lethargy, and recurring fever. Skin and mucous membrane infections increase. Oral fungal infections such as thrush and chronic infection caused by the herpes simplex virus are also common.

As this stage progresses, the immune system collapses. OIs move deeper into the body. It is not uncommon for a parasitic infection called toxoplasmosis to attack the brain, while the cryptococcosis fungus attacks the nervous system, liver, bones, and skin. Cytomegalovirus can cause pneumonia, encephalitis, and retinitis. The latter, an inflammation of the retina, can cause blindness. Many other infections can occur. The consequences and complications of compromised immune function are many, and death is usually the result of the OIs and cancers that arise due to the impaired immune system—not HIV. Once a dangerous OI develops, life expectancy is about one year without treatment.

Dementia

HIV-associated dementia (also called HIV-associated neurocognitive disorders) is now recognized as a declining cognitive (thinking) function that generally occurs during the late stages of HIV infection. The dementia is caused by HIV infection of the central nervous system, which includes the brain, and is different from the forgetfulness and difficulty in concentrating that can be the consequences of depression and fatigue. Lewis John Haddow et al. estimate in "A Systematic Review of the Screening Accuracy of the HIV Dementia Scale and International HIV Dementia Scale" (*PLoS One*, vol. 8, no. 4, April 16, 2013) that up to 50% of people infected with HIV will develop a neurological disorder, such as dementia.

Selected Cancers

Historically, the diagnosis of specific AIDS-defining cancers—non-Hodgkin's lymphoma, Kaposi's sarcoma, and cervical cancer—was attributed to compromised immune systems, and the occurrence of other cancers was thought to result from the fact that people with HIV/AIDS were living longer because of the widespread use of ART. In "Incidence and Timing of Cancer in HIV-Infected Individuals following Initiation of Combination Antiretroviral Therapy" (*Clinical Infectious Diseases*, vol. 57, no. 5, September 2013), Elizabeth L. Yanik et al. discuss the results of their study, which considered the incidence and timing of cancer diagnoses among 11,485 patients beginning combination ART between 1996 and 2011. The researchers find that Kaposi's sarcoma and lymphoma rates were highest immediately following ART initiation, especially among patients with low CD4 cell counts. By contrast, other cancers increased with time on ART, which Yanik et al. posit may reflect increased cancer risk with advancing age.

Although investigators do not yet know exactly why the rates of the cancers are higher among people with HIV infection, they hypothesize that:

- HIV or another as yet undetected virus may increase the risk of developing cancer

- ART may increase the risk of developing cancer

- People with HIV may have lifestyle or other environmental exposures that increase their risk, such as smoking or excessive alcohol consumption

In "Risk of Cancer among HIV-Infected Individuals Compared to the Background Population: Impact of Smoking and HIV" (*AIDS*, vol. 28, no. 10, June 19, 2014), Marie Helleberg et al. observe that as the HIV-infected population ages, the incidence of non-AIDS-defining cancers has outpaced that of AIDS-defining cancers. Helleberg et al. compared the rates of cancer in an HIV-infected population to those in an uninfected population and classified cancers as smoking-related, related to viral infections, or other. The researchers find that HIV patients had increased risk of cancers that are considered related to smoking or viral infections but did not have increased risk of other cancers compared with the uninfected population.

TRANSMISSION OF HIV

When AIDS was first identified, it was compared to the plague pandemic (also known as the Black Death) of the 14th century, in terms of the public panic surrounding the disease and its possible spread. The comparison is not a good one. The bacterium that caused the Black Death (and that still causes bubonic plague) is highly contagious, largely because it is readily transmitted via food, water, and air. HIV is not nearly as contagious. Moreover, by observing precautions that prevent the sharing of bodily fluids, the transmission of HIV can be almost entirely prevented.

The accumulated knowledge of more than 30 years of research has definitively established that HIV can only be transmitted by the following routes:

- Oral, anal, or vaginal sex with an infected person. Sexual intercourse—particularly heterosexual sex—is the most common mode of HIV transmission worldwide.

- Sharing drug needles or syringes with an infected person.

- Maternal transmission to a baby at the time of birth and through breast milk. Paul J. Weidle and Steven Nesheim report in "HIV Drug Resistance and Mother-to-Child Transmission of HIV" (*Clinics in Perinatology*, vol. 37, no. 4, December 2010) that pregnant women who develop HIV drug resistance may transmit this resistance to their infants via breast-feeding. Although breast-feeding is a known source of HIV transmission, in many developing countries where alternative sources of nutrition are unavailable, the benefits of breast-feeding outweigh the risks. For this reason, the WHO recommends in *Guidelines on HIV and Infant Feeding 2010* (2010, http://whqlibdoc.who.int/publications/2010/97892415 99535_eng.pdf?ua=1) that where ART is available "mothers known to be HIV-infected are now recommended to breast-feed until 12 months of age and replacement feeding should not be used unless it is acceptable, feasible, affordable, sustainable and safe."

- Transplantation of HIV-infected organs or transfusion of infected bodily fluids, such as blood or blood products. During the mid-1980s the transfusion of HIV-infected blood caused thousands of cases of AIDS and led to many deaths in Europe, the United States, and Canada. The blood agencies of the affected countries have revamped their blood-testing policies so that molecular assay techniques, which detect HIV genetic material, are used to screen donated blood.

Confirming the involvement of bodily fluids in HIV transmission, high concentrations of HIV have been found in blood, semen, and cerebrospinal fluid. Not all bodily fluids seem to be involved equally, because HIV concentrations 1,000 times less have been found in saliva, tears, vaginal secretions, breast milk, and feces. However, there have been no reports of HIV transmission from tears or human bites. In fact, Diane C. Shugars et al. report in "Endogenous Salivary Inhibitors of Human Immunodeficiency Virus" (*Archives of Oral Biology*, vol. 44, no. 6, June 1999) that HIV is rarely transmitted through salivary secretions because a protein found in human saliva actually blocks the virus from entering the system.

Figure 2.3 shows the number of AIDS cases in adolescents and adults by year of diagnosis and transmission category in the United States between 1985 and 2012.

Casual Contact

Although HIV is an infectious, contagious disease, it is not spread in the same manner as a common cold. It is not spread by sneezing or coughing, as are airborne illnesses. HIV is not spread by sharing a bathroom, by swimming in a pool, or by hugging or shaking hands. Studies of family members who lived with and cared for AIDS patients have not found definitive evidence that

FIGURE 2.3

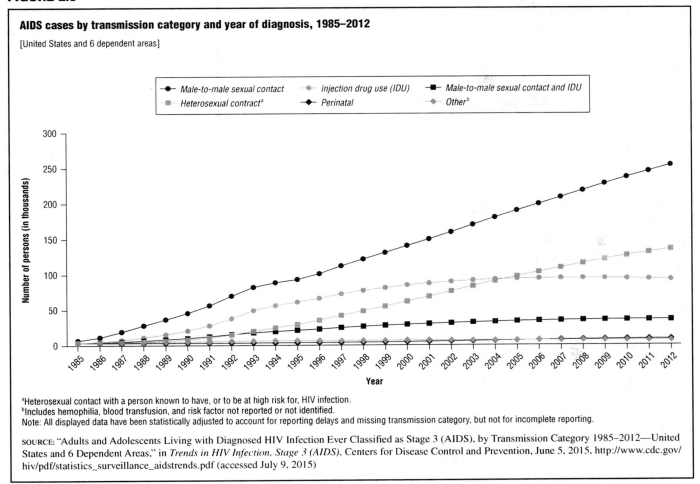

AIDS cases by transmission category and year of diagnosis, 1985–2012

[United States and 6 dependent areas]

[a]Heterosexual contact with a person known to have, or to be at high risk for, HIV infection.
[b]Includes hemophilia, blood transfusion, and risk factor not reported or not identified.
Note: All displayed data have been statistically adjusted to account for reporting delays and missing transmission category, but not for incomplete reporting.

SOURCE: "Adults and Adolescents Living with Diagnosed HIV Infection Ever Classified as Stage 3 (AIDS), by Transmission Category 1985–2012—United States and 6 Dependent Areas," in *Trends in HIV Infection, Stage 3 (AIDS)*, Centers for Disease Control and Prevention, June 5, 2015, http://www.cdc.gov/hiv/pdf/statistics_surveillance_aidstrends.pdf (accessed July 9, 2015)

anyone has become infected through casual contact. Still, myths abound. To combat misinformation, the U.S. surgeon general and public health education initiatives continue to stress that HIV is not spread by:

- Bites from mosquitoes or other insects

- Bites from animals

- Food handled, prepared, or served by HIV-infected people

- Forks, spoons, knives, or drinking glasses used by HIV-infected people

- Casual contact such as touching, hugging, or kissing a person who is HIV positive (open-mouth kissing with a person who is HIV positive is not recommended because of potential exposure to blood)

Donating Blood

Health officials agree that donating blood poses no danger of HIV infection for blood donors. The needles used to draw blood from donors are new and are thrown away after one use. Therefore, contact with HIV from donating blood is impossible.

SAFETY OF BLOOD AND TRANSPLANT PROCEDURES

To safeguard the nation's transplant recipients, the CDC suggests that all donors of blood products, tissues, and organs be screened and tested. The recommendations include screening for behaviors (risk factors) associated with the acquisition of HIV infection, a physical examination for signs and symptoms related to HIV infection, and laboratory screening for antibodies to HIV. It is important to remember that the CDC does not regulate medical protocol; its main function is to offer health care guidelines and information to the nation and its health care providers.

The U.S. Blood Supply

Before HIV-antibody testing began in 1985, an estimated 70% of hemophiliacs (people with inherited bleeding disorders) who received blood products were given tainted blood-clotting factor (a concentrate of blood used to stem bleeding) and were therefore infected with HIV. According to Steve Sternberg, in "A Legacy of Tainted Blood" (USAToday.com, July 11, 2006), approximately 10,000 of these patients developed AIDS, and by 2006 approximately 5,000 of them had died.

The widespread use of two blood-screening tests, both of which are also used on plasma and other blood products, has strengthened the safety of the U.S. blood and plasma supply. Since 1992 the U.S. Public Health Service, an arm of the HHS, has required that all blood and plasma donations be screened for the rare HIV-2 antibody, as well as for the more common HIV-1 antibody.

In 2001 the FDA approved the first nucleic acid test (NAT) system to screen plasma donors for HIV. Rather than relying on the identification of antigens or antibodies, the NAT provides extremely sensitive detection of RNA from HIV-1. Even with this system, however, there is still some risk due to the "window period," during which a person who has acquired the HIV-1 infection may still test negative. For HIV-1 antigen and antibody detection, the window period is 16 and 21 days, respectively, following infection. NAT systems reduce the window period to 12 days. Put another way, anyone who is infected with HIV and who donates blood more than 12 days after exposure to the virus will register HIV positive.

In "New Technologies Promise to Improve Blood Supply Safety" (*Nature Medicine*, vol. 17, no. 5, May 5, 2011), Michelle Pflumm explains that to further improve the safety of the blood supply, U.S. blood banks have introduced new technologies that use deoxyribonucleic acid–based screening to detect previously undetectable levels of HIV and other pathogens in blood. Although officials assert that the U.S. blood supply is "safer than it's ever been," they concede that "transfusion is still associated with [a] risk of transmission."

Blood and Organ Donation Guidelines Revised in 2015

Since 1998 the FDA has recommended that men who have ever had sex with men not donate blood because in addition to HIV, they are at increased risk for hepatitis B and C infections. In May 2015 the FDA released draft guidelines that would allow men who have had sex with men to donate blood if they have abstained from sex for one year. In "As Promised, FDA to Lift Ban on Gay Blood Donation" (NBCNews.com, May 12, 2015), Maggie Fox reports that the American Red Cross and America's Blood Centers agree that the lifetime ban is not necessary, and the CDC estimates the risk of contracting HIV from a transfusion is a scant one in 1.5 million.

Foreign Blood Supplies

Historically, HIV infection from contaminated blood was much more common in other countries. According to Craig R. Whitney, in "Top French Officials Cleared over Blood with AIDS Virus" (NYTimes.com, March 10, 1999), a French court ruled in 1998 that a former prime minister and two former cabinet members would be tried on charges that they allowed HIV-contaminated blood to be used for transfusions between 1984 and 1985. Relatives of the patients argued that the French government had refused U.S. technology that would have detected antibodies in the tainted blood in favor of a French procedure that was in development. Approximately 4,400 people acquired HIV as a result of this action. Many of the victims were hemophiliacs, and about 40% of the total number infected had died of AIDS. The former French officials, Prime Minister Laurent Fabius

(1946–), Minister of Social Affairs Georgina Dufoix (1942–), and Minister of Health Edmond Hervé (1942–), faced charges of involuntary homicide and went to trial in 1999. Hervé was convicted without a penalty, and Dufoix and Fabius were acquitted. The tragedy resulted in the overhaul of the blood supply and donation networks in France.

Jane Perlez notes in "Parents Sue Romania over Child's H.I.V. Infection" (NYTimes.com, August 31, 1995) that the WHO reported in 1995 that 3,000 children in Romania—home to thousands of abandoned babies left in squalid institutions after the fall of the Romanian dictator Nicolae Ceauşescu (1918–1989)—were infected by contaminated blood and syringes during the late 1980s. The WHO estimated that 1,000 of those children had died. According to Perlez, "Romania has more than half of the juvenile AIDS cases in Europe. More than 90% of the country's reported AIDS cases are among children, most of whom were infected by contaminated needles and syringes." The Romanian Health Ministry faced litigation for causing the spread of HIV.

According to the article "Another German Trial for H.I.V.-Tainted Blood" (Reuters, November 30, 1995), Gunter Kurt Eckert, the owner of a German drug laboratory, was charged in 1995 with nearly 6,000 counts of murder or attempted murder for selling HIV-tainted blood products to German hospitals in 1987. Nearly 90% of the 6,000 batches had not been tested for HIV. Testing has been mandatory in Germany since 1986. Eckert was found guilty and sentenced to six and a half years in prison.

The article "Canada's Tainted Blood Scandal: A Timeline" (CBC.ca, October 1, 2007) notes that the Canadian blood collection, testing, and distribution system was completely overhauled in the wake of the distribution of blood that was contaminated with HIV and the hepatitis C virus. In 1989 Ottawa established a $150 million fund to compensate the 1,250 Canadians who were infected with HIV as a result of contact with infected blood. It was discovered that 95% of hemophiliacs who received blood products prior to 1990 had been infected with hepatitis C. In 2001 the Canadian Supreme Court ruled that the negligence of the blood agency during the early years of the AIDS crisis entitled several thousand affected Canadians to a $1.2 billion federal-provincial government compensation offer. Legal wrangling in the intervening years delayed the implementation of the court's ruling.

Although the WHO has examined blood safety and all developed countries have strengthened their screening efforts, problems persist in developing countries. The WHO notes in the fact sheet "Blood Safety and Availability" (June 2015, http://www.who.int/mediacentre/factsheets/fs279/en) that 25 of the 100 countries reporting blood-screening data in 2012 were unable to screen all donated blood for one or more transmissible infections, including HIV.

Organ and Tissue Transplants

There are cases of HIV transmission through organ (kidney, liver, heart, lung, and pancreas) and other tissue transplants. The risk of such transmission, however, is low simply because there are far fewer transplant cases than blood transfusions.

In 1994 the FDA began regulating the sale of bone, skin, corneas, cartilage, tendons, and similar nonblood vessel–bearing tissues that are used for transplants. The FDA requires that all procurement agencies conduct behavioral screening and infectious-disease (HIV-1, HIV-2, hepatitis B virus, and hepatitis C virus) testing of donors.

In "HIV Transmitted from a Living Organ Donor— New York City, 2009" (*Morbidity and Mortality Weekly Report*, vol. 60, no. 10, March 18, 2011), the CDC reports the first documented case in the United States of HIV transmission through the transplantation of an organ from a living donor, despite screening. The recipient of the kidney tested negative for HIV 12 days before the transplant. One year after the transplant, the recipient was hospitalized with candidiasis, and HIV infection was confirmed with a positive Western blot. Because the recipient had not engaged in any behaviors that would increase the risk for acquiring HIV, the donor was investigated. The donor was an adult male with a previous diagnosis of syphilis (a sexually transmitted infection) and a history of sex with male partners; however, he tested negative for HIV 79 days before the transplant. During the public health investigation, the donor reported unprotected sex with one male partner during the year before the transplant, including the time between his initial evaluation and organ donation. When advanced deoxyribonucleic acid testing was performed on a sample of the donor's blood that was drawn 11 days before the transplant, three HIV genes were identified.

In June 2015 the HHS lifted the ban that prevented donation of organs from HIV-infected patients to other HIV-infected patients. In "HHS Lifts HIV Organ-Donor Ban" (ModernHealthcare.com, May 12, 2015), Sabriya Rice notes that according to the CDC, about 30% of HIV-infected people in the United States might eventually need a kidney transplant, and lifting the organ donor ban will enable more of these patients to receive transplants.

TESTING PEOPLE FOR HIV

A person who is infected with HIV produces antibodies specific to the virus as part of the body's immune response. Although the antibodies are not enough to successfully fight HIV, they are of diagnostic value, as they indicate the presence of the virus.

Antibody-based HIV testing is done, rather than a direct test for the virus itself, because it is too difficult to isolate the virus from the blood. Testing serves to determine if there is a viral infection in donated blood, tissues, or organs. This protects the recipients of the donated material and can be used to identify HIV-infected donors.

An antibody-based test cannot detect all HIV-positive blood. It typically takes between four and 12 weeks following HIV infection for antibodies to appear, although in rare cases this period can be up to one year. The introduction of tests that detect the viral nucleic acid rather than the HIV antibodies has markedly increased the detection sensitivity of blood screening. Still, even nucleic acid detection has a window period, albeit a shorter one, of about 12 days.

The fact that detection is not absolute from the moment of HIV infection means that the possibility exists that some HIV-infected donors may not be diagnosed, and their blood may enter the nation's blood supply. However, the number of predicted contaminated blood samples is extremely small. To further reduce the chances of contaminated blood entering the blood supply, blood banks routinely question potential donors about high-risk behaviors. Donors whose behavior might indicate an increased risk of HIV infection (such as injection drug use or unsafe sex) are automatically excluded from donating blood.

Tests for HIV Screening and Diagnosis

Conventional HIV testing involves testing a blood sample or oral fluid sample collected at a laboratory; depending on the test, results may be available in less than an hour or several days. Urine samples collected by a health care provider and tested at a laboratory produce results in a few days or up to two weeks. Rapid tests may be performed in a laboratory, clinic, or college. Home tests may be purchased in stores and online.

There are three types of HIV diagnostic tests—antigen/antibody tests, antibody tests, and RNA tests, which look for the virus RNA directly. Antigen/antibody and RNA tests detect HIV infection earlier than antibody tests (as quickly as three weeks after exposure to the virus). Additional testing is performed if an initial test result is positive. HIV tests are generally very accurate, but follow-up testing of the same specimen confirms the diagnosis. Confirmatory tests include the enzyme immunoassay (EIA, formerly known as ELISA) and the Western blot.

Introduced in 1985, EIA uses purified HIV antigens to probe for the presence of complementary antibodies in a sample such as blood. If anti-HIV antibodies are present in the sample, they attach themselves to the viral proteins that have been immobilized on a plastic surface. A second antibody that has been raised against the anti-HIV antibody (antibodies are proteins, too, so they can function as antigens, stimulating the formation of antibodies) is bound to the anti-HIV antibodies. The second antibody contains a chemical that can be made to change color. The color change reveals the presence of the anti-HIV antibody. If no color change appears, no anti-HIV antibody is present in the blood sample. This test is reliable, simple to conduct, and inexpensive.

The Western blot, introduced in 1987, is a confirmatory test. This means it is commonly used to verify the results of the less-specific assays. The Western blot technique separates various HIV proteins from one another, based on their speed of movement through a gel under the influence of electricity. The separated proteins are transferred from the gel to a membrane made of a material such as nitrocellulose. When the nitrocellulose is exposed to a blood sample, antibodies that recognize one of the proteins on the nitrocellulose will bind to the particular protein. As with EIA, a color reaction indicates the site of the bound antibodies. The Western blot provides a positive, negative, or intermediate result. The presence of three or more of the color bands confirms HIV infection. If fewer (one or two) bands appear, the test is considered intermediate, and retesting is performed six months later. If no color bands appear, the test is considered negative with no HIV present, although many people who test negative also repeat the test six months later.

The FDA ensures that diagnostic and blood-screening assays for HIV accurately detect and/or measure HIV in blood and other bodily fluids, including urine and saliva. The EIA and Western blot antibody tests diagnose HIV exposure or infection. Other tests, such as polymerase chain reaction (PCR) viral load and HIV genotyping, are used to monitor patients' progress. PCR uses a heat-resistant bacterial enzyme to amplify the copies of target stretches of genetic material to detectable amounts. HIV genotyping tests blood from HIV-infected people for HIV strains associated with certain patterns of resistance. A variety of screening tests are used to prevent infected blood from entering blood banks.

Rapid-Response Tests

The FDA has approved a number of rapid-response tests that are designed for use in clinical and nonclinical settings. The tests detect the presence of HIV antibodies in 20 minutes or less and are as accurate as the standard Western blot test. In 2013 the FDA approved the first rapid antigen-antibody test, which also distinguishes between acute and established HIV-1 infections.

Figure 2.4 lists the rapid HIV tests that had been approved by the FDA as of December 2014. It also shows the bodily fluids that can be used and the sensitivity and specificity of each of the rapid HIV tests. (Antigen/antibody and RNA tests are not available for oral fluid.) Sensitivity is the ability or extent to which a diagnostic

FIGURE 2.4

FDA-approved rapid HIV tests, December 2014

Test name	Time to test result	Indications for use	Sensitivity for established HIV-1 infection	Specificity	Approved specimen types and volumes	Test kit shelf life
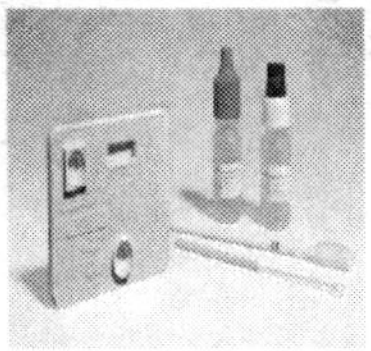 Chembio DPP HIV-1/2	15 min	Antibodies to HIV-1 and 2	Finger stick whole blood 99.8 (99.2–99.9) oral fluid 98.9 (98.0–99.4) Venous whole blood 99.9 (99.4–99.9)	Finger stick whole blood 100 (99.8–100) oral fluid/ venous whole blood 99.9 (99.7–99.9)	Finger stick or venous whole blood 10 µl or oral fluid swab	23 months
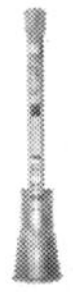 Clearview COMPLETE HIV 1/2	15 min	Antibodies to HIV-1 and 2	Finger stick or venous whole blood 99.7 (98.9–100.0)	Finger stick or venous whole blood 99.9 (99.6–100.0)	Finger stick or venous whole blood 2.5 µL	24 months
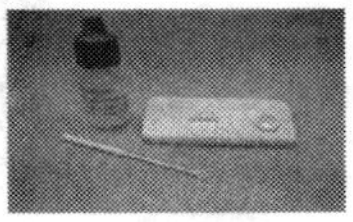 Clearview HIV 1/2 STAT-PAK	15 min	Antibodies to HIV-1 and 2	Finger stick or venous whole blood 99.7 (98.9–100)	Finger stick or venous whole blood 99.9 (99.6–100.0)	Finger stick or venous whole blood 5 µL	24 months
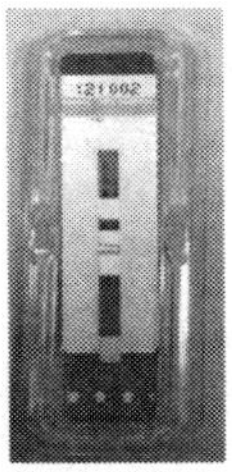 Determine HIV-1/2 Ag/Ab Combo Test	20 min	Antibodies to HIV-1 and HIV-2, detects HIV-1 p24 Antigen	Venous/finger stick whole blood 99.9 (99.4–100)	Venous whole blood: low risk subjects 100 (99.6–100) high risk subjects: 99.2 (98.2–99.7) Finger stick whole blood: low risk subjects 100 (99.5–100), high risk subjects 99.7 (98.9–100)	Finger stick or venous whole blood 50 µL	14 months
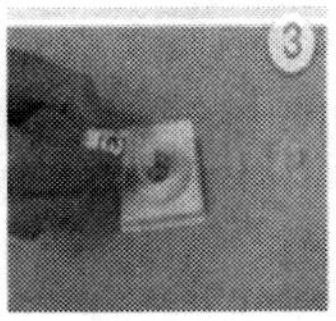 INSTI HIV-1 Antibody Test	<2 min	Validated for HIV-1 antibodies only but contains HIV-2 proteins	Finger stick whole blood 99.8 (99.3–99.9), venous whole blood 99.9 (99.5–100)	Finger stick whole blood 99.0 (97.9–99.6), venous whole blood 100 (99.7–100)	Finger stick or venous whole blood 50 µl	12 months
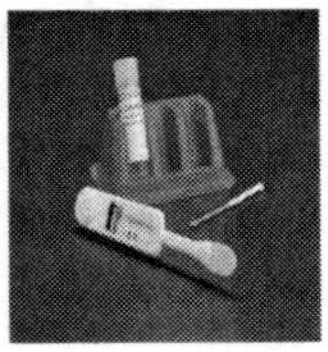 OraQuick ADVANCE Rapid HIV-1/2 Antibody Test	20 min	Antibodies to HIV-1 and 2	Oral fluid 99.3 (98.4–99.7) finger stick whole blood (venous whole blood not evaluated) 99.6 (98.5–99.9)	Oral fluid 99.8 (99.6–99.9), finger stick whole blood (venous whole blood not evaluated) 100 (99.7–100)	Finger stick or venous whole blood 5 µl or oral fluid swab	12 months

test detects a disease when it is truly present. Specificity is the ability or extent to which a diagnostic test excludes the presence of a disease when it is truly not present. In other words, a sensitive test will produce a positive test

FIGURE 2.4

FDA-approved rapid HIV tests, December 2014 [CONTINUED]

Test name	Time to test result	Indications for use	Sensitivity for established HIV-1 infection	Specificity	Approved specimen types and volumes	Test kit shelf life
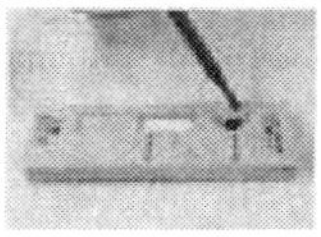 Uni-Gold Recombigen HIV-1/2	10 min	Antibodies to HIV-1 and HIV-2	Finger stick or venous whole blood 100 (99.5–100.0)	Finger stick or venous whole blood 99.7 (99.0–100)	Finger stick or venous whole blood 50 µL	12 months

SOURCE: Adapted from "Rapid HIV Tests Suitable for Use in Non-Clinical Settings (CLIA-Waived)," in *HIV Testing in Non-Clinical Settings*, Centers for Disease Control and Prevention, December 16, 2014, http://www.cdc.gov/hiv/pdf/testing_listnonclinicalsettings.pdf (accessed July 20, 2015)

TABLE 2.4

FDA-approved home HIV tests, June 2015

Trade name	Infectious agent	Format	Specimen	Use	Manufacturer	Approval date
Home access HIV-1 test system	HIV-1	Dried blood spot collection device	Dried blood spot	In vitro diagnostic: self-use by people who wish to obtain anonymous HIV testing.	Home Access Health Corp., Hoffman Estates, IL	7/22/1996
OraSure HIV-1 oral specimen collection device	HIV-1	Oral specimen collection device	Oral fluid	For use with HIV diagnostic assays that have been approved for use with this device.	OraSure Technologies Bethlehem, PA	12/23/1994
OraQuick in-home HIV test	HIV-1, HIV-2	Immunoassay	Oral fluid	Over-the-counter (OTC) diagnostic home-use test. A positive result is preliminary and follow-up confirmatory testing is needed.	OraSure Technologies Bethlehem, PA	07/03/2012

SOURCE: Adapted from "Anti-HIV Specimen Collection Devices, Testing Services, and Home Test Kits," in *Complete List of Donor Screening Assays for Infectious Agents and HIV Diagnostic Assays*, U.S. Food and Drug Administration, June 18, 2015, http://www.fda.gov/BiologicsBloodVaccines/BloodBlood Products/ApprovedProducts/LicensedProductsBLAs/BloodDonorScreening/InfectiousDisease/ucm080466.htm#anti_HIV_CollectionTestingHomeUseKits (accessed July 20, 2015)

result when the patient has the disease, whereas a specific test will give a negative result when the patient does not have the disease.

Home Testing

The CDC explains in "Testing" (June 30, 2015, http://www.cdc.gov/hiv/basics/testing.html) that as of October 2015, that there were two FDA-approved home tests for HIV: the Home Access Express HIV-1 Test System, produced by the Home Access Health Corporation, and the OraQuick In-Home HIV Test. (See Table 2.4; note that the second item listed in the table is a collection device used in the insurance industry for risk assessment.) The Home Access Express HIV-1 Test System entails a finger prick to collect a blood sample, which is then sent to a licensed laboratory. The results may be available via phone as early as the next business day. If the test is positive, then a follow-up test is performed immediately. The manufacturer provides confidential counseling and referral to treatment. The test conducted on the blood sample collected at home detects infection later than most tests that analyze blood drawn from a vein but earlier than tests performed on oral fluid.

The OraQuick In-Home HIV Test does not require sending a sample to a laboratory for analysis. Using a saliva sample, the kit provides a test result in 20 minutes and is approved for over-the-counter sale in stores and online. Positive test results using this home test must be confirmed by follow-up laboratory-based testing. Because the level of antibody in oral fluid is lower than it is in blood, oral fluid tests detect infection later after exposure than do blood tests. The test also can give a false negative result (reporting no infection when HIV infection is present) for a number of reasons, including HIV infection within three months or less before testing.

Proponents of home testing state that it offers the advantages of privacy and ease of use. Critics of home testing point out that it is expensive; a kit costs as much as $65 and may be prohibitively expensive for poorer populations—for whom such a test is most needed. Critics also question the impersonal practice of communicating HIV-positive results and follow-up counseling by telephone.

Rapid Home Testing May Change Behavior

In "Attitude and Behavior Changes among Gay and Bisexual Men after Use of Rapid Home HIV Tests to Screen Sexual Partners" (*AIDS and Behavior*, vol. 18, no. 5, May 2014), Timothy Frasca et al. observe that rapid home tests can help to determine a partner's HIV status with a greater degree of reliability than simply by asking. As a result, prospective partners could use home tests to make informed decisions about the health risks associated with a particular sexual encounter or partner. Frasca et al. posit that routine use of home tests might have other longer-lasting benefits such as changing home test users' attitudes toward their sexual practices and choice of partners. To test their hypothesis the researchers gave a three-month supply of home test kits to men who reported multiple male partners and little or no condom use for anal intercourse. At the end of the study, about half of the participants described changes in their attitudes and/or behaviors related to sexual risk. These changes included increased awareness of risk, increased discussion of sexually transmitted infections and HIV safety measures, and changes in partner choice. Frasca et al. conclude, "access to home tests not only may affect how they evaluate risk to self and others, but also lead them to value their own HIV-negative status as they reaffirm it with each new testing opportunity. It emerges as a potential vehicle for stimulating a more autonomous, user-directed process of self-examination and adaptation."

Promoting HIV Testing

National HIV Testing Day (2015, http://aids.gov/ news-and-events/awareness-days/hiv-testing-day) has been celebrated on June 27 of each year since 1995. AIDS.gov describes how to plan various HIV/AIDS awareness activities and directs people to HIV information and resources, including testing sites and other services. The CDC has an information and referral website (http://hivtest.cdc.gov) that answers frequently asked questions about HIV and AIDS and locates test centers by zip code.

Choosing Not to Be Tested

Despite efforts to encourage HIV testing, the CDC reports in "HIV in the United States: At a Glance" (July 1, 2015, http://www.cdc.gov/hiv/statistics/basics/ataglance .html) that nearly 13% of people living with HIV infection are unaware of their status because they have not been tested. The reasons for not being tested include denial of HIV risk factors, stigma and fear of testing positive, and lack of access to testing. In "Why Youths Aren't Getting Tested for HIV" (CNN.com, February 19, 2013), Sari Zeidler offers another reason: physicians' difficulty talking about sexually transmitted infections, especially with gay, bisexual, and transgendered men. This discomfort may result in missed opportunities to test people who are at risk for HIV infection.

Revised Recommendations for HIV Testing

In 2006 the CDC revised its recommendations for HIV testing, which were published by Bernard M. Branson et al. in "Revised Recommendations for HIV Testing of Adults, Adolescents, and Pregnant Women in Health-Care Settings" (*Morbidity and Mortality Weekly Report*, vol. 55, no. RR-14, September 22, 2006). The 2006 recommendations updated and replaced guidelines issued in 1993. The 2006 guidelines advise routine HIV screening of adults, adolescents, and pregnant women in health care settings in the United States; to screen people who are at high risk for HIV infection at least annually; to eliminate the requirement for separate written consent for HIV testing, making general consent sufficient to permit HIV testing; and to remove the requirement to provide prevention counseling as part of HIV screening and testing in health care settings. The 2006 guidelines also advise that HIV screening be part of routine prenatal screening for all pregnant women and that repeat screening during the third trimester of pregnancy be performed in areas where there are high rates of HIV infection among pregnant women.

In 2013 the CDC urged community health centers to implement routine HIV testing consistent with the 2006 recommendations. In *Implementation of Routine HIV Testing in Health Care Settings: Issues for Community Health Centers* (January 2011, http://www.cdc.gov/hiv/ topics/testing/resources/guidelines/pdf/routinehivtesting .pdf), the CDC explains that community health centers provide primary care for more than 16 million people, including vulnerable populations that may be at high risk for HIV infection. The CDC developed a plan as well as tools and resources that community health centers can use to institute routine HIV screening. Figure 2.5 shows a road map for implementing routine HIV testing and following up on test results.

Test Tracks HIV/AIDS Progression

In June 1996 the FDA approved a test to help determine how fast an HIV infection will progress to full-blown AIDS. Developed by Roche Diagnostic Systems Inc., the Amplicor HIV-1 monitor test is not intended to screen for HIV or to confirm an HIV diagnosis. Instead, the test detects the amount of HIV in the blood (the viral load) by measuring HIV genetic material. An increased viral load indicates the advancement of the infection toward AIDS and an increasing predisposition to develop OIs. The test is based on the PCR technique, which can be completed in less than one hour, and it was the first PCR-based test to be approved.

FDA approval was granted in 1997 to expand the use of the test as an aid in managing HIV in patients undergoing ART. In 1999 a more sensitive version of the test became available, and this test has been widely used

FIGURE 2.5

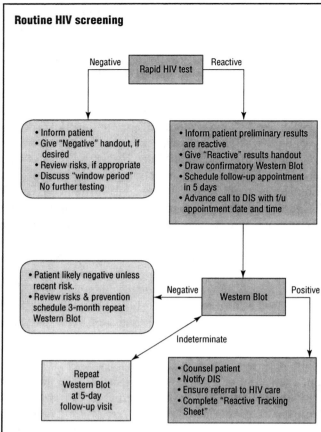

Routine HIV screening

DIS = Disease intervention specialist.

SOURCE: Jeff Bosshart, Kathleen McNamara, and Cheryl Bodica, "Routine HIV Screening," in *Implementation of Routine HIV Testing in Health Care Settings: Issues for Community Health Centers*, Centers for Disease Control and Prevention, National Center for HIV/AIDS, Viral Hepatitis, Sexual Transmitted Diseases, and Tuberculosis Prevention, Division of HIV/AIDS Prevention, and National Association for Community Health Centers, 2015, http://stacks.cdc.gov/view/cdc/20849 (accessed July 20, 2015)

since then to help evaluate and track the progression of HIV infection and disease and to predict the risk of complications and OIs.

In "Detection of Drug Resistance Mutations at Low Plasma HIV-1 RNA Load in a European Multicentre Cohort Study" (*Journal of Antimicrobial Chemotherapy*, vol. 66, no. 8, August 2011), Mattia C. F. Prosperi et al. report that although there are not yet conclusive data to support the clinical utility of this approach, "testing at low viral load may identify emerging antiretroviral drug resistance at an early stage," when prompt treatment changes may most effectively reduce the accumulation of resistance and viral adaptive changes.

World Health Organization and U.S. Preventive Services Task Force Guidelines

In 2015 the WHO published new guidelines on HIV testing services, *Consolidated Guidelines on HIV Testing Services* (July 2015, http://www.who.int/hiv/pub/guidelines/hiv-testing-services/en), which aim to ensure the quality of HIV testing and recommend testing by trained lay providers in areas where there is a shortage of health workers. The WHO asserts that lay providers "can, using rapid diagnostic tests, independently conduct safe and effective HIV testing services."

The U.S. Preventive Services Task Force updated its HIV screening guidelines in 2013. In "Screening for HIV" (April 2013, http://www.uspreventiveservicestask force.org/uspstf13/hiv/hivfinalrs.htm), the task force recommends that clinicians screen all adolescents and adults aged 15 to 65 years for HIV infection. Younger adolescents and older adults who are at increased risk should also be screened. Furthermore, the task force advises clinicians to screen all pregnant women for HIV.

CHAPTER 3
PATTERNS AND TRENDS IN HIV/AIDS SURVEILLANCE

DETERMINING THE NUMBER OF PEOPLE INFECTED WITH HIV

The U.S. Centers for Disease Control and Prevention (CDC) keeps track of the number of people in the United States who are infected with HIV, the virus that causes AIDS. The historical continuity of CDC data permits trend analyses—when viewed over a number of years, the figures provide a reasonable indication of the progress of the disease in the United States.

Estimates of HIV infection are important because they directly influence public health and medical resource allocation as well as political and economic decisions. However, definitive figures are difficult to obtain because laws prevent testing for HIV without consent and permission. Furthermore, many people are understandably reluctant to participate in community or household surveys because of confidentiality concerns.

Health officials contend that knowing the prevalence of HIV infections (prevalence is a measure of all cases of illness existing at a given point in time) is not as crucial as knowing whether the number of HIV infections is rising or falling. The rate at which people develop HIV/AIDS during a specified period is known as the incidence rate. The CDC explains in "Surveillance Systems" (May 11, 2015, http://www.cdc.gov/hiv/statistics/surveillance/systems/index.html) that before April 2008 estimates were based on reports from states that mandated confidential reporting of HIV cases, along with other small studies and surveys. Beginning in April 2008 all jurisdictions implemented universal, confidential, name-based HIV infection reporting. Beginning with its annual report covering the year 2011, the CDC has reported data on the diagnoses of HIV from all 50 states and six U.S. dependent areas.

CDC data indicate that an estimated 896,621 adults and adolescents were living with a diagnosed HIV infection in 2011. (See Figure 3.1.) That same year, 2,653 children aged 12 years and under were living with a diagnosed HIV infection. (See Figure 3.2.)

The prevalence rate of HIV infection among adults and adolescents was estimated at 342.1 per 100,000 population at the end of 2011. Figure 3.1 shows that the rates of HIV infection varied widely from state to state, from 33.2 per 100,000 in North Dakota to 770.6 per 100,000 in New York.

More than half of all adults and adolescents with a diagnosed HIV infection at yearend 2011 were suffering from AIDS. Figure 3.3 shows 504,957 adults and adolescents were living with diagnosed AIDS at that time. The CDC reports in *Epidemiology of HIV Infection through 2012* (2015, http://www.cdc.gov/hiv/pdf/statistics_surveillance _epi-hiv-infection.pdf) that 362 children aged 12 years and under were living with diagnosed AIDS at the end of 2011.

AIDS CASE NUMBERS

The first cases of what came to be recognized as AIDS were reported in the United States in June 1981. Five young, homosexual males in California were diagnosed with *Pneumocystis carinii* pneumonia and other opportunistic infections. The CDC notes in *HIV/AIDS Surveillance Report: U.S. HIV and AIDS Cases Reported through December 1997* (1997, http://www.cdc.gov/hiv/pdf/statistics_hivsur92.pdf) that by August 1989 approximately 100,000 cases of AIDS had been reported to the agency. By December 1997 that number had risen to 641,086; of these, 390,692 people had died. Cumulatively, through 2013 there were 1,182,528 reported cases of AIDS in the United States. (See Table 3.1.) Of these, 1,173,129 were among adults and adolescents and 9,399 were among children aged 12 years and under. In *HIV Surveillance Report: Diagnoses of HIV Infection in the United States and Dependent Areas, 2013* (February 2015, http://www.cdc.gov/hiv/pdf/g-l/hiv_surveillance _report_vol_25.pdf), the CDC reports that, as of 2012, a cumulative total of 683,076 people had died of the disease in the United States.

FIGURE 3.1

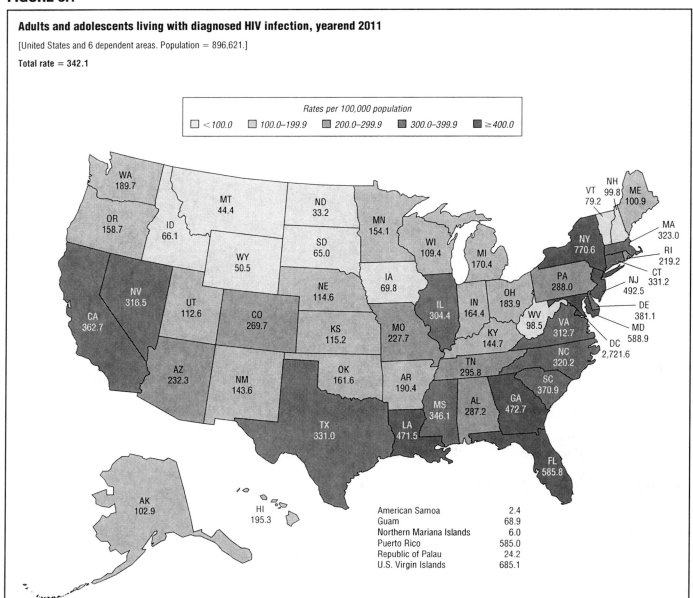

Adults and adolescents living with diagnosed HIV infection, yearend 2011

[United States and 6 dependent areas. Population = 896,621.]

Total rate = 342.1

Rates per 100,000 population

☐ <100.0   ▨ 100.0–199.9   ▨ 200.0–299.9   ▨ 300.0–399.9   ■ ≥400.0

American Samoa	2.4
Guam	68.9
Northern Mariana Islands	6.0
Puerto Rico	585.0
Republic of Palau	24.2
U.S. Virgin Islands	685.1

Note: Data include persons with a diagnosis of HIV infection regardless of stage of disease at diagnosis. All displayed data have been statistically adjusted to account for reporting delays, but not for incomplete reporting.

SOURCE: "Rates of Adults and Adolescents Living with Diagnosed HIV Infection, Year-end 2011—United States and 6 Dependent Areas," in *Epidemiology of HIV Infection through 2012*, Centers for Disease Control and Prevention, National Center for HIV/AIDS, Viral Hepatitis, Sexual Transmitted Diseases, and Tuberculosis Prevention, Division of HIV/AIDS Prevention, July 9, 2015, http://www.cdc.gov/hiv/pdf/statistics_surveillance_epi-hiv-infection.pdf (accessed July 22, 2015)

During the mid-1990s the number of AIDS cases rose dramatically. This surge was not an actual numerical increase, but was due to the expanded 1993 AIDS surveillance definition, which added diseases and conditions that had not been part of the previous definition of AIDS. By the late 1990s the number of AIDS cases leveled off and began to decline, probably as a result of the increasing use of antiretroviral therapy, which delays the progression of HIV infection. Between 2009 and 2013 the number of cases diagnosed each year decreased, from 45,999 in 2009 to 41,387 in 2013, and the rate per 100,000 population

decreased slightly from 15.3 in 2009 to 15 in 2013. (See Table 3.2.) The numbers of new AIDS cases diagnosed annually also decreased during this same period, from 30,498 in 2009 to 23,850 in 2013, with the AIDS prevalence rate per 100,000 population falling from 10.2 in 2009 to 8.4 in 2013. (See Table 3.1.)

THE NATURE OF THE EPIDEMIC

Changes in the distribution of HIV infection illustrate the increasing diversity of those affected by the epidemic.

FIGURE 3.2

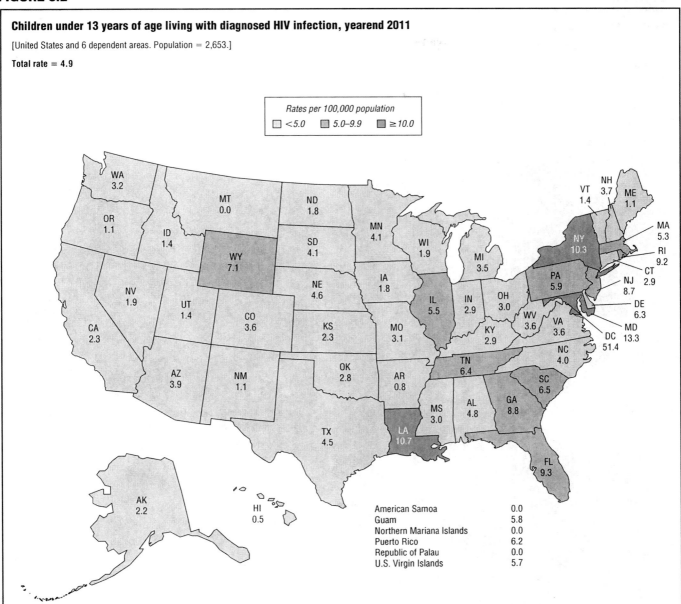

Children under 13 years of age living with diagnosed HIV infection, yearend 2011

[United States and 6 dependent areas. Population = 2,653.]

Total rate = 4.9

Rates per 100,000 population

☐ <5.0   ▨ 5.0–9.9   ▨ ≥10.0

American Samoa	0.0
Guam	5.8
Northern Mariana Islands	0.0
Puerto Rico	6.2
Republic of Palau	0.0
U.S. Virgin Islands	5.7

Note: Data include persons with a diagnosis of HIV infection regardless of stage of disease at diagnosis. All displayed data have been statistically adjusted to account for reporting delays, but not for incomplete reporting.

SOURCE: "Rates of Children Aged <13 Years Living with Diagnosed HIV Infection, Year-end 2011—United States and 6 Dependent Areas," in *Epidemiology of HIV Infection through 2012*, Centers for Disease Control and Prevention, National Center for HIV/AIDS, Viral Hepatitis, Sexual Transmitted Diseases, and Tuberculosis Prevention, Division of HIV/AIDS Prevention, July 9, 2015, http://www.cdc.gov/hiv/pdf/statistics_surveillance_epi-hiv-infection.pdf (accessed July 22, 2015)

The CDC notes in "Current Trends Update: Acquired Immunodeficiency Syndrome—United States, 1981–1990" (*Morbidity and Mortality Weekly Report*, vol. 40, no. 22, June 7, 1991) that all of the 189 AIDS cases reported in 1981 in the United States were males. Three-fourths (76%) of them were men who had sex with men (MSM) living in New York and California. In 1990, of the 43,339 AIDS cases reported by all states, approximately 30% were from New York and California, 11.5% were women, and about 2% were children. In 1999 the proportions of reported cases among women, African Americans, Hispanics, and people exposed through heterosexual contact all increased. By contrast, the percentage of reported cases among whites and MSM declined somewhat.

Table 3.1 and Table 3.2 show that between 2009 and 2013 MSM sexual contact continued to account for

FIGURE 3.3

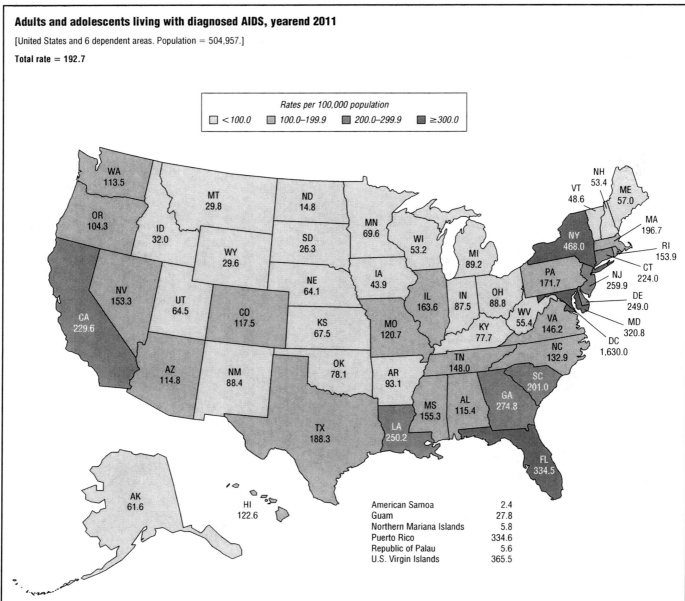

Adults and adolescents living with diagnosed AIDS, yearend 2011

[United States and 6 dependent areas. Population = 504,957.]

Total rate = 192.7

Rates per 100,000 population

☐ <100.0 ▨ 100.0–199.9 ▨ 200.0–299.9 ■ ≥300.0

WA 113.5
OR 104.3
ID 32.0
MT 29.8
ND 14.8
MN 69.6
WI 53.2
MI 89.2
NY 468.0
VT 48.6
NH 53.4
ME 57.0
MA 196.7
RI 153.9
CT 224.0
NV 153.3
UT 64.5
WY 29.6
SD 26.3
IA 43.9
IL 163.6
IN 87.5
OH 88.8
PA 171.7
NJ 259.9
DE 249.0
MD 320.8
CA 229.6
CO 117.5
NE 64.1
KS 67.5
MO 120.7
KY 77.7
WV 55.4
VA 146.2
DC 1,630.0
NC 132.9
AZ 114.8
NM 88.4
OK 78.1
AR 93.1
TN 148.0
SC 201.0
AK 61.6
HI 122.6
TX 188.3
LA 250.2
MS 155.3
AL 115.4
GA 274.8
FL 334.5

American Samoa	2.4
Guam	27.8
Northern Mariana Islands	5.8
Puerto Rico	334.6
Republic of Palau	5.6
U.S. Virgin Islands	365.5

Note: All displayed data have been statistically adjusted to account for reporting delays, but not for incomplete reporting.

SOURCE: "Rates of Adults and Adolescents Living with Diagnosed HIV Infection Ever Classified as Stage 3 (AIDS), Year-end 2011—United States and 6 Dependent Areas," in *Epidemiology of HIV Infection through 2012*, Centers for Disease Control and Prevention, National Center for HIV/AIDS, Viral Hepatitis, Sexual Transmitted Diseases, and Tuberculosis Prevention, Division of HIV/AIDS Prevention, July 9, 2015, http://www.cdc.gov/hiv/pdf/ statistics_surveillance_epi-hiv-infection.pdf (accessed July 22, 2015)

the largest proportion of diagnosed cases; however, there were also substantial numbers of HIV and AIDS diagnoses attributable to injection drug use or to heterosexual contact.

Regional Differences

AIDS cases have been reported throughout the United States and its dependent areas. The distribution of cases, however, is far from even. In 2012 the highest rate by far was in the District of Columbia, where the rate was 67.4 per 100,000 population. (See Figure 3.4.) Among U.S. states,

rates were highest in Georgia (26.6), Louisiana (18.4), and Maryland (17). The lowest rates were in Vermont (0), North Dakota (0.9), and Idaho (1.2). Figure 3.5 shows the corresponding AIDS rates for children under the age of 13 years at the end of 2011. The estimated rates for children living with AIDS ranged from 0 per 100,000 population in Arkansas, Maine, Missouri, Montana, New Hampshire, Oregon, Vermont, Washington, and Wyoming to 15.6 per 100,000 population in the District of Columbia.

RATES IN MAJOR METROPOLITAN AREAS. AIDS cases tend to be concentrated in urban areas. Table 3.3 gives

TABLE 3.1

AIDS diagnoses by selected characteristics, 2009–13 and cumulative

	2009			2010			2011			2012			2013			Cumulative[b]	
		Estimated[a]			Estimated[a]			Estimated[a]			Estimated[a]			Estimated[a]			
	No.	No.	Rate	No.	No.	Rate	No.	No.	Rate	No.	No.	Rate	No.	No.	Rate	No.	Est. No.[a]
Age at diagnosis (yr)																	
<13	14	14	0.0	23	24	0.0	15	16	0.0	10	10	0.0	7	8	0.0	9,399	9,421
13–14	45	46	0.6	47	49	0.6	37	39	0.5	28	29	0.4	25	30	0.4	1,442	1,461
15–19	439	450	2.1	454	470	2.1	428	447	2.1	340	361	1.7	381	435	2.1	8,636	8,793
20–24	1,947	1,996	9.3	1,987	2,062	9.5	1,971	2,064	9.3	1,863	1,982	8.8	1,996	2,239	9.8	50,040	50,787
25–29	3,140	3,220	14.9	2,884	2,993	14.2	2,763	2,896	13.6	2,701	2,877	13.4	2,787	3,123	14.5	138,724	139,957
30–34	3,651	3,743	18.8	3,302	3,423	17.1	3,129	3,276	16.0	3,218	3,424	16.4	2,927	3,268	15.4	222,750	224,308
35–39	4,335	4,442	21.6	3,708	3,844	19.1	3,179	3,329	17.0	2,891	3,074	15.8	2,869	3,200	16.3	241,443	243,169
40–44	4,989	5,116	24.4	4,304	4,463	21.3	3,753	3,930	18.7	3,424	3,640	17.3	3,121	3,496	16.8	202,176	204,006
45–49	4,813	4,935	21.6	4,273	4,431	19.6	3,953	4,138	18.7	3,614	3,843	17.7	3,386	3,781	17.8	137,405	139,062
50–54	3,492	3,578	16.4	3,180	3,298	14.8	2,900	3,043	13.5	2,863	3,045	13.5	2,803	3,135	13.9	81,518	82,718
55–59	1,939	1,987	10.5	1,759	1,826	9.2	1,793	1,874	9.2	1,756	1,872	9.0	1,789	1,998	9.4	44,927	45,628
60–64	917	939	5.9	933	967	5.7	910	950	5.3	984	1,049	5.9	1,019	1,144	6.3	23,899	24,274
≥65	777	796	2.0	741	767	1.9	724	754	1.8	721	766	1.8	740	831	1.9	20,169	20,455
Race/ethnicity																	
American Indian/Alaska Native	104	106	4.5	119	122	5.4	114	117	5.1	101	105	4.5	96	104	4.5	3,486	3,514
Asian[c]	374	384	2.8	365	380	2.6	367	384	2.5	358	382	2.4	374	415	2.6	9,560	9,712
Black/African American	14,326	14,687	39.0	13,440	13,951	36.7	12,353	12,946	33.7	11,949	12,735	32.9	11,678	13,172	33.7	491,715	497,267
Hispanic/Latino[d]	6,454	6,629	13.7	5,599	5,817	11.5	5,215	5,469	10.5	4,981	5,307	10.0	4,814	5,336	9.9	213,246	215,685
Native Hawaiian/other Pacific Islander	37	38	8.4	39	40	8.1	32	33	6.5	30	32	6.1	34	37	6.9	845	855
White	7,917	8,097	4.1	6,979	7,208	3.7	6,505	6,786	3.4	6,079	6,429	3.3	6,090	6,759	3.4	433,681	436,557
Multiple races	1,286	1,322	29.0	1,054	1,097	19.4	969	1,020	17.5	915	984	16.4	764	867	14.0	29,995	30,448
Transmission category																	
Male adult or adolescent																	
Male-to-male sexual contact	12,574	15,530	—	11,635	14,575	—	11,157	13,958	—	10,700	13,821	—	10,542	14,611	—	520,784	577,403
Injection drug use	1,741	2,432	—	1,482	2,152	—	1,242	1,825	—	1,105	1,705	—	932	1,610	—	164,750	187,218
Male-to-male sexual contact and injection drug use	1,322	1,595	—	1,130	1,389	—	977	1,232	—	860	1,115	—	716	1,026	—	77,304	83,828
Heterosexual contact[e]	2,626	3,549	—	2,239	3,155	—	2,093	2,918	—	1,891	2,790	—	1,774	2,865	—	64,842	82,447
Other[f]	4,398	125	—	4,138	116	—	3,696	122	—	3,821	115	—	4,164	144	—	106,136	11,545
Subtotal	22,661	23,232	18.7	20,624	21,387	17.1	19,165	20,055	15.9	18,377	19,546	15.3	18,128	20,256	15.7	933,816	942,440
Female adult or adolescent																	
Injection drug use	1,160	1,734	—	959	1,472	—	839	1,313	—	755	1,225	—	645	1,143	—	74,970	89,790
Heterosexual contact[e]	4,108	6,156	—	3,584	5,599	—	3,265	5,240	—	3,003	5,077	—	2,696	5,109	—	111,561	146,521
Other[f]	2,555	125	—	2,405	136	—	2,271	132	—	2,268	114	—	2,374	172	—	52,782	5,868
Subtotal	7,823	8,016	6.2	6,948	7,206	5.5	6,375	6,684	5.0	6,026	6,417	4.8	5,715	6,424	4.8	239,313	242,178
Child (<13 yrs at diagnosis)																	
Perinatal	13	13	—	17	18	—	12	13	—	9	9	—	6	7	—	8,532	8,553
Other[g]	1	1	—	6	6	—	3	3	—	1	1	—	1	1	—	867	869
Subtotal	14	14	0.0	23	24	0.0	15	16	0.0	10	10	0.0	7	8	0.0	9,399	9,421
Region of residence																	
Northeast	6,516	6,750	12.2	5,639	5,923	10.7	5,119	5,449	9.8	4,771	5,173	9.3	4,301	4,872	8.7	348,674	352,167
Midwest	3,652	3,714	5.6	3,369	3,456	5.2	3,249	3,356	5.0	3,130	3,283	4.9	2,944	3,221	4.8	125,360	126,372
South	14,718	15,036	13.3	13,715	14,183	12.3	12,908	13,466	11.6	12,382	13,109	11.2	12,769	14,345	12.1	473,007	477,964
West	5,612	5,761	8.0	4,872	5,054	7.0	4,279	4,484	6.2	4,130	4,408	6.0	3,836	4,251	5.7	235,487	237,536
Total[h]	30,498	31,262	10.2	27,595	28,616	9.3	25,555	26,755	8.6	24,413	25,973	8.3	23,850	26,688	8.4	1,182,528	1,194,039

[a]Estimated numbers resulted from statistical adjustment that accounted for reporting delays and missing transmission category, but not for incomplete reporting. Rates are per 100,000 population. Rates are not calculated by transmission category because of the lack of denominator data.
[b]From the beginning of the epidemic through 2013.
[c]Includes Asian/Pacific Islander legacy cases.
[d]Hispanics/Latinos can be of any race.
[e]Heterosexual contact with a person known to have, or to be at high risk for, HIV infection.
[f]Includes hemophilia, blood transfusion, perinatal exposure, and risk factor not reported or not identified.
[g]Includes hemophilia, blood transfusion, and risk factor not reported or not identified.
[h]Because column totals for estimated numbers were calculated independently of the values for the subpopulations, the values in each column may not sum to the column total.
Note: Reported numbers less than 12, as well as estimated numbers (and accompanying rates and trends) based on these numbers, should be interpreted with caution because the numbers have underlying relative standard errors greater than 30% and are considered unreliable.

SOURCE: "Table 2a. Stage 3 (AIDS), by Year of Diagnosis and Selected Characteristics, 2009–2013 and Cumulative—United States," in *HIV Surveillance Report: Diagnoses of HIV Infection in the United States and Dependent Areas, 2013*, vol. 25, Centers for Disease Control and Prevention, National Center for HIV/AIDS, Viral Hepatitis, Sexual Transmitted Diseases, and Tuberculosis Prevention, Division of HIV/AIDS Prevention, February 2015, http://www.cdc.gov/hiv/pdf/g-l/hiv_surveillance_report_vol_25.pdf#Page=56f (accessed July 22, 2015)

TABLE 3.2

HIV infection by year of diagnosis and selected characteristics, 2009–13

	2009			2010			2011			2012			2013		
		Estimated[a]			Estimated[a]			Estimated[a]			Estimated[a]			Estimated[a]	
	No.	No.	Rate	No.	No.	Rate	No.	No.	Rate	No.	No.	Rate	No.	No.	Rate
Age at diagnosis (yr)															
<13	218	223	0.4	225	232	0.4	187	196	0.4	232	250	0.5	164	187	0.4
13–14	30	31	0.4	40	41	0.5	44	47	0.6	49	53	0.6	39	45	0.5
15–19	2,187	2,228	10.3	2,069	2,123	9.7	1,988	2,074	9.6	1,846	1,989	9.3	1,652	1,863	8.8
20–24	6,741	6,875	31.9	7,064	7,265	33.5	7,066	7,386	33.3	7,196	7,752	34.3	7,059	8,053	35.3
25–29	6,510	6,641	30.6	6,342	6,533	30.9	6,366	6,658	31.3	6,556	7,083	33.1	6,844	7,825	36.3
30–34	5,714	5,835	29.3	5,481	5,652	28.2	5,262	5,508	26.9	5,589	6,037	28.9	5,404	6,165	29.0
35–39	5,659	5,779	28.1	5,028	5,184	25.8	4,456	4,673	23.8	4,264	4,611	23.7	4,246	4,858	24.8
40–44	5,991	6,120	29.2	5,233	5,402	25.8	4,800	5,032	23.9	4,554	4,923	23.4	4,217	4,820	23.1
45–49	5,297	5,413	23.7	4,860	5,014	22.1	4,628	4,859	21.9	4,449	4,822	22.2	4,311	4,961	23.4
50–54	3,659	3,742	17.2	3,512	3,629	16.2	3,364	3,532	15.6	3,274	3,554	15.7	3,254	3,747	16.6
55–59	2,163	2,212	11.7	2,065	2,137	10.8	1,992	2,095	10.3	1,975	2,146	10.3	2,151	2,467	11.6
60–64	1,007	1,031	6.5	1,073	1,109	6.5	1,069	1,123	6.3	1,066	1,164	6.5	1,150	1,316	7.3
≥65	823	842	2.1	789	815	2.0	812	858	2.1	825	901	2.1	896	1,045	2.3
Race/ethnicity															
American Indian/Alaska Native	167	169	7.2	180	183	8.1	172	177	7.8	194	202	8.8	197	218	9.4
Asian	718	734	5.4	717	742	5.0	787	827	5.4	833	901	5.8	862	973	6.0
Black/African American	21,661	22,136	58.7	20,510	21,148	55.6	19,453	20,436	53.3	19,079	20,803	53.7	18,803	21,836	55.9
Hispanic/Latino[b]	9,411	9,620	19.9	9,009	9,317	18.4	8,852	9,299	17.9	8,980	9,710	18.3	8,878	10,117	18.7
Native Hawaiian/other Pacific Islander	64	65	14.5	59	61	12.1	56	59	11.5	71	75	14.4	61	67	12.7
White	12,518	12,750	6.4	11,957	12,290	6.2	11,465	11,923	6.0	11,593	12,372	6.3	11,672	13,101	6.6
Multiple races	1,460	1,497	32.8	1,349	1,395	24.7	1,249	1,318	22.6	1,125	1,223	20.4	914	1,039	16.8
Transmission category															
Male adult or adolescent															
Male-to-male sexual contact	21,811	27,394	—	21,712	27,106	—	21,791	27,357	—	21,962	28,967	—	21,498	30,689	—
Injection drug use	1,507	2,501	—	1,306	2,205	—	1,076	1,879	—	922	1,799	—	887	1,942	—
Male-to-male sexual contact and injection drug use	1,251	1,611	—	1,177	1,507	—	1,024	1,346	—	978	1,316	—	851	1,270	—
Heterosexual contact[c]	3,120	4,501	—	2,871	4,176	—	2,725	3,959	—	2,452	3,776	—	2,199	3,887	—
Other[d]	7,625	56	—	6,935	55	—	6,415	53	—	6,953	79	—	7,745	99	—
Subtotal	**35,314**	**36,062**	**29.1**	**34,001**	**35,049**	**28.0**	**33,031**	**34,595**	**27.4**	**33,267**	**35,937**	**28.2**	**33,180**	**37,887**	**29.4**
Female adult or adolescent															
Injection drug use	931	1,687	—	777	1,426	—	661	1,288	—	599	1,227	—	510	1,154	—
Heterosexual contact[c]	5,014	8,943	—	4,669	8,382	—	4,200	7,905	—	3,800	7,811	—	3,446	8,031	—
Other[d]	4,522	56	—	4,109	46	—	3,955	57	—	3,977	61	—	4,087	93	—
Subtotal	**10,467**	**10,686**	**8.3**	**9,555**	**9,855**	**7.5**	**8,816**	**9,250**	**7.0**	**8,376**	**9,099**	**6.8**	**8,043**	**9,278**	**6.9**
Child (<13 yrs at diagnosis)															
Perinatal	175	179	—	175	180	—	135	142	—	154	165	—	93	107	—
Other[e]	43	44	—	50	52	—	52	54	—	78	85	—	71	80	—
Subtotal	**218**	**223**	**0.4**	**225**	**232**	**0.4**	**187**	**196**	**0.4**	**232**	**250**	**0.5**	**164**	**187**	**0.4**
Region of residence															
Northeast	9,006	9,209	16.7	8,421	8,711	15.7	7,865	8,307	14.9	7,829	8,629	15.5	7,499	8,908	15.9
Midwest	5,812	5,917	8.9	5,559	5,698	8.5	5,444	5,634	8.4	5,608	5,906	8.8	5,600	6,109	9.0
South	23,032	23,513	20.7	21,895	22,564	19.6	21,244	22,285	19.2	20,804	22,629	19.3	21,066	24,323	20.5
West	8,149	8,332	11.6	7,906	8,163	11.3	7,481	7,814	10.7	7,634	8,122	11.0	7,222	8,013	10.8
Total[f]	**45,999**	**46,971**	**15.3**	**43,781**	**45,136**	**14.6**	**42,034**	**44,040**	**14.1**	**41,875**	**45,287**	**14.4**	**41,387**	**47,352**	**15.0**

[a]Estimated numbers resulted from statistical adjustment that accounted for reporting delays and missing transmission category, but not for incomplete reporting. Rates are per 100,000 population. Rates are not calculated by transmission category because of the lack of denominator data.
[b]Hispanics/Latinos can be of any race.
[c]Heterosexual contact with a person known to have, or to be at high risk for, HIV infection.
[d]Includes hemophilia, blood transfusion, perinatal exposure, and risk factor not reported or not identified.
[e]Includes hemophilia, blood transfusion, and risk factor not reported or not identified.
[f]Because column totals for estimated numbers were calculated independently of the values for the subpopulations, the values in each column may not sum to the column total.
Note: Data include persons with a diagnosis of HIV infection regardless of stage of disease at diagnosis.

SOURCE: "Table 1a. Diagnoses of HIV Infection, by Year of Diagnosis and Selected Characteristics, 2009–2013—United States," in *HIV Surveillance Report: Diagnoses of HIV Infection in the United States and Dependent Areas, 2013*, vol. 25, Centers for Disease Control and Prevention, National Center for HIV/ AIDS, Viral Hepatitis, Sexual Transmitted Diseases, and Tuberculosis Prevention, Division of HIV/AIDS Prevention, February 2015, http://www.cdc.gov/hiv/ pdf/g-l/hiv_surveillance_report_vol_25.pdf#Page=56f (accessed July 22, 2015)

statistics on the prevalence of AIDS among the populations of metropolitan statistical areas (MSAs; large cities and their surrounding areas as delineated by the federal government). Across all MSAs there was a prevalence of 204.8 people living with AIDS per 100,000 population at yearend 2012, much higher than the rate of 60.6 in nonmetropolitan areas. Out of all the MSAs tracked, Miami–Ft. Lauderdale–West Palm Beach (486.8), New York–Newark–Jersey City

FIGURE 3.4

Rates of AIDS in adults and adolescents by state, 2012

[United States and 6 dependent areas. Population = 28,319.]

Total rate = 8.9

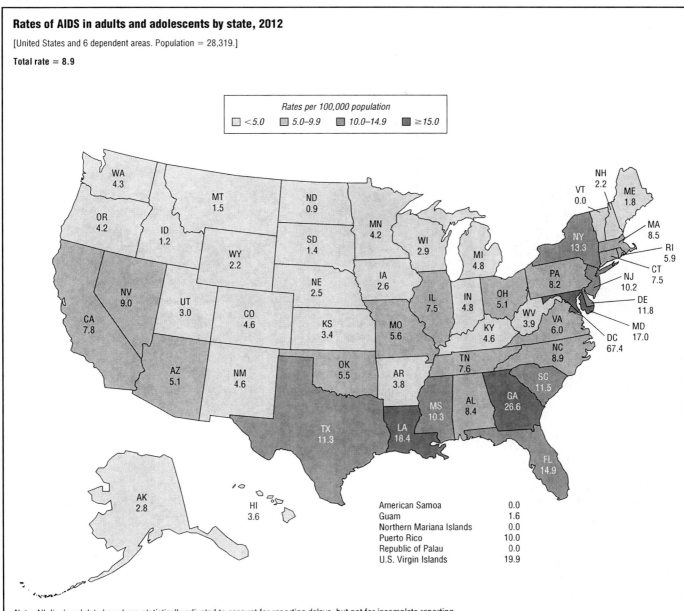

American Samoa 0.0
Guam 1.6
Northern Mariana Islands 0.0
Puerto Rico 10.0
Republic of Palau 0.0
U.S. Virgin Islands 19.9

Note: All displayed data have been statistically adjusted to account for reporting delays, but not for incomplete reporting.

SOURCE: "Rates of Stage 3 (AIDS) Classifications among Persons with HIV Infection, 2012—United States and 6 Dependent Areas," in *Epidemiology of HIV Infection through 2012*, Centers for Disease Control and Prevention, National Center for HIV/AIDS, Viral Hepatitis, Sexual Transmitted Diseases, and Tuberculosis Prevention, Division of HIV/AIDS Prevention, July 9, 2015, http://www.cdc.gov/hiv/pdf/statistics_surveillance_epi-hiv-infection.pdf (accessed July 22, 2015)

(434.4), and San Francisco–Oakland–Hayward (366.6) had the highest prevalence of AIDS.

There are several reasons for the higher prevalence of AIDS in urban areas. First, metropolitan areas are often more tolerant of lesbians, gays, and bisexuals, including MSM. Second, large metropolitan areas tend to have greater numbers of people who use injection drugs, which is another risk factor for HIV infection. Third, although HIV infection and transmission are not restricted to heavily populated

areas, people seeking treatment may migrate to these areas for better access to medical care and social services.

Current Age and Sex Distribution

Of the estimated 1,194,039 cumulative total reported cases of AIDS in 2013, 1,184,618 (99.2% of the cumulative total) were among adults and adolescents. (See Table 3.1.) The remaining 9,421 cases (0.8%) were children aged 12 years and under. According to the CDC, in 2012 more people aged 45 to 49 years (103,599) and 50 to 54 years (100,925)

FIGURE 3.5

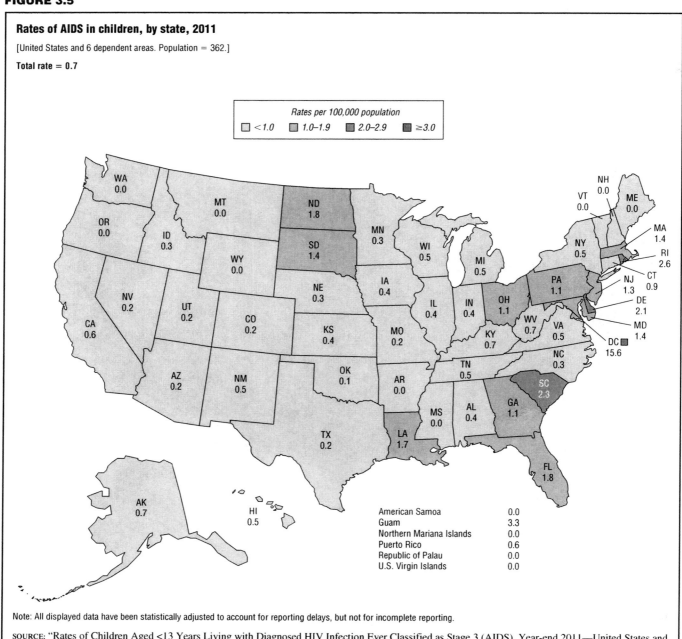

Rates of AIDS in children, by state, 2011

[United States and 6 dependent areas. Population = 362.]

Total rate = 0.7

Rates per 100,000 population

☐ <1.0   ▨ 1.0–1.9   ▨ 2.0–2.9   ▨ ≥3.0

WA 0.0
OR 0.0
ID 0.3
MT 0.0
ND 1.8
SD 1.4
WY 0.0
NV 0.2
UT 0.2
CA 0.6
CO 0.2
NE 0.3
MN 0.3
WI 0.5
IA 0.4
MI 0.5
NY 0.5
NH 0.0
VT 0.0
ME 0.0
MA 1.4
RI 2.6
CT 0.9
NJ 1.3
PA 1.1
OH 1.1
IL 0.4
IN 0.4
DE 2.1
MD 1.4
DC 15.6
KS 0.4
MO 0.2
KY 0.7
WV 0.7
VA 0.5
NC 0.3
AZ 0.2
NM 0.5
OK 0.1
AR 0.0
TN 0.5
SC 2.3
GA 1.1
MS 0.0
AL 0.4
LA 1.7
TX 0.2
FL 1.8
AK 0.7
HI 0.5

American Samoa	0.0
Guam	3.3
Northern Mariana Islands	0.0
Puerto Rico	0.6
Republic of Palau	0.0
U.S. Virgin Islands	0.0

Note: All displayed data have been statistically adjusted to account for reporting delays, but not for incomplete reporting.

SOURCE: "Rates of Children Aged <13 Years Living with Diagnosed HIV Infection Ever Classified as Stage 3 (AIDS), Year-end 2011—United States and 6 Dependent Areas," in *Epidemiology of HIV Infection through 2012*, Centers for Disease Control and Prevention, National Center for HIV/AIDS, Viral Hepatitis, Sexual Transmitted Diseases, and Tuberculosis Prevention, Division of HIV/AIDS Prevention, July 9, 2015, http://www.cdc.gov/hiv/pdf/statistics_surveillance_epi-hiv-infection.pdf (accessed July 22, 2015)

were living with AIDS (204,524, or 39.5% of all cases) than the members of any other age categories. (See Table 3.4.)

Cumulatively, as of 2013 an estimated 80% of all adults and adolescents ever diagnosed with AIDS in the United States (942,440) were men. (See Table 3.1.) Women accounted for an estimated 242,178 cumulative cases (20% of the cumulative total).

Race and Ethnicity

The changing racial and ethnic profile and characteristics of people in the United States with HIV/AIDS

reflect a shift in the population at risk for the disease over the years. In *HIV/AIDS Surveillance Report: U.S. HIV and AIDS Cases Reported through December 2001* (2001, http://www.cdc.gov/hiv/pdf/statistics_2001_HIV _Surveillance_Report_vol_13_no2.pdf), the CDC indicates that in 1993 nearly half (46.1%) of all people living with AIDS in the United States were white. By 2012 this group's share had fallen to 30.9%. (See Table 3.4.) In 1993, African Americans accounted for 34.9% of people living with AIDS. In 2012, they made up 41.1% of people with AIDS, a larger share than any other racial or ethnic

TABLE 3.3

Reported AIDS cases and annual rates, by metropolitan area of residence and age category, 2013, and cumulative

MSA of residence	Diagnosis, 2013				Diagnosis, cumulative[a]			Prevalence of stage 3 (AIDS), year-end 2012		
		Estimated[b]			Adults or adolescents Estimated[b]	Children	Total		Estimated[b]	
	No.	No.	Rate[c]	Rank[d]	No.	No.	No.	No.	No.	Rate[c]
Akron, OH	13	15	2.1	101	905	1	906	401	403	57.1
Albany–Schenectady–Troy, NY	41	44	5.0	78	2,637	26	2,663	1,167	1,139	130.1
Albuquerque, NM	37	41	4.5	81	1,798	3	1,801	799	799	88.8
Allentown–Bethlehem–Easton, PA–NJ	47	50	6.1	60	1,723	20	1,743	846	828	100.1
Atlanta–Sandy Springs–Roswell, GA	837	1,020	18.5	7	31,680	148	31,828	14,568	14,348	263.1
Augusta–Richmond County, GA–SC	52	64	11.0	24	2,548	23	2,571	1,092	1,076	186.7
Austin–Round Rock, TX	136	150	8.0	40	6,090	26	6,116	2,845	2,871	156.5
Bakersfield, CA	44	49	5.7	66	2,086	9	2,095	1,218	1,227	143.5
Baltimore–Columbia–Towson, MD	468	618	22.3	6	25,666	222	25,888	10,050	10,024	364.0
Baton Rouge, LA	198	208	25.4	3	5,373	24	5,397	2,432	2,436	299.0
Birmingham–Hoover, AL	149	188	16.5	11	3,311	25	3,336	1,325	1,327	117.0
Boise City, ID	8	9	1.4	103	413	—	413	213	213	33.3
Boston–Cambridge–Newton, MA–NH[e]	200	264	5.6	67	16,903	154	17,057	7,603	7,961	171.5
Boston Division	124	164	8.4	—	10,486	93	10,579	4,537	4,749	246.5
Cambridge Division	73	97	4.2	—	6,043	60	6,103	2,916	3,062	133.5
Bridgeport–Stamford–Norwalk, CT	55	60	6.3	56	4,279	58	4,337	1,838	1,846	197.8
Buffalo–Cheektowaga–Niagara Falls, NY	64	67	5.9	64	2,958	21	2,979	1,228	1,192	105.2
Cape Coral–Fort Myers, FL	75	79	12.0	21	2,207	25	2,232	971	969	150.3
Charleston–North Charleston, SC	81	87	12.3	19	2,652	24	2,676	1,222	1,227	175.9
Charlotte–Concord–Gastonia, NC–SC	334	357	15.3	12	5,605	27	5,632	2,738	2,755	120.1
Chattanooga, TN–GA	32	36	6.6	51	1,291	3	1,294	619	601	111.8
Chicago–Naperville–Elgin, IL–IN–WI	796	905	9.5	29	37,743	260	38,003	16,104	16,412	172.5
Chicago Division	717	818	11.1	—	34,576	239	34,814	14,636	14,936	204.2
Elgin Division	16	18	2.8	—	773	8	781	367	371	59.2
Gary Division	42	47	6.6	—	1,383	8	1,391	591	590	83.6
Lake County Division	21	23	2.7	—	1,012	5	1,017	510	515	59.2
Cincinnati, OH–KY–IN	100	107	5.0	77	3,668	20	3,688	1,772	1,779	83.6
Cleveland–Elyria, OH	121	129	6.3	58	5,140	49	5,189	2,319	2,325	112.6
Colorado Springs, CO	17	18	2.6	98	712	5	717	327	327	48.9
Columbia, SC	103	110	13.8	14	4,348	27	4,375	2,264	2,269	289.2
Columbus, OH	157	167	8.5	33	4,515	22	4,537	2,082	2,093	107.6
Dallas–Fort Worth–Arlington, TX	712	805	11.8	23	26,356	63	26,419	11,958	12,228	182.4
Dallas Division	560	638	14.2	—	20,878	37	20,915	9,532	9,778	220.9
Fort Worth Division	152	166	7.2	—	5,478	26	5,504	2,426	2,450	107.7
Dayton, OH	40	43	5.3	71	1,547	14	1,561	739	742	92.4
Deltona–Daytona Beach–Ormond Beach, FL	61	64	10.7	25	2,023	19	2,042	879	876	147.2
Denver–Aurora–Lakewood, CO	133	142	5.2	74	8,387	23	8,410	3,869	3,872	146.3
Des Moines–West Des Moines, IA	31	33	5.5	68	731	4	735	360	360	61.1
Detroit–Warren–Dearborn, MI	322	349	8.1	36	13,079	77	13,156	5,254	5,131	119.5
Detroit Division	237	257	14.5	—	10,256	60	10,316	3,910	3,804	212.2
Warren Division	85	92	3.7	—	2,823	17	2,840	1,344	1,326	53.1
Durham–Chapel Hill, NC	27	28	5.3	73	1,522	10	1,532	666	669	127.3
El Paso, TX	77	81	9.7	28	2,033	10	2,043	1,062	1,071	128.8
Fresno, CA	57	62	6.5	54	2,079	11	2,090	989	997	105.3
Grand Rapids–Wyoming, MI	40	44	4.4	83	1,174	6	1,180	567	559	55.6
Greensboro–High Point, NC	54	57	7.7	41	1,728	19	1,747	786	789	107.2
Greenville–Anderson–Mauldin, SC	57	60	7.1	45	1,965	4	1,969	908	910	108.1
Harrisburg–Carlisle, PA	34	38	6.8	50	1,586	9	1,595	760	736	132.7
Hartford–West Hartford–East Hartford, CT	83	92	7.6	42	5,874	46	5,920	2,349	2,362	194.5
Honolulu (Urban), HI	37	43	4.4	84	2,366	13	2,379	999	1,004	102.9
Houston–The Woodlands–Sugar Land, TX	842	928	14.7	13	33,360	172	33,532	13,821	14,017	227.0
Indianapolis–Carmel–Anderson, IN	125	133	6.8	49	5,149	25	5,174	2,472	2,478	128.5
Jackson, MS	161	170	29.6	2	3,390	30	3,420	1,546	1,526	264.8
Jacksonville, FL	234	246	17.6	9	7,928	78	8,006	3,586	3,575	259.4
Kansas City, MO–KS	123	135	6.6	52	5,901	15	5,916	2,736	2,730	133.9
Knoxville, TN	41	46	5.4	69	1,306	7	1,313	623	605	71.4
Lakeland–Winter Haven, FL	76	81	13.0	17	2,438	22	2,460	1,094	1,090	176.9
Lancaster, PA	14	15	2.8	96	880	22	902	406	396	75.2
Las Vegas–Henderson–Paradise, NV	224	242	11.9	22	6,223	28	6,251	3,028	3,020	151.2
Little Rock–North Little Rock–Conway, AR	69	77	10.6	26	1,797	12	1,809	866	874	121.8
Los Angeles–Long Beach–Anaheim, CA	1,064	1,194	9.1	31	70,713	306	71,019	30,522	31,043	238.1
Anaheim Division	144	160	5.1	—	8,334	44	8,378	3,870	3,933	127.5
Los Angeles Division	920	1,034	10.3	—	62,379	262	62,641	26,652	27,111	272.4
Louisville/Jefferson County, KY–IN	93	103	8.2	35	3,130	27	3,157	1,476	1,469	117.4
Madison, WI	14	15	2.4	99	663	5	668	311	312	50.2
McAllen–Edinburg–Mission, TX	63	69	8.4	34	1,000	12	1,012	557	566	70.3
Memphis, TN–MS–AR	360	420	31.3	1	7,185	19	7,204	3,303	3,224	240.5

TABLE 3.3

Reported AIDS cases and annual rates, by metropolitan area of residence and age category, 2013, and cumulative [CONTINUED]

MSA of residence	Diagnosis, 2013 No.	Estimated[b] No.	Estimated[b] Rate[c]	Rank[d]	Diagnosis, cumulative[a] Adults or adolescents Estimated[b] No.	Children Estimated[b] No.	Total No.	Prevalence of stage 3 (AIDS), year-end 2012 No.	Estimated[b] No.	Estimated[b] Rate[c]
Miami–Fort Lauderdale–West Palm Beach, FL	1,362	1,435	24.6	4	67,716	1,002	68,718	28,149	28,058	486.8
Fort Lauderdale Division	443	471	25.6	—	20,737	264	21,002	9,135	9,109	501.9
Miami Division	685	718	27.4	—	35,416	512	35,928	14,152	14,104	544.0
West Palm Beach Division	234	247	18.0	—	11,563	225	11,788	4,862	4,845	357.3
Milwaukee–Waukesha–West Allis, WI	75	78	5.0	76	3,171	20	3,191	1,473	1,476	94.3
Minneapolis–St. Paul–Bloomington, MN–WI	134	142	4.1	87	5,649	24	5,673	2,846	2,847	83.2
Modesto, CA	10	11	2.0	102	827	6	833	388	389	74.6
Nashville–Davidson–Murfreesboro–Franklin, TN	132	149	8.5	32	5,040	23	5,063	2,553	2,488	144.1
New Haven–Milford, CT	64	69	8.0	39	5,162	74	5,236	2,178	2,188	253.3
New Orleans–Metairie, LA	271	286	23.0	5	10,955	75	11,030	4,326	4,320	351.9
New York–Newark–Jersey City, NY–NJ–PA[e]	2,386	2,648	13.3	15	228,961	3,028	231,989	85,111	86,181	434.4
Nassau County Division	123	129	4.5	—	9,332	117	9,449	3,568	3,479	122.2
New York Division	1,948	2,160	15.2	—	193,508	2,539	196,047	73,009	74,055	524.9
Newark Division	298	340	13.6	—	24,093	360	24,453	7,772	7,901	317.7
North Port–Sarasota–Bradenton, FL	52	55	7.5	43	2,407	29	2,436	1,041	1,039	144.3
Ogden–Clearfield, UT	5	5	0.9	104	316	4	320	165	166	27.0
Oklahoma City, OK	88	98	7.4	44	2,907	5	2,912	1,205	1,218	93.9
Omaha–Council Bluffs, NE–IA	33	39	4.4	82	1,360	5	1,365	691	691	78.1
Orlando–Kissimmee–Sanford, FL	357	381	16.8	10	11,418	95	11,513	5,443	5,430	244.2
Oxnard–Thousand Oaks–Ventura, CA	23	26	3.1	95	1,229	5	1,234	538	539	64.6
Palm Bay–Melbourne–Titusville, FL	37	38	7.0	46	1,807	11	1,818	806	802	146.6
Philadelphia–Camden–Wilmington, PA–NJ–DE–MD	621	726	12.0	20	34,504	315	34,819	15,160	15,032	249.7
Camden Division	76	88	7.0	—	3,855	42	3,897	1,554	1,581	126.0
Montgomery County Division	79	88	4.5	—	2,800	11	2,811	1,148	1,112	57.3
Philadelphia Division	391	466	22.0	—	24,206	240	24,446	10,928	10,806	512.3
Wilmington Division	75	85	11.8	—	3,643	22	3,665	1,530	1,533	214.8
Phoenix–Mesa–Scottsdale, AZ	255	269	6.1	59	9,808	32	9,840	4,629	4,626	106.9
Pittsburgh, PA	90	99	4.2	86	3,912	21	3,933	1,664	1,615	68.4
Portland–South Portland, ME	16	20	3.9	90	722	1	723	353	358	69.2
Portland–Vancouver–Hillsboro, OR–WA	99	108	4.7	79	5,838	9	5,847	2,615	2,625	114.7
Providence–Warwick, RI–MA	86	102	6.4	55	4,763	42	4,805	2,113	2,163	135.1
Provo–Orem, UT	2	2	0.4	105	148	3	151	85	85	15.5
Raleigh, NC	93	98	8.1	37	2,925	16	2,941	1,628	1,636	137.7
Richmond, VA	78	85	6.8	48	4,337	34	4,371	2,021	2,036	165.1
Riverside–San Bernardino–Ontario, CA	233	265	6.0	61	10,854	59	10,913	5,136	5,226	120.3
Rochester, NY	55	58	5.3	72	3,690	17	3,707	1,664	1,623	150.0
Sacramento–Roseville–Arden-Arcade, CA	91	102	4.6	80	4,925	28	4,953	2,157	2,170	98.9
St. Louis, MO–IL	158	168	6.0	62	7,527	43	7,570	3,426	3,421	122.3
Salt Lake City, UT	34	37	3.2	93	1,986	9	1,995	1,068	1,069	95.1
San Antonio–New Braunfels, TX	173	183	8.0	38	6,631	31	6,663	3,040	3,069	137.3
San Diego–Carlsbad, CA	267	296	9.2	30	15,463	69	15,532	7,199	7,316	230.3
San Francisco–Oakland–Hayward, CA[e]	393	442	9.8	27	45,839	99	45,939	16,216	16,327	366.6
Oakland Division	180	205	7.7	—	11,925	51	11,976	5,054	5,150	195.6
San Francisco Division	203	226	14.3	—	32,212	44	32,256	10,550	10,567	674.7
San Jose–Sunnyvale–Santa Clara, CA	69	75	3.9	89	4,721	15	4,736	2,271	2,284	120.7
San Juan–Carolina–Caguas, PR	221	290	12.7	18	24,606	278	24,884	7,519	7,254	314.5
Scranton–Wilkes-Barre–Hazelton, PA	11	13	2.3	100	693	7	700	321	310	55.0
Seattle–Tacoma–Bellevue, WA	169	184	5.1	75	10,890	29	10,919	4,865	4,876	137.3
Seattle Division	154	167	6.0	—	9,633	19	9,652	4,309	4,319	157.6
Tacoma Division	15	17	2.0	—	1,257	10	1,267	556	557	68.6
Spokane–Spokane Valley, WA	15	17	3.2	94	650	1	651	269	270	50.7
Springfield, MA	27	36	5.7	65	2,481	28	2,509	1,001	1,053	168.3
Stockton–Lodi, CA	43	48	6.9	47	1,433	14	1,447	682	686	97.9
Syracuse, NY	27	28	4.2	85	1,555	9	1,564	669	651	98.5
Tampa–St. Petersburg–Clearwater, FL	360	377	13.1	16	14,129	115	14,244	6,080	6,062	213.1
Toledo, OH	20	22	3.6	91	1,026	14	1,040	467	469	77.0
Tucson, AZ	49	53	5.4	70	2,449	10	2,459	1,046	1,044	105.2
Tulsa, OK	52	57	5.9	63	1,928	10	1,938	824	831	87.3
Virginia Beach–Norfolk–Newport News, VA–NC	102	112	6.6	53	5,849	64	5,914	2,590	2,600	153.1
Washington–Arlington–Alexandria, DC–VA–MD–WV	879	1,098	18.5	8	40,026	324	40,351	18,251	18,523	316.0
Silver Spring Division	172	235	18.7	—	4,020	28	4,048	2,091	2,130	171.3
Washington Division	707	863	18.4	—	36,006	296	36,303	16,160	16,393	354.9
Wichita, KS	24	25	3.9	88	1,023	2	1,025	453	453	71.2
Winston-Salem, NC	39	41	6.3	57	1,286	9	1,295	620	624	96.4
Worcester, MA–CT	26	33	3.5	92	2,503	22	2,525	1,155	1,203	130.3
Youngstown–Warren–Boardman, OH–PA	14	15	2.7	97	710	—	710	315	315	56.4
Subtotal for MSAs (population of ≥500,000)	**19,353**	**21,702**	**10.1**	**—**	**1,030,521**	**8,518**	**1,039,039**	**433,020**	**435,421**	**204.8**

TABLE 3.3

Reported AIDS cases and annual rates, by metropolitan area of residence and age category, 2013, and cumulative [CONTINUED]

	Diagnosis, 2013				Diagnosis, cumulative[a]			Prevalence of stage 3 (AIDS), year-end 2012		
					Adults or adolescents	Children	Total			
		Estimated[b]				Estimated[b]			Estimated[b]	
MSA of residence	No.	No.	Rate[c]	Rank[d]	No.	No.	No.	No.	No.	Rate[c]
Metropolitan areas (population of 50,000–499,999)	2,992	3,349	5.7	—	119,509	828	120,338	52,711	52,556	89.8
Nonmetropolitan areas	1,662	1,846	4.0	—	62,793	426	63,219	28,181	28,103	60.6
Total[f]	**24,181**	**27,121**	**8.5**	**—**	**1,218,997**	**9,824**	**1,228,821**	**516,934**	**519,130**	**163.5**

MSA = metropolitan statistical area.

[a]From the beginning of the epidemic through 2013.

[b]Estimated numbers resulted from statistical adjustment that accounted for reporting delays, but not for incomplete reporting.

[c]Rates are per 100,000 population.

[d]Based on estimated rate.

[e]Counts of stage 3 (AIDS) classifications for the metropolitan divisions do not sum to the MSA total. MSA total includes data from 1 metropolitan division with population of ≤500,000.

[f]Includes persons whose county of residence is unknown. Because column totals for estimated numbers were calculated independently of the values for the subpopulations, the values in each column may not sum to the column total.

Note: Because of the lack of U.S. census information for all U.S. dependent areas, table includes data for only the United States and Puerto Rico. Reported numbers less than 12, as well as estimated numbers (and accompanying rates and trends) based on these numbers, should be interpreted with caution because the numbers have underlying relative standard errors greater than 30% and are considered unreliable.

SOURCE: "Table 23. Stage 3 (AIDS), 2013 and Cumulative, and Persons Living with Diagnosed HIV Infection Ever Classified as Stage 3 (AIDS) (Prevalence), Year-end 2012, by Metropolitan Statistical Area of Residence—United States and Puerto Rico," in *HIV Surveillance Report: Diagnoses of HIV Infection in the United States and Dependent Areas, 2013*, vol. 25, Centers for Disease Control and Prevention, National Center for HIV/AIDS, Viral Hepatitis, Sexual Transmitted Diseases, and Tuberculosis Prevention, Division of HIV/AIDS Prevention, February 2015, http://www.cdc.gov/hiv/pdf/g-l/hiv_surveillance_report_vol_25.pdf#Page=56f (accessed July 22, 2015)

group. The percentage of people living with AIDS who are Hispanic also grew over this period, from 17.8% in 1993 to 23% in 2012. Table 3.1 shows that African Americans accounted for 491,715 AIDS diagnoses between the beginning of recordkeeping and 2013, again more than any other racial or ethnic group.

As of 2013, new AIDS cases were occurring among African Americans at a much higher rate than they were among other racial and ethnic groups in the United States. In 2013 there were an estimated 13,172 new cases of AIDS cases among African American adults and adolescents, a rate of 33.7 cases per 100,000 people in this population. (See Table 3.1.) The corresponding figures for whites were 6,759 cases for a rate of 3.4 per 100,000 people; for Hispanics they were 5,336 cases for a rate of 9.9 per 100,000.

Table 3.5 shows that there was a similar disparity in new HIV cases among children in 2013. That year, the rate of HIV infection per 100,000 African American children (1.7) was substantially higher than the rates for children in any other racial or ethnic group. Across all groups, most new HIV cases among children that year were transmitted from HIV-positive mothers to their children while they were still in the womb.

Causes of Racial Disparities

In "HIV among African Americans" (July 8, 2015, http://www.cdc.gov/hiv/risk/racialethnic/aa/facts/index.html), the CDC explores why African Americans account for a disproportionate share of HIV/AIDS cases. The CDC describes a number of factors that affect the African American community and may contribute to the situation. Among them is the fact

that African Americans tend to have sex with partners of the same race, and as there is a relatively high prevalence of HIV in the African American population this puts them at greater risk of exposure than other groups. There is also a disproportionately high rate of other sexually transmitted infections (STI) among African Americans, and having an STI can increase the chance of getting or transmitting HIV. In addition, the poverty rate is higher among African Americans than most other racial and ethnic groups. This affects their access to quality health care, housing, and education in ways that increase their chances of contracting HIV.

The CDC's "HIV among Hispanics/Latinos" (October 15, 2015, http://www.cdc.gov/hiv/group/racialethnic/hispaniclatinos/index.html) discusses the high rate of HIV in this ethnic group. As with African Americans, HIV and other STIs are relatively prevalent in the Hispanic population. This group also has a relatively high poverty rate. In addition, the CDC notes that traditional gender roles and cultural norms among Hispanics may discourage them from seeking testing and treatment. Illegal immigrants in the Hispanic community might also avoid testing and treatment out of fear of discovery and deportation.

To reduce disparities in the incidence and prevalence of HIV infection, the CDC supports prevention and intervention programs for African Americans, Hispanics, and other hard-hit populations. The "Act against AIDS Campaign" (2015, http://www.cdc.gov/actagainstaids) aims to improve knowledge and dispel misperceptions about HIV in the United States. The campaign consists of a number of programs, several of which assist minority groups. "Take

TABLE 3.4

Numbers of persons living with AIDS, by year and selected characteristics, 2009–12

| | 2009 | | | 2010 | | | 2011 | | | 2012 | | |
| | | Estimated[a] | | | Estimated[a] | | | Estimated[a] | | | Estimated[a] | |
	No.	No.	Rate	No.	No.	Rate	No.	No.	Rate	No.	No.	Rate
Age at end of year												
<13	539	543	1.0	448	452	0.8	366	370	0.7	305	309	0.6
13–14	472	475	5.7	325	328	3.9	253	255	3.1	192	194	2.3
15–19	2,700	2,721	12.4	2,555	2,582	11.6	2,297	2,330	10.6	1,972	2,009	9.3
20–24	7,023	7,114	32.6	7,616	7,753	35.3	8,106	8,297	37.0	8,292	8,539	37.3
25–29	15,664	15,856	72.1	16,008	16,273	76.0	16,344	16,693	77.5	16,683	17,138	79.2
30–34	27,900	28,165	139.5	28,164	28,515	140.2	28,402	28,857	138.9	28,661	29,227	138.1
35–39	49,572	49,901	239.5	45,668	46,064	226.4	42,917	43,397	218.5	41,315	41,881	212.1
40–44	83,602	83,972	394.5	79,380	79,831	377.0	74,569	75,096	352.5	70,161	70,739	332.2
45–49	105,662	105,943	458.1	107,429	107,765	470.3	106,738	107,139	477.5	103,599	103,979	473.5
50–54	83,229	83,337	378.2	89,688	89,826	397.1	95,328	95,479	418.2	100,925	100,976	442.1
55–59	53,868	53,878	280.2	59,189	59,183	295.3	65,398	65,362	318.7	71,829	71,662	340.9
60–64	27,404	27,400	170.7	31,910	31,880	185.1	36,310	36,225	200.7	40,936	40,707	225.6
≥65	20,971	20,926	52.1	24,082	23,999	58.5	27,759	27,614	65.8	32,441	32,138	73.4
Race/ethnicity												
American Indian/Alaska Native	1,352	1,356	—	1,412	1,417	—	1,477	1,483	—	1,539	1,544	—
Asian[b]	4,883	4,927	—	5,191	5,249	—	5,486	5,557	—	5,788	5,878	—
Black/African American	193,674	194,277	—	200,417	201,203	—	206,409	207,362	—	212,686	213,559	—
Hispanic/Latino[c]	109,361	109,872	—	112,762	113,380	—	115,839	116,570	—	119,029	119,846	—
Native Hawaiian/other Pacific Islander	381	384	—	415	419	—	439	444	—	468	474	—
White	152,027	152,391	—	154,964	155,376	—	157,505	157,956	—	159,883	160,187	—
Multiple races	16,928	17,024	—	17,301	17,406	—	17,632	17,743	—	17,918	18,010	—
Transmission category												
Male adult or adolescent												
Male-to-male sexual contact	203,865	227,712	—	211,110	236,842	—	217,903	245,335	—	224,666	253,865	—
Injection drug use	50,858	59,621	—	50,208	59,199	—	49,535	58,663	—	48,931	58,127	—
Male-to-male sexual contact and injection drug use	30,416	33,113	—	30,512	33,330	—	30,492	33,418	—	30,457	33,436	—
Heterosexual contact[d]	33,768	41,109	—	34,973	42,843	—	36,097	44,398	—	37,085	45,849	—
Perinatal	2,144	2,151	—	2,230	2,238	—	2,300	2,310	—	2,346	2,355	—
Other[e]	43,780	2,283	—	46,246	2,262	—	48,355	2,246	—	50,777	2,238	—
Subtotal	**364,831**	**365,989**	**291.2**	**375,279**	**376,714**	**297.4**	**384,682**	**386,369**	**302.2**	**394,262**	**395,870**	**306.7**
Female adult or adolescent												
Injection drug use	26,477	33,265	—	26,329	33,355	—	26,050	33,275	—	25,851	33,197	—
Heterosexual contact[d]	60,090	77,018	—	62,090	80,370	—	63,860	83,429	—	65,495	86,367	—
Perinatal	2,227	2,236	—	2,348	2,360	—	2,445	2,459	—	2,512	2,526	—
Other[e]	24,442	1,180	—	25,968	1,199	—	27,384	1,212	—	28,886	1,230	—
Subtotal	**113,236**	**113,699**	**86.7**	**116,735**	**117,283**	**88.1**	**119,739**	**120,375**	**89.7**	**122,744**	**123,320**	**91.1**
Child (<13 yrs at end of year)												
Perinatal	518	521	—	428	432	—	344	348	—	288	292	—
Other[e]	21	21	—	20	20	—	22	22	—	17	17	—
Subtotal	**539**	**543**	**1.0**	**448**	**452**	**0.8**	**366**	**370**	**0.7**	**305**	**309**	**0.6**
Region of residence												
Northeast	132,381	133,326	241.2	134,265	135,322	244.4	135,858	137,035	246.5	137,523	138,725	248.7
Midwest	50,643	50,793	76.0	52,479	52,664	78.6	54,268	54,486	81.1	56,098	56,295	83.6
South	189,674	189,829	167.5	196,909	197,202	171.7	203,565	203,980	175.8	210,291	210,539	179.6
West	95,226	95,875	134.0	98,015	98,784	137.0	100,207	101,083	138.8	102,357	103,285	140.5
U.S. dependent areas	10,682	10,408	236.9	10,794	10,477	254.5	10,889	10,531	258.1	11,042	10,655	263.5
Total[f]	**478,606**	**480,231**	**154.2**	**492,462**	**494,449**	**157.7**	**504,787**	**507,115**	**160.7**	**517,311**	**519,500**	**163.4**

[a]Estimated numbers resulted from statistical adjustment that accounted for reporting delays and missing transmission category, but not for incomplete reporting. Rates are per 100,000 population. Rates by race/ethnicity are not provided because U.S. census information for U.S. dependent areas is limited. Rates are not calculated by transmission category because of the lack of denominator data.
[b]Includes Asian/Pacific Islander legacy cases.
[c]Hispanics/Latinos can be of any race.
[d]Heterosexual contact with a person known to have, or to be at high risk for, HIV infection.
[e]Includes hemophilia, blood transfusion, and risk factor not reported or not identified.
[f]Because column totals for estimated numbers were calculated independently of the values for the subpopulations, the values in each column may not sum to the column total.

SOURCE: "Table 15b. Persons Living with Diagnosed HIV Infection Ever Classified as Stage 3 (AIDS), by Year and Selected Characteristics, 2009–2012—United States and 6 Dependent Areas," in *HIV Surveillance Report: Diagnoses of HIV Infection in the United States and Dependent Areas, 2013*, vol. 25, Centers for Disease Control and Prevention, National Center for HIV/AIDS, Viral Hepatitis, Sexual Transmitted Diseases, and Tuberculosis Prevention, Division of HIV/AIDS Prevention, February 2015, http://www.cdc.gov/hiv/pdf/g-l/hiv_surveillance_report_vol_25.pdf#Page=56f (accessed July 22, 2015)

TABLE 3.5

Diagnosed HIV infection, by race/ethnicity and selected characteristics, 2013

	American Indian/Alaska Native No.	Estimated[b] No.	Rate	Asian No.	Estimated[b] No.	Rate	Black/African American No.	Estimated[b] No.	Rate	Hispanic/Latino[a] No.	Estimated[b] No.	Rate	Native Hawaiian/other Pacific Islander No.	Estimated[b] No.	Rate	White No.	Estimated[b] No.	Rate	Multiple races No.	Estimated[b] No.	Rate	Total No.	Estimated[b] No.[c]	Rate
Age at diagnosis (yr)																								
<13	0	0	0.0	14	15	0.6	108	122	1.7	11	13	0.1	0	0	0.0	23	26	0.1	8	10	0.5	164	187	0.4
13–14	1	1	1.4	1	1	0.3	26	30	2.6	4	4	0.2	0	0	0.0	6	7	0.2		1	0.4	39	45	0.5
15–19	3	4	2.2	9	10	1.1	1,107	1,257	41.1	305	340	7.4	1	1	2.6	184	202	1.7	43	49	7.6	1,652	1,863	8.8
20–24	34	37	18.4	126	145	12.2	4,004	4,611	135.3	1,384	1,575	33.7	7	8	16.2	1,327	1,481	11.6	177	196	36.1	7,059	8,053	35.3
25–29	33	36	20.8	152	174	13.0	3,220	3,741	131.4	1,659	1,887	42.9	12	13	26.7	1,606	1,793	14.5	162	181	44.1	6,844	7,825	36.3
30–34	35	39	24.5	144	161	11.7	2,151	2,489	91.4	1,435	1,635	37.4	14	15	32.9	1,502	1,682	13.8	123	144	39.7	5,404	6,165	29
35–39	17	18	12.6	124	140	10.6	1,681	1,955	79.0	1,112	1,268	31.3	5	5	13.6	1,208	1,360	12.1	99	112	37.7	4,246	4,858	24.8
40–44	21	22	15.2	125	137	10.3	1,598	1,868	71.6	958	1,090	29.1	5	5	18.4	1,435	1,609	12.7	75	86	31.6	4,217	4,820	23.1
45–49	20	22	14.2	81	90	7.8	1,723	2,027	76.5	826	946	28.8	8	9	26.5	1,564	1,765	12.9	89	102	42.7	4,311	4,961	23.4
50–54	19	23	14.3	34	39	3.7	1,370	1,609	59.3	569	652	23.3	7	7	22.4	1,198	1,351	8.7	57	66	27.7	3,254	3,747	16.6
55–59	5	6	3.9	29	35	3.6	936	1,088	44.8	340	388	17.7	1	1	4.2	799	903	5.9	41	46	22.4	2,151	2,467	11.6
60–64	4	4	3.6	12	13	1.6	494	580	30.2	147	168	10.4	1	1	4.9	470	523	3.9	22	26	16.6	1,150	1,316	7.3
≥65	5	6	2.6	11	12	0.7	385	458	11.9	128	150	4.5	0	0	0.0	350	398	1.1	17	21	6.8	896	1,045	2.3
Transmission category																								
Male adult or adolescent																								
Male-to-male sexual contact	91	120	—	487	703	—	7,902	12,069	—	5,273	7,199	—	33	47	—	7,212	9,853	—	500	699	—	21,498	30,689	—
Injection drug use	19	22	—	17	26	—	265	903	—	230	480	—	0	0	—	337	473	—	19	37	—	887	1,942	—
Male-to-male sexual contact and injection drug use	6	10	—	8	12	—	139	331	—	188	271	—	2	3	—	488	611	—	20	32	—	851	1,270	—
Heterosexual contact[d]	14	17	—	38	56	—	1,254	2,493	—	483	718	—	1	2	—	360	530	—	49	71	—	2,199	3,887	—
Other[e]	24	0	—	157	2	—	4,092	52	—	1,461	16	—	11	0	—	1,851	28	—	149	0	—	7,745	99	—
Subtotal	154	169	18.4	707	799	12.5	13,652	15,847	105.7	7,635	8,686	41.8	47	52	24.1	10,248	11,495	13.8	737	839	44.1	33,180	37,887	29.4
Female adult or adolescent																								
Injection drug use	7	14	—	1	7	—	151	532	—	75	175	—	2	3	—	259	393	—	15	31	—	510	1,154	—
Heterosexual contact[d]	12	34	—	67	150	—	2,182	5,268	—	559	1,232	—	5	13	—	551	1,174	—	70	159	—	3,446	8,031	—
Other[e]	24	0	—	73	2	—	2,710	67	—	598	11	—	7		—	591	13	—	84	0	—	4,087	93	—
Subtotal	43	49	5.1	141	159	2.2	5,043	5,867	34.8	1,232	1,419	7.0	14	15	7.3	1,401	1,579	1.8	169	190	9.3	8,043	9,278	6.9
Child (<13 yrs at diagnosis)																								
Perinatal	0	0	—	7	8	—	60	68	—	8	10	—	0	0	—	14	16	—	4	5	—	93	107	—
Other[f]	0	0	—	7	7	—	48	54	—	3	4	—	0	0	—	9	10	—	4	5	—	71	80	—
Subtotal	0	0	0.0	14	15	0.6	108	122	1.7	11	13	0.1	0	0	0.0	23	26	0.1	8	10	0.5	164	187	0.4
Region of residence																								
Northeast	11	11	9.1	165	192	5.7	3,127	3,704	59.2	2,012	2,402	31.8	2	2	10.3	1,897	2,267	6.0	285	329	38.4	7,499	8,908	15.9
Midwest	25	27	6.8	84	92	4.7	2,764	3,016	43.3	614	698	14.0	2	2	7.2	1,968	2,121	4.1	143	153	12.9	5,600	6,109	9
South	56	69	8.9	231	263	7.2	11,616	13,669	60.8	3,634	4,080	20.6	12	15	18.2	5,162	5,814	8.4	355	412	20.5	21,066	24,323	20.5
West	105	111	10.7	382	426	6.0	1,296	1,447	43.0	2,618	2,937	13.5	45	49	12.1	2,645	2,898	7.5	131	145	6.8	7,222	8,013	10.8
Total[g]	197	218	9.4	862	973	6.0	18,803	21,836	55.9	8,878	10,117	18.7	61	67	12.7	11,672	13,101	6.6	914	1,039	16.8	41,387	47,352	15

TABLE 3.5

Diagnosed HIV infection, by race/ethnicity and selected characteristics, 2013 [CONTINUED]

[a]Hispanics/Latinos can be of any race.

[b]Estimated numbers resulted from statistical adjustment that accounted for reporting delays and missing transmission category, but not for incomplete reporting. Rates are per 100,000 population. Rates are not calculated by transmission category because of the lack of denominator data.

[c]Because the estimated totals were calculated independently of the corresponding values for each subpopulation, the subpopulation values may not sum to the totals shown here.

[d]Heterosexual contact with a person known to have, or to be at high risk for, HIV infection.

[e]Includes hemophilia, blood transfusion, perinatal exposure, and risk factor not reported or not identified.

[f]Includes hemophilia, blood transfusion, and risk factor not reported or not identified.

[g]Because column totals for estimated numbers were calculated independently of the values for the subpopulations, the values in each column may not sum to the column total.

Note: Data include persons with a diagnosis of HIV infection regardless of stage of disease at diagnosis.

Reported numbers less than 12, as well as estimated numbers (and accompanying rates and trends) based on these numbers, should be interpreted with caution.

SOURCE: "Table 3a. Diagnoses of HIV Infection, by Race/Ethnicity and Selected Characteristics, 2013—United States," in *HIV Surveillance Report: Diagnoses of HIV Infection in the United States and Dependent Areas, 2013*, vol. 25, Centers for Disease Control and Prevention, National Center for HIV/AIDS, Viral Hepatitis, Sexual Transmitted Diseases, and Tuberculosis Prevention, Division of HIV/AIDS Prevention, February 2015, http://www.cdc.gov/hiv/pdf/g-l/hiv_surveillance_report_vol_25.pdf#Page=56f (accessed July 22, 2015)

FIGURE 3.6

AIDS diagnoses by transmission category, 1985–2012

[United States and 6 dependent areas]

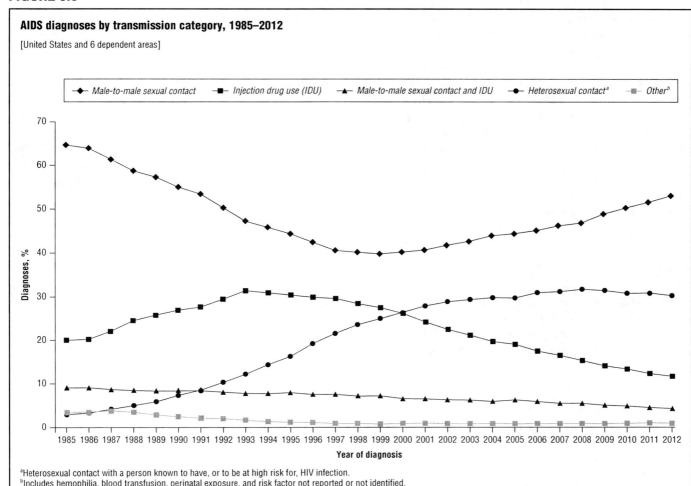

^aHeterosexual contact with a person known to have, or to be at high risk for, HIV infection.
^bIncludes hemophilia, blood transfusion, perinatal exposure, and risk factor not reported or not identified.
Note: All displayed data have been statistically adjusted to account for reporting delays and missing transmission category, but not for incomplete reporting.

SOURCE: "Percentages of Stage 3 (AIDS) Classifications among Adults and Adolescents with HIV Infection, by Transmission Category and Year of Diagnosis, 1985–2012—United States and 6 Dependent Areas," in *Epidemiology of HIV Infection through 2012*, Centers for Disease Control and Prevention, National Center for HIV/AIDS, Viral Hepatitis, Sexual Transmitted Diseases, and Tuberculosis Prevention, Division of HIV/AIDS Prevention, July 9, 2015, http://www.cdc.gov/hiv/pdf/statistics_surveillance_epi-hiv-infection.pdf (accessed July 22, 2015)

Charge. Take the Test" encourages African American women to get HIV testing. "Testing Makes Us Stronger" aims to increase HIV testing among gay and bisexual African American men. "Reasons/Razones" encourages gay and bisexual Hispanic men to get tested for HIV. The CDC is also a partner in the "Act against AIDS Leadership Initiative" (AAALI; April 2015, http://www.cdc.gov/act againstaids/partnerships/aaali.html). This is a network of organizations committed to intensifying HIV prevention efforts in African American and Hispanic communities.

HOW HIV IS TRANSMITTED

HIV can be transmitted by sexual contact with an infected person; by needle sharing among infected injection drug users; through the receipt of infected blood, blood products, or tissue; and directly from an infected mother to her infant during pregnancy, delivery, or breast-feeding.

In the United States the most common transmission route for HIV is MSM. This has been the case throughout the epidemic. As shown in Figure 3.6, in 1985 MSM accounted for about two-thirds of all AIDS diagnoses. By 1999 MSM as a means of transmission had declined to roughly 40% of cases, but its share soon began to increase again. In 2013 an estimated 54.7% of all new AIDS diagnoses among adults and adolescents were transmitted via MSM, including 72.1% of cases among men. (See Table 3.1.)

AIDS diagnoses attributable to injection drug use (IDU) grew from 20% to 31% between 1985 and 1993, but then began a steady decline. (See Figure 3.6.) IDU accounted for only 10.3% of diagnoses in 2013. (See Table 3.1.) AIDS diagnoses attributable to a combination of MSM and injection drug use declined from 9% in 1985 to 3.8% in 2013.

Heterosexual contact (with a person known to have, or at be at a high risk of having, HIV) as a means of HIV transmission has increased dramatically since the early days of the epidemic. In 1985 an estimated 3% of new AIDS diagnoses among adults and adolescents in the United States were due to heterosexual contact. (See Figure 3.6.) In 2013, 29.9% of new cases were attributed to this means of transmission. (Table 3.1.) Researchers suggest that one reason for steadily increasing HIV infection and AIDS among heterosexuals is that an increased proportion report multiple sex partners, which is a risk factor for HIV infection.

Transmission to Women

In 2013 newly reported AIDS cases among women that were attributable to injection drug use (estimated at 1,143) accounted for 17.8% of the total number of cases (6,424). (See Table 3.1.) When considering the role of heterosexual contact in the acquisition of AIDS, the proportion was far higher for women in 2013 (an estimated 5,109 cases, representing 79.5% of the total of 6,424) than for men (an estimated 2,865, representing 14.1% of the total of 20,256).

Blood Transfusions

As a result of screening procedures for blood and blood products that began in 1985, the CDC indicates that the number of AIDS cases among adult and adolescent transfusion recipients decreased between 1995 (664 cases) and 1997 (409 cases). A pronounced decrease in 1999 (256 cases) was followed by a steady decline. By 2008 the numbers had dropped so low that the CDC began reporting cases attributable to blood transfusion along with hemophilia, perinatal exposure, and other unidentified risk factors in a category called "Other." which accounted for 316 cases in 2013. (See Table 3.1.)

MORTALITY FROM AIDS

The CDC states in *HIV/AIDS Surveillance Report: U.S. HIV and AIDS Cases Reported through December 2001* that the number of deaths due to AIDS peaked at 51,670 in 1995. Since then, the number of deaths each year has been dropping. In 2012 the disease killed 12,317 people in the United States. (See Table 3.6.) As a result of more effective treatment, fewer people are dying from AIDS. As fewer people become infected with HIV, the death rate in subsequent years is expected to drop proportionally.

TABLE 3.6

AIDS deaths, 2009–12 and cumulative

	2009 No.	2009 Estimated[a] No.	2009 Rate	2010 No.	2010 Estimated[a] No.	2010 Rate	2011 No.	2011 Estimated[a] No.	2011 Rate	2012 No.	2012 Estimated[a] No.	2012 Rate	Cumulative[b] No.	Cumulative[b] Est. No.[a]
Age at death (yr)														
<13	3	3	0.0	0	0	0.0	0	0	0.0	1	1	0.0	5,191	5,202
13–14	2	2	0.0	2	2	0.0	1	1	0.0	1	1	0.0	302	304
15–19	30	31	0.1	29	30	0.1	21	22	0.1	15	17	0.1	1,358	1,370
20–24	150	154	0.7	146	152	0.7	147	156	0.7	124	143	0.6	10,225	10,296
25–29	420	434	2.0	318	333	1.6	319	343	1.6	303	347	1.6	48,854	49,088
30–34	731	756	3.7	632	662	3.3	559	595	2.9	531	615	2.9	105,423	105,911
35–39	1,352	1,399	6.7	1,028	1,076	5.3	901	958	4.8	729	833	4.2	132,279	133,024
40–44	2,247	2,326	10.9	1,823	1,911	9.0	1,560	1,663	7.8	1,245	1,424	6.7	124,986	126,005
45–49	3,013	3,116	13.5	2,771	2,914	12.7	2,537	2,707	12.1	2,104	2,412	11.0	96,079	97,308
50–54	2,835	2,932	13.3	2,667	2,791	12.3	2,665	2,842	12.4	2,410	2,749	12.0	64,723	65,833
55–59	2,175	2,248	11.7	2,104	2,201	11.0	2,183	2,320	11.3	2,036	2,313	11.0	39,838	40,634
60–64	1,279	1,315	8.2	1,406	1,472	8.5	1,405	1,493	8.3	1,382	1,579	8.7	23,285	23,787
≥65	1,365	1,407	3.5	1,347	1,405	3.4	1,431	1,517	3.6	1,436	1,625	3.7	23,818	24,314
Race/ethnicity														
American Indian/Alaska Native	51	52	—	59	61	—	49	51	—	39	43	—	1,852	1,867
Asian[c]	63	65	—	57	59	—	73	77	—	56	61	—	3,455	3,477
Black/African American	7,546	7,802	—	6,706	7,035	—	6,368	6,794	—	5,683	6,549	—	267,815	271,004
Hispanic/Latino[d]	2,943	3,048	—	2,719	2,847	—	2,626	2,796	—	2,205	2,486	—	123,727	125,051
Native Hawaiian/other Pacific Islander	6	6	—	7	7	—	10	11	—	2	2	—	359	361
White	4,284	4,416	—	4,044	4,225	—	3,964	4,205	—	3,703	4,200	—	267,828	269,732
Multiple races	709	735	—	681	715	—	639	684	—	629	717	—	11,325	11,583
Transmission category														
Male adult or adolescent														
Male-to-male sexual contact	4,811	5,881	—	4,503	5,564	—	4,481	5,591	—	4,054	5,424	—	291,451	314,907
Injection drug use	2,539	3,001	—	2,260	2,709	—	2,013	2,470	—	1,789	2,332	—	128,099	140,940
Male-to-male sexual contact and injection drug use	1,216	1,357	—	1,061	1,200	—	1,016	1,165	—	912	1,115	—	48,618	51,881
Heterosexual contact[e]	1,144	1,568	—	1,130	1,524	—	1,072	1,475	—	976	1,422	—	29,851	37,707
Perinatal	22	23	—	25	26	—	33	36	—	37	43	—	389	404
Other[f]	1,786	79	—	1,625	79	—	1,542	80	—	1,357	67	—	51,160	8,785
Subtotal	11,518	11,909	9.5	10,604	11,102	8.8	10,157	10,816	8.5	9,125	10,403	8.1	549,568	554,623
Female adult or adolescent														
Injection drug use	1,315	1,611	—	1,137	1,414	—	1,145	1,422	—	976	1,328	—	51,447	58,483
Heterosexual contact[e]	1,862	2,528	—	1,706	2,377	—	1,608	2,303	—	1,465	2,255	—	48,711	60,544
Perinatal	44	45	—	30	32	—	44	47	—	40	46	—	505	523
Other[f]	860	28	—	796	25	—	775	29	—	710	25	—	20,939	3,700
Subtotal	4,081	4,212	3.2	3,669	3,847	2.9	3,572	3,802	2.8	3,191	3,655	2.7	121,602	123,251
Child (<13 yrs at death)														
Perinatal	3	3	—	0	0	—	0	0	—	1	1	—	4,714	4,724
Other[f]	0	0	—	0	0	—	0	0	—	0	0	—	477	478
Subtotal	3	3	0.0	0	0	0.0	0	0	0.0	1	1	0.0	5,191	5,202
Region of residence														
Northeast	4,013	4,141	7.5	3,755	3,927	7.1	3,526	3,737	6.7	3,106	3,482	6.2	206,850	208,570
Midwest	1,594	1,631	2.4	1,533	1,585	2.4	1,460	1,535	2.3	1,300	1,474	2.2	66,318	66,856
South	7,235	7,494	6.6	6,480	6,810	5.9	6,252	6,688	5.8	5,656	6,550	5.6	249,947	253,080
West	2,256	2,299	3.2	2,083	2,145	3.0	2,087	2,184	3.0	1,980	2,206	3.0	129,294	130,001
U.S. dependent areas	504	559	12.7	422	482	11.7	404	475	11.6	275	346	8.6	23,952	24,569
Total[g]	15,602	16,124	5.2	14,273	14,950	4.8	13,729	14,618	4.6	12,317	14,059	4.4	676,361	683,076

TABLE 3.6

AIDS deaths, 2009–12 and cumulative [CONTINUED]

ᵃEstimated numbers resulted from statistical adjustment that accounted for reporting delays and missing transmission category, but not for incomplete reporting. Rates are per 100,000 population. Rates by race/ethnicity are not provided because U.S. census information for U.S. dependent areas is limited. Rates are not calculated by transmission category because of the lack of denominator data.
ᵇFrom the beginning of the epidemic through 2012.
ᶜIncludes Asian/Pacific Islander legacy cases (see Technical Notes).
ᵈHispanics/Latinos can be of any race.
ᵉHeterosexual contact with a person known to have, or to be at high risk for, HIV infection.
ᶠIncludes hemophilia, blood transfusion, and risk factor not reported or not identified.
ᵍBecause column totals for estimated numbers were calculated independently of the values for the subpopulations, the values in each column may not sum to the column total.
Note: Deaths of persons with diagnosed HIV infection may be due to any cause. Reported numbers less than 12, as well as estimated numbers (and accompanying rates and trends) based on these numbers, should be interpreted with caution.

SOURCE: "Table 11b. Deaths of Persons with Diagnosed HIV Infection Ever Classified as Stage 3 (AIDS), by Year of Death and Selected Characteristics, 2009–2012 and Cumulative—United States and 6 Dependent Areas," in *HIV Surveillance Report: Diagnoses of HIV Infection in the United States and Dependent Areas, 2013*, vol. 25, Centers for Disease Control and Prevention, National Center for HIV/AIDS, Viral Hepatitis, Sexual Transmitted Diseases, and Tuberculosis Prevention, Division of HIV/AIDS Prevention, February 2015, http://www.cdc.gov/hiv/pdf/g-l/hiv_surveillance_report_vol_25.pdf#Page=56f (accessed July 22, 2015)

CHAPTER 4
POPULATIONS AT RISK

This chapter examines the prevalence rates of HIV infection; that is, the total number of people with HIV/AIDS in a population at a specified time. Prevalence rates are based on surveys of selected segments of the general population and of people in high-risk groups. They are not absolute numbers. Prevalence rates identify trends such as the geographic distribution of disease or changes in how the disease is transmitted. The Centers for Disease Control and Prevention (CDC) conducts HIV surveillance—collecting, analyzing, and publicizing prevalence rates and other information about new and existing cases of HIV/AIDS.

INCREASE IN HIV INFECTION AND AIDS AMONG HETEROSEXUALS

The increase in the number and proportion of HIV/AIDS cases among heterosexuals signals a major shift in the patterns of the epidemic. In 2013 an estimated 47,352 new cases of HIV infection among adults and adolescents were reported to the CDC. Approximately 25% (11,918) were attributed to heterosexual contact. (See Table 4.1.) In comparison, the CDC reports in *Weekly Surveillance Report, 1985* (December 30, 1985, http://stacks.cdc.gov/view/cdc/32530/Email) that 1% of all AIDS cases were attributable to heterosexual transmission in 1985.

The CDC notes that between 1997 and 2001 the number of new AIDS cases dropped significantly and that the proportions of those infected in each exposure category also changed. Cases attributed to male-to-male sexual contact (MSM) represented 35% of all cases in 1997 and 1998; thereafter, they dropped to 31% in 2001. In 2003 the MSM rate rebounded to 35%, and by 2013 it accounted for an estimated 65% (30,689) of new cases among adult and adolescent males. (See Table 4.1.) As estimated by the CDC, the MSM category continued to represent in 2013 the largest proportion (49%, or 577,403 of 1,184,620) of cumulative AIDS cases since 1981. (See Table 4.2.)

According to the CDC, in *HIV Surveillance in Women* (June 5, 2015, http://www.cdc.gov/hiv/pdf/q-z/cdc-hiv-surveillance-in-women-2013.pdf), there were 9,278 cases of HIV infection among adult and adolescent females reported by the 50 states, the District of Columbia, and six U.S. dependent areas in 2013. The majority of the cases were attributable to high-risk heterosexual contact, which accounted for between 84% and 87.7% of cases in adult and adolescent females. (See Table 4.3.) The percentage of cases attributable to injection drug use increased with advancing age, from 6.1% of females aged 13 to 19 years to 14.8% of females aged 45 years and older.

The proportion of women who contracted AIDS through heterosexual contact remained relatively constant at 37% in 2001 and 38% in 2002. In 2003, however, the proportion increased to 45%, and in 2013 it had risen to between 39.3% and 85.4% of cases in adult and adolescent females. (See Table 4.4.)

In 2013 the largest number of HIV infections in adult and adolescent females was among African American females—63% (5,867 of 9,278) of HIV diagnoses were in African American females (see Table 4.5), although African Americans accounted for just 12% of the U.S. female population. By contrast, white females made up 66% of the U.S. female adult and adolescent population but accounted for just 17% (1,579) of HIV infection diagnoses among females.

POPULATIONS AT RISK FOR HIV

Although men who have sex with men (whether homosexual or bisexual) continue to be most affected by HIV, injection drug users (IDUs) and transgender people also are at increased risk. In "Populations at Higher Risk for HIV: Route of Transmission" (September 11, 2014, http://198.246.124.22/nchhstp/newsroom/HIVFactSheets/Epidemic/Transmission.htm), the CDC observes that in 2010, 8% of new infections and 16% of

TABLE 4.1

HIV infections by transmission category, 2013

Transmission category	Estimated number of diagnoses of HIV infection, 2013		
	Adult and adolescent males	Adult and adolescent females	Total
Male-to-male sexual contact	30,689	NA	30,689
Injection drug use	1,942	1,154	3,096
Male-to-male sexual contact and injection drug use	1,270	NA	1,270
Heterosexual contact[a]	3,887	8,031	11,918
Other[b]	99	93	192

The distribution of the estimated number of diagnoses of HIV infection among children aged less than 13 years at the time of diagnosis in the United States, by transmission category, follows:

Perinatal	107
Other[c]	80

[a]Heterosexual contact with a person known to have, or to be at high risk for, HIV infection.
[b]Includes hemophilia, blood transfusion, perinatal exposure, and risk factor not reported or not identified.
[c]Includes hemophilia, blood transfusion, and risk factor not reported or not identified.

SOURCE: "Diagnoses of HIV Infection, by Transmission Category," in *Statistics Overview*, Centers for Disease Control and Prevention, National Center for HIV/AIDS, Viral Hepatitis, Sexual Transmitted Diseases, and Tuberculosis Prevention, Division of HIV/AIDS Prevention, June 30, 2015, http://www.cdc.gov/hiv/statistics/basics/index.html (accessed July 24, 2015)

TABLE 4.2

AIDS by transmission category, 2013 and cumulative through 2013

Transmission category	Estimated number of persons with diagnosed HIV infection ever classified as stage 3 (AIDS), 2013		
	Adult and adolescent males	Adult and adolescent females	Total
Male-to-male sexual contact	14,611	NA	14,611
Injection drug use	1,610	1,143	2,753
Male-to-male sexual contact and injection drug use	1,026	NA	1,026
Heterosexual contact[a]	2,865	5,109	7,974
Other[b]	144	172	316

Transmission category	Cumulative estimated number of persons with diagnosed HIV infection ever classified as stage 3 (AIDS), through 2013		
Male-to-male sexual contact	577,403	NA	577,403
Injection drug use	187,218	89,790	277,008
Male-to-male sexual contact and injection drug use	83,828	NA	83,828
Heterosexual contact[a]	82,447	146,521	228,968
Other[b]	11,545	5,868	17,413

[a]Heterosexual contact with a person known to have, or to be at high risk for, HIV infection.
[b]Includes hemophilia, blood transfusion, perinatal exposure, and risk factor not reported or not identified.

SOURCE: Adapted from "Estimated Number of Persons with Diagnosed HIV infection Ever Classified as Stage 3 (AIDS), 2013," and "Cumulative Estimated Number of Persons with Diagnosed HIV Infection Ever Classified as Stage 3 (AIDS), through 2013," in *Statistics Overview*, Centers for Disease Control and Prevention, National Center for HIV/AIDS, Viral Hepatitis, Sexual Transmitted Diseases, and Tuberculosis Prevention, Division of HIV/AIDS Prevention, June 30, 2015, http://www.cdc.gov/hiv/statistics/basics/index.html (accessed July 24, 2015)

people living with HIV were IDUs. A 2008 study reported that more than one-quarter of transgender women (28%) tested positive for HIV.

African Americans and Hispanics are disproportionately affected by HIV. The CDC reports in "Populations at Higher Risk for HIV: Racial and Ethnic Health Inequities" (December 9, 2014, http://198.246.124.22/nchhstp/newsroom/HIVFactSheets/Epidemic/Inequities.htm) that although African Americans constitute just 14% of the U.S. population, they account for 44% of new infections and 41% of those living with HIV. About 17% of the U.S. population is Hispanic, but 21% of new infections and 20 percent of people living with HIV are Hispanic.

These racial and ethnic disparities are largely due to socioeconomic factors, including poverty, language barriers, and concern about immigration status and higher rates of incarceration of men of color. Poverty can impede access to preventive care, testing and treatment as can language barriers, discrimination, stigma, and homophobia. Reduced access to care means there are higher rates of undiagnosed and untreated sexually transmitted infections (STIs; also known as STDs) including HIV, which further increases risk.

INJECTION DRUG USERS

During the 1990s the proportions of both HIV infection and AIDS deaths that were attributable to injection drug use among adults and adolescents increased. According to the CDC, in 1995 injection drug use was the exposure category for 25% of male and 47% of female AIDS deaths. Since 1995 the percentage of HIV/AIDS cases attributable to injection drug use has been steadily decreasing. By 2013 injection drug use accounted for an estimated 5% (1,942 of 37,887) of cases of HIV infection in adult and adolescent males and an estimated 12% (1,154 of 9,278) of cases in adult and adolescent females. (See Table 4.1.)

How HIV Is Transmitted through Injection Drug Use

HIV can be transmitted through injection drug use when the blood of an HIV-infected drug user is transferred to a drug user who is not yet infected with HIV. This transfer occurs almost exclusively through the sharing of injecting equipment, primarily needles and syringes.

Blood enters and makes contact with the needle and syringe in two ways. The first occurs when blood is drawn into the syringe to verify that the needle is inside a vein before the injection of the drug. The second occurs following the injection, when the syringe is refilled several times with blood from the vein to "wash out" any heroin, cocaine, or other drug left in the syringe after the first injection. Even the smallest amount of HIV-infected blood left in the syringe can cause the virus to be transmitted to the next user of the contaminated syringe and needle.

TABLE 4.3

HIV infection among females, by transmission category and age at diagnosis, 2013

	Age at diagnosis (in years)				
	13–19	20–24	25–34	35–44	≥45
	Population = 376	Population = 923	Population = 2,378	Population = 2,257	Population = 3,544
Transmission category	%	%	%	%	%
Injection drug use	6.1	9.8	11.6	12.2	14.8
Heterosexual contact[a]	84.0	87.7	87.6	87.6	84.9
Other[b]	9.9	2.5	0.8	0.2	0.3
Total	**100.0**	**100.0**	**100.0**	**100.0**	**100.0**

[a]Heterosexual contact with a person known to have, or to be at high risk for, HIV infection.
[b]Includes blood transfusion, perinatal exposure, and risk factor not reported or not identified.
Note: Data include persons with a diagnosis of HIV infection regardless of stage of disease at diagnosis. All displayed data have been statistically adjusted to account for reporting delays and missing transmission category, but not for incomplete reporting.

SOURCE: "Diagnoses of HIV Infection among Adult and Adolescent Females, by Transmission Category and Age at Diagnosis 2013—United States and 6 Dependent Areas," in *HIV Surveillance in Women*, Centers for Disease Control and Prevention, June 5, 2015, http://www.cdc.gov/hiv/pdf/q-z/cdc-hiv-surveillance-in-women-2013.pdf (accessed July 24, 2015).

TABLE 4.4

AIDS diagnoses among females, by transmission category and age at diagnosis, 2013

	Age at diagnosis (in years)				
	13–19	20–24	25–34	35–44	≥45
	Population = 147	Population = 348	Population = 1,308	Population = 1,821	Population = 2,915
Transmission category	%	%	%	%	%
Injection drug use	2.4	5.2	13.0	16.4	23.1
Heterosexual contact[a]	39.3	79.0	85.4	83.4	76.6
Other[b]	58.3	15.8	1.6	0.2	0.3
Total	**100.0**	**100.0**	**100.0**	**100.0**	**100.0**

[a]Heterosexual contact with a person known to have, or to be at high risk for, HIV infection.
[b]Includes blood transfusion, perinatal exposure, and risk factor not reported or not identified.
Note: All displayed data have been statistically adjusted to account for reporting delays and missing transmission category, but not for incomplete reporting.

SOURCE: "Stage 3 (AIDS) Classifications among Adult and Adolescent Females, by Transmission Category and Age at Diagnosis, 2013—United States and 6 Dependent Areas," in *HIV Surveillance in Women*, Centers for Disease Control and Prevention, June 5, 2015, http://www.cdc.gov/hiv/pdf/q-z/cdc-hiv-surveillance-in-women-2013.pdf (accessed July 24, 2015).

TABLE 4.5

HIV diagnoses among adult and adolescent females by race/ethnicity, 2013

Race/ethnicity	No.	Rate
American Indian/Alaska Native	49	5.1
Asian	159	2.2
Black/African American	5,867	34.8
Hispanic/Latino[a]	1,419	7.0
Native Hawaiian/other Pacific Islander	15	7.3
White	1,579	1.8
Multiple races	190	9.3
Total[b]	**9,278**	**6.9**

[a]Hispanics/Latinos can be of any race.
[b]Because column totals for estimated numbers were calculated independently of the values for the subpopulations, the values in each column may not sum to the column total.
Note: Data include persons with a diagnosis of HIV infection regardless of stage of disease at diagnosis. All displayed data have been statistically adjusted to account for reporting delays, but not for incomplete reporting. Rates are per 100,000 population.

SOURCE: "Diagnoses of HIV Infection among Adult and Adolescent females, by Race/Ethnicity—United States," in *HIV Surveillance in Women*, Centers for Disease Control and Prevention, June 5, 2015, http://www.cdc.gov/hiv/pdf/q-z/cdc-hiv-surveillance-in-women-2013.pdf (accessed July 24, 2015).

Among IDUs the risk of HIV infection increases in proportion to the duration of injection drug use—the longer the drug use, the greater the risk of infection. Diseases such as hepatitis show this same pattern. Risk also increases with the frequency of needle sharing and injection drug use in a geographic area, such as a large city, where there is a high prevalence of HIV infection.

General Trends

Table 4.1 shows that in 2013 injection drug use was responsible for an estimated 3,096 HIV infections (6.5% of the 47,352 infections) and an additional estimated 1,270 HIV infections (2.6%) were attributable to MSM in conjunction with injection drug use.

HIV is also spread among non-IDUs who trade sex for drugs, especially crack cocaine, as well as the partners of these users. Those who trade sex for drugs often engage in unprotected sex and have multiple sex partners. People who exchange sex for drugs and have an STI that causes ulcers or sores on the genitals, such as syphilis or herpes simplex, are at a higher risk for HIV infection. Drug and/or alcohol users may also be at greater risk for infection because these substances often lessen inhibitions and reduce the reluctance to have unsafe, unprotected sex.

WOMEN AND HIV/AIDS

The proportion of women among AIDS cases increased steadily, from a reported 7% in 1985 to 24% in 2013. (See Figure 4.1.) The CDC indicates that 74,970 reported cases (31%) of the 239,313 cumulative AIDS cases from 1981 through 2013 among females were associated either directly or indirectly with injection drug use. (See Table 3.1 in Chapter 3.)

The racial and ethnic differences among females with HIV/AIDS are striking. In *HIV Surveillance in Women*, the CDC notes that although African American and Hispanic females made up 12% and 15%, respectively, of all females in the United States in 2013, they accounted for 63% (5,867) and 15% (1,419), respectively, of the 9,278 adult and adolescent females diagnosed with HIV infection in 2013. (See Table 4.5.) In contrast, white females made up 66% of the U.S. female population but just 17% (1,579) of adult and adolescent females diagnosed with HIV.

Women can infect their unborn children with HIV during the course of pregnancy, during delivery, or by breast-feeding after birth. The dramatic decrease in the number of women who gave birth to HIV-infected babies during the 1990s was largely attributable to the introduction of antiretroviral therapy (ART). Women of childbearing age can be tested for HIV, and, if they are positive, they have the option of receiving ART before they become pregnant to decrease the chances of transmitting the virus to their unborn children.

Along with ART, which lowers the mother's viral load to undetectable levels, deliveries via elective cesarean section (the surgical delivery of a baby) rather than vaginal births may also help reduce mother-to-child transmission. In "Pregnant Women, Infants, and Children" (June 23, 2015, http://www.cdc.gov/hiv/risk/gender/pregnantwomen/index .html), the CDC states that with treatment perinatal transmission can be reduced to less than 1%.

Geographic Data on HIV/AIDS in Women

Most HIV/AIDS cases occur among women who live in large metropolitan areas with populations of greater than 500,000. However, the number of HIV/AIDS cases is increasing in rural areas, especially through heterosexual transmission. Figure 4.2 reveals that at the end of 2012 the highest rates of women living with AIDS were reported in the District of Columbia (843.2 cases per 100,000 population), New York (275.1), the U.S. Virgin Islands (254.3), Maryland (229.7), Florida (193.7) and Puerto Rico (195.9). In contrast, the lowest rates were reported by states in the Midwest.

Sexually Transmitted Diseases

Preventing, identifying, and promptly treating STIs is vitally important for the health of young women. Most HIV in women is spread through heterosexual sex (see Table 4.3), and the increase in STIs parallels that of HIV/AIDS.

FIGURE 4.1

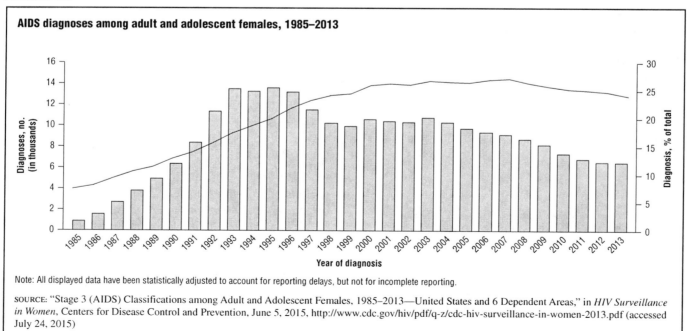

AIDS diagnoses among adult and adolescent females, 1985–2013

Note: All displayed data have been statistically adjusted to account for reporting delays, but not for incomplete reporting.

SOURCE: "Stage 3 (AIDS) Classifications among Adult and Adolescent Females, 1985–2013—United States and 6 Dependent Areas," in *HIV Surveillance in Women*, Centers for Disease Control and Prevention, June 5, 2015, http://www.cdc.gov/hiv/pdf/q-z/cdc-hiv-surveillance-in-women-2013.pdf (accessed July 24, 2015)

FIGURE 4.2

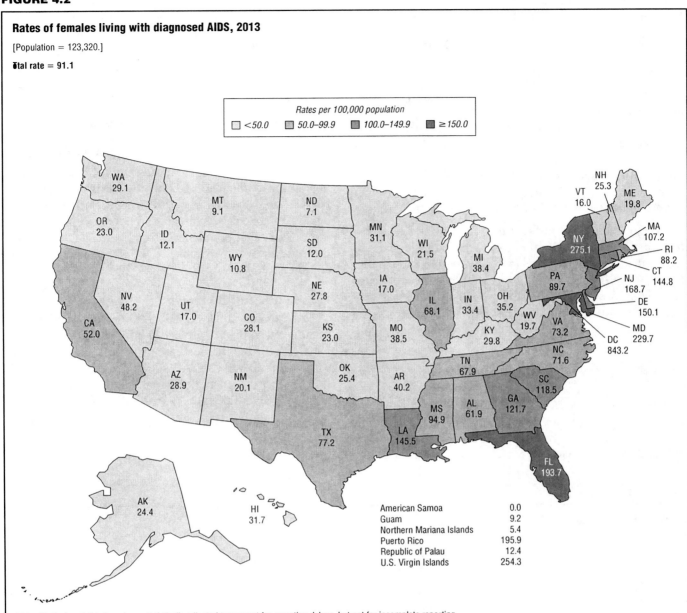

Rates of females living with diagnosed AIDS, 2013

[Population = 123,320.]

Total rate = 91.1

Rates per 100,000 population

□ <50.0   ▨ 50.0–99.9   ▨ 100.0–149.9   ▨ ≥150.0

WA 29.1	
MT 9.1	
OR 23.0	
ID 12.1	
ND 7.1	
MN 31.1	
NH 25.3	
VT 16.0	
ME 19.8	
WY 10.8	
SD 12.0	
WI 21.5	
MI 38.4	
NY 275.1	
MA 107.2	
NV 48.2	
UT 17.0	
NE 27.8	
IA 17.0	
IL 68.1	
IN 33.4	
OH 35.2	
PA 89.7	
RI 88.2	
CT 144.8	
CA 52.0	
CO 28.1	
KS 23.0	
MO 38.5	
KY 29.8	
WV 19.7	
VA 73.2	
NJ 168.7	
DE 150.1	
MD 229.7	
AZ 28.9	
NM 20.1	
OK 25.4	
AR 40.2	
TN 67.9	
NC 71.6	
DC 843.2	
TX 77.2	
LA 145.5	
MS 94.9	
AL 61.9	
GA 121.7	
SC 118.5	
FL 193.7	
AK 24.4	
HI 31.7	

American Samoa	0.0
Guam	9.2
Northern Mariana Islands	5.4
Puerto Rico	195.9
Republic of Palau	12.4
U.S. Virgin Islands	254.3

Note: All displayed data have been statistically adjusted to account for reporting delays, but not for incomplete reporting.

SOURCE: "Rates of Adult and Adolescent Females Living with Diagnosed HIV Infection Ever Classified as Stage 3 (AIDS) Year-end 2012—United States and 6 Dependent Areas," in *HIV Surveillance in Women*, Centers for Disease Control and Prevention, June 5, 2015, http://www.cdc.gov/hiv/pdf/q-z/cdc-hiv-surveillance-in-women-2013.pdf (accessed July 24, 2015)

In "STDs and HIV—CDC Fact Sheet" (April 23, 2015, http://www.cdc.gov/std/Hiv/STDFact-STD-HIV.htm), the CDC explains that people with STIs are more likely than people who do not have STIs to get HIV. Women with STIs have an increased number of HIV target cells (CD4+ T cells) present in their cervical secretions. These cells facilitate the entrance of HIV into the body. Furthermore, women with STIs are more likely to shed HIV in both ulcer-forming and inflammatory genital secretions. They are also more likely to shed HIV in greater amounts than people infected with HIV alone, which contributes to the spread of HIV. By treating an STI, the shedding of HIV on sexual contact is lessened, which in turn reduces the spread of HIV infection.

MSM SEXUAL CONTACT

MSM is still the major risk category for HIV infection. However, epidemiologists (public health researchers who analyze the extent and types of illnesses in a population and the factors that influence their distribution) believe that HIV/AIDS among MSM may have peaked in 1992. As in previous years, in 2013 MSM contact accounted for two-thirds of all HIV exposure and transmission for males with or without injection drug use (22,349, or 67%, of the 33,180 reported cases). (See Table 3.5 in Chapter 3.)

OLDER ADULTS

The CDC reports in "HIV among People Aged 50 and Over" (May 12, 2015, http://www.cdc.gov/hiv/group/age/olderamericans/index.html) that adults aged 50 years and older accounted for 8,575 (18%) of the estimated 47,352 new diagnoses of HIV infection in 2013, 7,108 (27%) of the estimated 26,688 AIDS diagnoses, and 312,000 (26%) of the estimated 1.2 million people living with HIV in 2013. (See Figure 4.3.)

Older adults may not feel they are at risk and therefore may engage in unsafe sex. Older adults are more likely than younger adults to be diagnosed late in the course of HIV infection, in part because health care providers do not always test older patients and because older adults may mistakenly assume that symptoms of HIV infection are normal, age-related changes.

PRISONERS AND AIDS

According to Laura M. Maruschak of the Bureau of Justice Statistics, in *HIV in Prisons, 2001–2010* (March 2015, http://www.bjs.gov/content/pub/pdf/hivp10.pdf), the number of HIV-positive state and federal prisoners declined 3% each year between 2001 and 2010. Likewise,

among inmates with HIV/AIDS the number of AIDS-related deaths declined an average of 13% per year, and among all inmates it dropped 16% per year. (See Figure 4.4.) The number of state inmates with HIV/AIDS decreased from 19,290 in 2009 to 18,515 in 2010. The number of federal inmates with HIV/AIDS declined from 1,590 to 1,578 during the same period.

Every year since statistics have been gathered, AIDS-related conditions have been the second-leading cause of death for state prison inmates, behind "illness/natural causes." Nevertheless, the proportion of deaths attributable to AIDS declined markedly between 1995 and 2010. Maruschak notes that as of 2008 the rate of AIDS-related deaths for state prison inmates dropped below the rate for the U.S. general population. (See Figure 4.5.) This sharp drop is likely attributable to effective treatment with combination ART.

Sex and Racial Differences

At yearend 2010, 20,093 U.S. inmates were reported as infected with HIV or had confirmed cases of AIDS, which was a slight decrease from the previous year's estimate of 20,880 HIV/AIDS cases. AIDS-related deaths in U.S. prisons also decreased slightly—from 102 in 2008, to 101 in 2009, to 79 in 2010. (See Table 4.6.)

Male inmates make up the overwhelming majority of HIV-infected or confirmed cases of AIDS among inmates in state and federal prisons. In 2010 an estimated 18,337

FIGURE 4.3

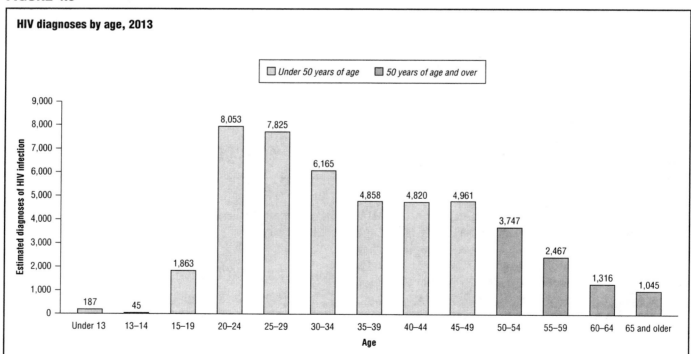

SOURCE: "Estimated Diagnoses of HIV Infection by Age, 2013, United States," in *HIV among People Aged 50 and Over,* Centers for Disease Control and Prevention, National Center for HIV/AIDS, Viral Hepatitis, Sexual Transmitted Diseases, and Tuberculosis Prevention, Division of HIV/AIDS Prevention, May 12, 2015, http://www.cdc.gov/hiv/group/age/olderamericans/index.html (accessed July 24, 2015)

FIGURE 4.4

Rate of HIV/AIDS cases and AIDS-related deaths among prison inmates, 2001–10

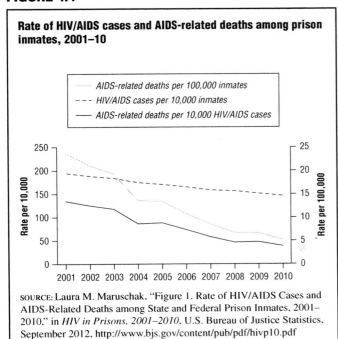

SOURCE: Laura M. Maruschak, "Figure 1. Rate of HIV/AIDS Cases and AIDS-Related Deaths among State and Federal Prison Inmates, 2001–2010," in *HIV in Prisons, 2001–2010*, U.S. Bureau of Justice Statistics, September 2012, http://www.bjs.gov/content/pub/pdf/hivp10.pdf (accessed July 24, 2015)

FIGURE 4.5

AIDS-related deaths in state prisons and in the U.S. general population, 2001–09

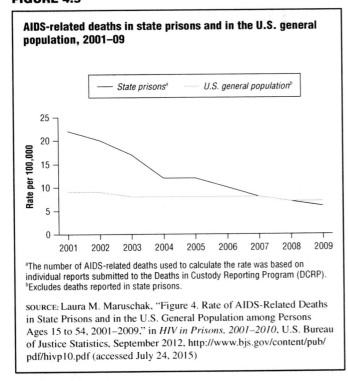

ᵃThe number of AIDS-related deaths used to calculate the rate was based on individual reports submitted to the Deaths in Custody Reporting Program (DCRP).
ᵇExcludes deaths reported in state prisons.

SOURCE: Laura M. Maruschak, "Figure 4. Rate of AIDS-Related Deaths in State Prisons and in the U.S. General Population among Persons Ages 15 to 54, 2001–2009," in *HIV in Prisons, 2001–2010*, U.S. Bureau of Justice Statistics, September 2012, http://www.bjs.gov/content/pub/pdf/hivp10.pdf (accessed July 24, 2015)

male inmates were known to be HIV positive or diagnosed with AIDS, compared with 1,756 female inmates. However, as a percentage of the U.S. inmate population, a higher percentage of female inmates were reported with HIV/AIDS (1.9% compared with 1.4% of male inmates).

TABLE 4.6

AIDS-related deaths among state and federal prison inmates, 2008–10

Jurisdiction	Number			Rate per 100,000 inmates		
	2008	2009	2010	2008	2009	2010
U.S. total	102	101	79	7	7	5
Federal	13	7	7	6	3	3
State	89	94	72	7	7	5

Note: Includes deaths in private facilities.

SOURCE: Laura M. Maruschak, "Table 4. AIDS-Related Deaths among State Prison Inmates in Custody, 2008–2010," in *HIV in Prisons, 2001–2010*, U.S. Bureau of Justice Statistics, September 2012, http://www.bjs.gov/content/pub/pdf/hivp10.pdf (accessed July 24, 2015)

Drug and Needle Use among Prisoners

Public education campaigns about the "safer" use of drugs and syringes appear to be reducing HIV infection in the general public. These measures, however, seem to be having little effect in prisons. Many incarcerated IDUs continue to inject while in prison, often sharing needles because injection equipment is in short supply.

This is a dilemma for prisons, where syringes and needles are prohibited, as are illegal drugs, and chemicals for disinfecting the illicit needles are not readily available. Although state and federal prison officials in the United States want to stop the spread of HIV among inmates, most cannot keep pace with or stem the flow of illegal drugs into prisons. To minimize the spread of HIV in prisons, countries such as Switzerland and the United Kingdom provide prisoners with disinfectant or clean needles. U.S. officials believe these actions endorse illegal drug use. Instead, they focus on providing treatment and rehabilitation programs for drug-addicted prisoners.

Nonetheless, many observers believe that prison systems can and should do more to prevent HIV transmission related to injection drug use. They assert that needle and syringe programs and drug substitution therapy, such as methadone maintenance (the use of methadone as treatment for a person who is addicted to heroin), sharply reduce the sharing of injecting equipment and the spread of HIV and other blood-borne pathogens. For example, Sheryl L. Catz et al. describe in "Prevention Needs of HIV-Positive Men and Women Awaiting Release from Prison" (*AIDS and Behavior*, vol. 16, no. 1, January 2012) a Wisconsin prison system initiative that offers health education classes to inmates who are HIV negative or positive. Among the topics covered is the transmission of STIs, including HIV. The researchers note that needle exchange programs are crucial for reducing the risk of transmission, that there are not enough of these programs, and that clean needles are neither affordable nor legal.

U.S. Prison Systems Take Action to Prevent HIV Infection

In "Integrated Prevention Services for HIV Infection, Viral Hepatitis, Sexually Transmitted Diseases, and Tuberculosis for Persons Who Use Drugs Illicitly: Summary Guidance from CDC and the U.S. Department of Health and Human Services" (*Morbidity and Mortality Weekly Report*, vol. 61, no. 5, November 9, 2012), Hrishikesh Belani et al. assert that prevention services are vital in jails, prisons, and juvenile detention centers. The researchers recommend a comprehensive range of services that can be delivered in correctional settings to people who use illicit drugs, including routine HIV testing, access to sterile drug injection or clean preparation equipment, and referral to appropriate care upon release. (See Table 4.7.) Figure 4.6 shows Belani et al.'s recommendations for monitoring and evaluating services that are delivered to people who use drugs illicitly across all settings and underscores the importance of integrated prevention and treatment services to improve how IDUs fare in terms of their health.

TABLE 4.7

Recommended prevention services for inmates who use illicit drugs, 2012

Correctional institution

Examples of integrated prevention services

Routine HIV testing, TB screening, and vaccination for viral hepatitis A and B
Screening of young women in jails and juvenile detention centers for gonorrhea and chlamydia
HCV testing conducted
HIV-infected inmates referred to HIV clinical services during and after incarceration, and progress tracked
Access to sterile drug injection or clean preparation equipment and condoms
Education on prevention of overdose
Persons addicted to opiates offered medication-assisted therapy while incarcerated or via referral at discharge
Comprehensive health risk assessment services for TB, HIV, STDs, and viral hepatitis as well as counseling for reproductive health, drug use, alcohol misuse, and mental health disorders
Case management for housing/drug/alcohol/mental health services and discharge planning to inmates for appropriate follow-up care in the community
Routine screening for syphilis, chlamydia, and gonorrhea
% of inmates screened for infection with HIV, TB, and viral hepatitis
No. of inmates diagnosed with syphilis, chlamydia, or gonorrhea
% of inmates receiving HAV/HBV vaccination
% of tested inmates who test positive for HIV, TB, or viral hepatitis
% of inmates with diagnosed HIV infection, syphilis, chlamydia, gonorrhea, TB, or viral hepatitis who receive comprehensive discharge planning and continued care

HAV = Hepatitis A Virus.
HBV = Hepatitis B Virus.
HIV = Human Immunodeficiency Virus.
STD = Sexually Transmitted Disease.
TB = Tuberculosis.

SOURCE: Adapted from Hrishikesh Belani et al., "Table. Examples of Integrated Prevention Services That Can Be Delivered in Different Settings to Persons Who Use Drugs Illicitly and Examples of Monitoring and Evaluation Indicators," in "Integrated Prevention Services for HIV Infection, Viral Hepatitis, Sexually Transmitted Diseases, and Tuberculosis for Persons Who Use Drugs Illicitly: Summary Guidance from CDC and the U.S. Department of Health and Human Services," *MMWR*, vol. 61, no. 5, November 9, 2012, http://www.cdc.gov/mmwr/pdf/rr/rr6105.pdf (accessed July 24, 2015)

The CDC recommends in "HIV in Correctional Settings" (June 2012, http://www.cdc.gov/hiv/resources/factsheets/pdf/correctional.pdf) that "HIV screening be provided upon entry into prison and before release and that voluntary HIV testing be offered periodically during incarceration." Operational, legal, and financial challenges have also hampered HIV testing in correctional settings. For example, the regular turnover of jail inmates has prompted many jurisdictions to use rapid HIV tests and to test within the first 24 hours of incarceration. Some jurisdictions do not provide HIV testing because it increases their laboratory and medical costs.

Just as state policies on HIV testing vary, so do policies regarding HIV-positive inmates. For example, in "Alabama to End Segregation of HIV-Positive Inmates" (WSJ.com, September 20, 2013), Arian Campo-Flores reports that the Alabama Department of Corrections ended isolation of HIV-infected inmates from other prisoners effective November 2014. Alabama began the practice during the 1980s to halt the spread of HIV (which may occur through consensual sex, rape, injection drug use, or even when inmates apply tattoos) and to control medical care costs. Alabama was the last state to abolish this once common practice.

SEX WORKERS

In "UNAIDS Terminology Guide" (October 2011, http://www.unaids.org/sites/default/files/media_asset/JC2118_terminology-guidelines_en_0.pdf), sex workers are defined as "female, male, and transgender adults and young people over the age of 18 who receive money or goods in exchange for sexual services, either regularly or occasionally." Because they have a high number of sexual partners and inconsistent condom use (often because of their clients' unwillingness), sex workers are at risk of being infected with HIV and can potentially transmit the virus to many clients. The clients of sex workers serve as a "bridge population" for the transmission of HIV—they convey the virus from this high-risk population to the general population.

In *Consolidated Guidelines on HIV Prevention, Diagnosis, Treatment and Care for Key Populations* (July 2014, http://apps.who.int/iris/bitstream/10665/128048/1/9789241507431_eng.pdf?ua=1ua=1), the World Health Organization (WHO) reports that globally, the average HIV prevalence among sex workers is about 12%, but prevalence varies between and within regions. The WHO asserts, "Legal issues, stigma, discrimination and violence pose barriers to HIV services for sex workers."

HEMOPHILIACS

Hemophilia is a group of genetic disorders in which defects in a number of genes located on the X chromosome disrupt the proper clotting of blood. The most common type

FIGURE 4.6

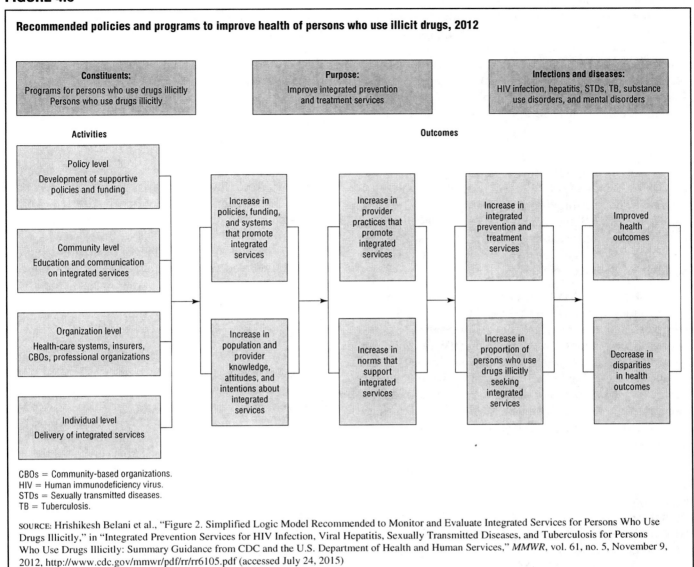

Recommended policies and programs to improve health of persons who use illicit drugs, 2012

CBOs = Community-based organizations.
HIV = Human immunodeficiency virus.
STDs = Sexually transmitted diseases.
TB = Tuberculosis.

SOURCE: Hrishikesh Belani et al., "Figure 2. Simplified Logic Model Recommended to Monitor and Evaluate Integrated Services for Persons Who Use Drugs Illicitly," in "Integrated Prevention Services for HIV Infection, Viral Hepatitis, Sexually Transmitted Diseases, and Tuberculosis for Persons Who Use Drugs Illicitly: Summary Guidance from CDC and the U.S. Department of Health and Human Services," *MMWR*, vol. 61, no. 5, November 9, 2012, http://www.cdc.gov/mmwr/pdf/rr/rr6105.pdf (accessed July 24, 2015)

of hemophilia (hemophilia A) is a deficiency of a clotting substance designated Factor VIII. Varying severities of hemophilia can occur, depending on the level of Factor VIII present in the patient's plasma. Treatment of hemophilia involves close attention to injury prevention and periodic intravenous administration of Factor VIII concentrates, commonly known as clotting factors.

Because screening for HIV antibodies was not available until 1985, many hemophiliacs were exposed to HIV-contaminated blood and clotting factors. The national distribution of clotting factor concentrates before 1985 led to a high prevalence of HIV infections among hemophiliacs. The prevalence of HIV infection differs by the type and severity of the coagulation (clotting) disorder.

According to the Hemophilia Federation of America (HFA), in "History of Hemophilia" (2015, http://www .hemophiliafed.org/bleeding-disorders/history-of-hemophilia),

during the early 1970s and 1980s about half of all people with hemophilia became infected with HIV through blood products. As a result, 50% of Americans with hemophilia were infected with HIV, and more than half of those infected died.

A Slow Reaction

Concentrated clotting factor, which is derived from human blood obtained from as many as 2,000 donors, became available during the mid-1970s. Its success at stopping bleeding was so dramatic that hemophilia changed from a disease that produced intense pain, disability, and the possibility of premature death to one that allowed sufferers to lead nearly normal lives. Hemophiliacs could infuse clotting factors into their own blood if they thought bleeding was about to start. Patients were advised by their physicians to "infuse early and often."

During the late 1970s and early 1980s some clotting factor concentrates were inadvertently infected with HIV. Even after the first cases of HIV/AIDS appeared in people with hemophilia and the CDC identified this new disease as being blood borne, physicians did not advise their patients to alter their clotting factor treatments. Hemophiliacs were encouraged to continue using their clotting factor because researchers and physicians were not sure there would be a major epidemic.

Anecdotal reports from hemophiliacs indicate that when many of them became infected, primary care doctors were slow to respond and supplied little information. There was no warning to practice safe sex to prevent the spread of HIV. Some hemophiliacs reported receiving more information from gay men's organizations than from their own hematologists (physicians who specialize in diseases and disorders of the blood).

ANGER AND COMPENSATION. Many hemophiliacs believed they were entitled to compensation or, at the very least, assistance in paying the overwhelming medical expenses they incurred as a result of HIV infection and AIDS treatment. They maintain that the companies that produced the clotting factors were slow to warn the public about HIV and slow to use heat treatment to eliminate the live virus from the clotting factors (although this procedure has not gained widespread acceptance among scientists as an adequate method to inactivate HIV).

Hemophilia foundations in some countries have persuaded government pharmaceutical or insurance companies to compensate HIV-infected hemophiliacs. Peter D. Weinberg et al. report in "Legal, Financial, and Public Health Consequences of HIV Contamination of Blood and Blood Products in the 1980s and 1990s" (*Annals of Internal Medicine*, vol. 136, no. 4, February 19, 2002) that Armour Pharmaceuticals agreed to pay six Canadians $1.5 million each; Germany offered people infected with HIV and those who became ill with AIDS annual compensation; and Switzerland extended annual compensation of $12,216 to people with AIDS. France gave one-time compensation of $87,735 to hemophiliacs

at the time they were diagnosed with AIDS due to tainted blood products. During the first decade of the 21st century, more than 20 developed countries acted to compensate HIV-infected hemophiliacs. By contrast, developing countries continued to grapple with blood-supply safety issues.

In 1995 the U.S. Supreme Court refused to hear a class action suit brought by hemophiliacs against a pharmaceutical company and other blood-product manufacturers (*Barton v. American Red Cross*, 826 F. Supp. 412 and 826 F. Supp. 407, append 43 F. 3rd 678, certiorari denied 116 S. Ct. 84). Regardless, some companies have reached out-of-court settlements with affected people. For example, according to the article "4 Drug Companies Ordered to Pay Hemophiliacs" (NYTimes.com, May 8, 1997), in 1997 four manufacturers of blood clotting products were ordered by a federal judge to pay approximately $670 million to settle cases on behalf of more than 6,000 hemophiliacs who were infected in the United States during the early 1980s. The settlement compensated each infected hemophiliac with an estimated $100,000 payment.

The international catastrophe of HIV/AIDS in the hemophilia community was recognized by the U.S. federal government in 1998 with passage of the Ricky Ray Hemophilia Relief Fund Act (May 31, 2000, https://www.federalregister.gov/articles/2000/05/31/00-13418/ricky-ray-hemophilia-relief-fund-program). Named for Ricky Ray (1977–1992), a boy with hemophilia who died from AIDS, the act provided "payments of $100,000 to any individual with HIV infection who has any blood-clotting disorder and was treated with antihemophilic factor at any time between July 1, 1982, and December 31, 1987." Payments were also extended to spouses, former spouses, and children of beneficiaries who became infected with HIV, and specified survivors were eligible to receive the payments on behalf of individuals who had died from the disease. When the program closed in October 2005, it had paid over $559 million to more than 7,171 eligible infected individuals and survivors.

CHAPTER 5
CHILDREN, ADOLESCENTS, AND HIV/AIDS

HIV/AIDS IN CHILDREN: DIFFERENT FROM HIV/AIDS IN ADULTS

HIV can cause AIDS in adults and children. The virus attacks and damages the immune and central nervous systems of all infected people. However, the development and course of the disease in children differs considerably from its progression in adults.

Before the use of highly active antiretroviral therapy (HAART) and early intervention strategies, there were two patterns of HIV progression among children. The National Institute of Allergy and Infectious Diseases (NIAID) reports in the fact sheet "HIV Infection in Infants and Children" (January 31, 2000, http://www.niaid.nih.gov/news/news releases/Archive/2000/Pages/drug_regimen_backgrounder .aspx) that serious illness developed in 20% of infected infants during their first year of life. The second pattern, which occurred in the other 80% of infected children, is more gradual and is similar to the development and progression of the disease that is observed in adults.

In "Children and HIV" (November 16, 2009; https://www.aids.gov/hiv-aids-basics/just-diagnosed-with-hiv-aids/overview/children) the U.S. Department of Health and Human Services (HHS) explains that infants require a special form of test in order to diagnose if they have HIV, one that can take several months to complete. This is because the usual tests for HIV used in adults involve the detection of antibodies formed by the body in response to HIV. Infants have often not developed the full capacity to produce antibodies at the time of testing. Furthermore, HIV-infected mothers may transmit antibodies alone, without the virus, to their babies. Thus infants with positive results from antibody tests at birth may later test negative, indicating that the mother transmitted the HIV antibodies to the baby, but not the virus itself.

Among infants and children, the disease is characterized by wasting syndrome and the failure to thrive. Unusually severe and frequent cases of typical childhood infections are common among children with HIV, which may result in extended hospital stays. The HHS states that children can be susceptible to the same opportunistic infections as adults, but additionally are vulnerable to a lung disease called *lymphocytic interstitial pneumonitis* that is rare in adults. The HHS also says, however, that "many children with HIV reach adolescence without issue, and maintain relatively intact immune systems."

Whether HIV positive or not, babies born to HIV-infected mothers appear to be predisposed to a variety of heart problems. In the landmark study "Cardiovascular Status of Infants and Children of Women Infected with HIV-1 (P2C2 HIV): A Cohort Study" (*Lancet*, vol. 360, no. 9330, August 3, 2002), Steven E. Lipshultz et al. examined more than 500 infants born to HIV-positive women. They discovered that the babies suffered from significantly higher rates of abnormalities, such as defects in the heart wall and valve and reduced pumping action. These defects occurred in less than 1% of healthy children whose mothers were not infected with HIV. Lipshultz et al. recognize that HIV alone did not necessarily cause these anomalies; a mother's alcohol, drug, or nutrition problems can also interfere with fetal heart development.

Hamisu M. Salihu et al. analyzed over 1.6 million birth records in Florida. In "Maternal HIV/AIDS Status and Neurological Outcomes in Neonates: A Population-Based Study" (*Maternal and Child Health Journal*, April 20, 2011), the researchers report that babies born to HIV-infected mothers are at higher risk of having feeding difficulties and seizures (sudden loss of consciousness).

A CASE DEFINITION FOR CHILDREN

Because data were limited during the first few years of HIV's acknowledged presence in the United States, the

U.S. Centers for Disease Control and Prevention's (CDC) definition of AIDS did not differentiate between adults and children until 1987, when the classification system was revised. The CDC's Division of HIV/AIDS Prevention, National Center for HIV/AIDS, Viral Hepatitis, STD, and TB Prevention updated the pediatric definition in 1994, 1999, 2008 and 2014 as more information about HIV and AIDS became available. Surveillance case definitions are primarily used to monitor the HIV infection at the population level rather than to guide clinical decisions for individual patients. The 2014 revision addresses changing diagnostic criteria in response to diagnostic testing procedures that involve multiple tests and do not necessarily use the Western blot or immunofluorescence HIV antibody assays.

Changes to the surveillance case definitions were published by Richard M. Selik et al. of the CDC in "Revised Surveillance Case Definitions for HIV Infection —United States, 2014" (*Morbidity and Mortality Weekly Report*, vol. 63, no. RR-03, April 11, 2014). The 2014 criteria:

- Distinguish between HIV-1 and HIV-2 infection and recognize early HIV infection. A confirmed case can be classified as stages 0, 1, 2, 3, or unknown. Early infection (stage 0) is a negative HIV test within 6 months of HIV diagnosis and AIDS is stage 3.

- No longer require distinguishing definitive (confirmed by advanced laboratory testing) from presumptive diagnoses (often made on the bases of physical examination or preliminary testing) of opportunistic illnesses for stage 3.

- Classifies stages 1 to 3 on the basis of the CD4+ T-lymphocyte count unless people have had a stage-3–defining opportunistic illness. The CD4+ T-lymphocyte percentage is used only when the CD4+ T-lymphocyte count is unknown to prevent overestimating the proportion of cases in stage 3. (See Table 5.1.)

Children Younger than 18 Months

As noted earlier, the screening and confirmatory blood tests that accurately diagnose HIV in adults are not reliable for detecting HIV in children younger than 18 months old due to the presence of passively acquired maternal antibodies. Early recognition of HIV infection in infants younger than 18 months is accomplished using virologic tests such as the HIV-1 DNA or RNA assays by polymerase chain reaction (PCR). PCR amplifies the amounts of viral genetic material to detectable levels by the direct isolation of the HIV virus using viral culture techniques or by the detection of the p24 viral antigen.

In *Guidelines for the Use of Antiretroviral Agents in Pediatric HIV Infection* the National Institutes of Health's Panel on Antiretroviral Therapy and Medical Management of HIV-Infected Children (NIH Panel) offers recommendations on the timing of diagnostic testing for infants at risk for HIV infection and for those with known perinatal HIV exposure. (See Table 5.2.) The guidelines also recommend that all HIV-infected expectant mothers be given antiretroviral therapy (ART) and that HIV-infected mothers be warned about the risks of transmission through breast-feeding. Infants with negative HIV tests at birth should be retested periodically during the first 18 months of life.

Classification System

The 2014 changes in diagnostic criteria did not alter the existing classification system that was developed in 1994 for HIV infection in children less than 18 months or children aged 18 months to less than 13 years old. Table 5.1 shows the three categories of HIV infection as defined by CD4+ T-lymphocyte counts and the percentage of total lymphocytes for children less than one year in age, those one to five years of age, and those aged six years and older.

PERINATAL INFECTION

In *HIV Surveillance Report: Diagnoses of HIV Infection and AIDS in the United States and Dependent Areas,*

TABLE 5.1

HIV infection stage by age and CD4+ T-lymphocyte count, 2014

| Stage* | Age on date of CD4 T-lymphocyte test | | | | | |
| | <1 year | | 1–5 years | | 6 years through adult | |
	Cells/μL	%	Cells/μL	%	Cells/μL	%
1	≥1,500	≥34	≥1,000	≥30	≥500	≥26
2	750–1,499	26–33	500–999	22–29	200–499	14–25
3	<750	<26	<500	<22	<200	<14

*The stage is based primarily on the CD4+ T-lymphocyte count; the CD4+ T-lymphocyte count takes precedence over the CD4 T-lymphocyte percentage, and the percentage is considered only if the count is missing.
Note: If none of the above apply (e.g., because of missing information on CD4 test results), the stage is U (unknown).

SOURCE: "Table. HIV infection Stage, Based on Age-Specific CD4+ T-Lymphocyte Count or CD4+ T-Lymphocyte Percentage of Total Lymphocytes," in *Terms, Definitions, and Calculations Used in CDC HIV Surveillance Publications*, Centers for Disease Control and Prevention, National Center for HIV/AIDS, Viral Hepatitis, Sexual Transmitted Diseases, and Tuberculosis Prevention, Division of HIV/AIDS Prevention, May 11, 2015, http://www.cdc.gov/hiv/statistics/surveillance/terms.html (accessed July 24, 2015)

TABLE 5.2

Diagnosis of HIV infection in infants and children, March 2015

Panel's recommendations

- Virologic assays that directly detect HIV must be used to diagnose HIV infection in infants younger than 18 months; antibody tests should not be used.
- HIV RNA and HIV DNA nucleic acid tests (NATs) are recommended as preferred virologic assays.
- Virologic diagnostic testing in infants with known perinatal HIV exposure is recommended at ages 14 to 21 days, 1 to 2 months, and 4 to 6 months.
- Virologic diagnostic testing at birth should be considered for infants at high risk of HIV infection.
- Virologic diagnostic testing should be considered 2 to 4 weeks after cessation of antiretroviral (ARV) prophylaxis for infants receiving combination ARV infant prophylaxis, if the results of prior virologic testing were negative while the infant was receiving prophylaxis.
- A positive virologic test should be confirmed as soon as possible by a repeat virologic test on a second specimen.
- Definitive exclusion of HIV infection in non-breastfed infants is based on two or more negative virologic tests, with one obtained at age ≥1 month and one at age ≥4 months, or two negative HIV antibody tests from separate specimens obtained at age ≥6 months.
- Some experts confirm the absence of HIV infection at 12 to 18 months of age in infants with prior negative virologic tests by performing an antibody test to document loss of maternal HIV antibodies.
- Children with perinatal HIV exposure aged 18 to 24 months may have residual maternal HIV antibodies; definitive exclusion or confirmation of HIV infection in children in this age group who are HIV antibody-positive should be based on a NAT.
- Diagnosis of HIV infection in children with non-perinatal exposure or children with perinatal exposure aged >24 months relies primarily on the use of HIV antibody tests; when acute HIV infection is suspected, testing with an HIV NAT may be necessary to diagnose HIV infection.

SOURCE: Adapted from Panel on Antiretroviral Therapy and Medical Management of HIV-Infected Children, "Diagnosis of HIV Infection in Infants and Children: Panel's Recommendations," in *Guidelines for the Use of Antiretroviral Agents in Pediatric HIV Infection*, AIDSinfo, U.S. Department of Health and Human Services, July 26, 2015, https://aidsinfo.nih.gov/guidelines/html/2/pediatric-arv-guidelines/55/diagnosis-of-hiv-infection-in-infants-and children (accessed July 27, 2015).

2013 (February 2015, http://www.cdc.gov/hiv/pdf/g-l/hiv_surveillance_report_vol_25.pdf), the CDC indicates that perinatal exposure accounts for the overwhelming majority (90.9%) of all AIDS diagnoses among children in the United States since recordkeeping began. A number of factors are associated with an increased risk of an HIV-positive mother passing the infection to her baby. They include a low CD4+ T-cell count, a high viral load (the concentration of the virus in the blood), advanced HIV progression, the presence of a particular HIV protein (p24) in serum, and placental membrane inflammation. Intrapartum (at the time of birth) events that result in increased exposure of the baby to maternal blood—breast-feeding, low vitamin A levels, premature rupture of membranes, prenatal use of illicit drugs, and premature delivery—also increase the risk of mother-to-child transmission. In addition, the risk of perinatal transmission increases when the mother does not know she is infected until late in the course of the illness.

Despite these potential routes of transmission, the number of HIV-infected infants has been declining as a result of the more widespread use of ART to prevent pregnant women from passing HIV infection to their offspring. Planned cesarean section delivery (the surgical delivery of a baby), the presence of neutralizing antibodies in the mother, and timely ART further reduce the chances of mother-to-infant HIV transmission. The CDC notes that among HIV-infected children survival is slightly lower for those with infection that is attributed to perinatal transmission.

Antiretroviral Therapy

The use of ART to prevent mother-to-child transmission (PMTCT) has substantially decreased this route

of HIV transmission. The CDC observes in "HIV among Pregnant Women, Infants, and Children" (June 23, 2015, http://www.cdc.gov/hiv/group/gender/pregnantwomen/index.html) that ART combined with timely, appropriate prenatal care can reduce the risk of transmission to less than 1%. In the United States the estimated numbers of perinatally acquired AIDS cases have dropped dramatically as a result of voluntary HIV testing of pregnant women, the use of ART for pregnant women and newborn infants, and the treatment of HIV infections that slow progression to AIDS.

In 2013, the number of HIV diagnoses attributable to perinatal exposure was highest among African Americans (60), compared with Hispanics (8), Asian Americans (7), and whites (14). (See Table 3.5 in Chapter 3.)

In *HIV/AIDS Data and Statistics* (2015, http://www.who.int/hiv/data/en), the World Health Organization (WHO) says that global efforts to reduce the rate of mother-to-child transmission have seen significant gains. In 2007 only 33% of HIV-positive pregnant women were getting drugs to prevent transmission, but as of 2014, 73% were receiving treatment. The percentage of HIV-exposed infants receiving ART rose from 20% in 2007 to 32% in 2014. On June 30, 2015, the WHO announced that Cuba became the first country to eliminate mother-to-child transmission of HIV and syphilis. In Cuba, less than 2% of children whose mothers are HIV-infected are born with the virus, the lowest rate possible with present prevention methods.

Changing Thinking about How to Prevent Mother-to-Child Transmission

When HIV-positive mothers breast-feed their babies they run a risk of transmitting the virus to them via their breast milk. However, advising HIV-infected mothers to forgo breast-feeding has had mixed results worldwide in terms of preventing HIV infection and the overall health of the infant. In some regions it can be difficult to get access to infant formula and to safe drinking water. Hoosen M. Coovadia et al. report in "Mother-to-Child Transmission of HIV-1 Infection during Exclusive Breastfeeding in the First 6 Months of Life: An Intervention Cohort Study" (*Lancet*, vol. 369, no. 9567, March 31, 2007) that in cases in which HIV-infected mothers chose to feed their babies a combination of breast milk and either formula or soft foods, there were actually higher rates of mother-to-infant transmission of HIV than in cases where infants were exclusively breast-fed.

Coovadia et al. indicate that exclusive breast-feeding reduced the risk of HIV transmission by nearly half compared with when formula was given with breast milk, and by more than 10 times compared with when solid foods were also part of the infants' diet. These findings are somewhat surprising. One might expect that the more breast milk the infants consumed, the greater the viral exposure and rate of infection. Coovadia et al. posit several ideas about how exclusive breast-feeding might lead to a lower rate of infection, including:

- Exclusive breast-feeding protects the integrity of the lining of the gastrointestinal tract (the mouth, esophagus, stomach, and intestines), and an intact gastrointestinal tract may prevent the HIV from entering the blood.

- The consumption of foreign proteins such as cows' milk protein as in formula milk might stimulate the large numbers of immune receptors that ordinarily line the gastrointestinal tract and enable the virus to better adhere to the lining of the gastrointestinal tract and enter into the underlying tissues.

- Exclusive breast-feeding is also associated with a lower amount of HIV virus in the milk, compared with when the mother combines breast-feeding and formula feeding. When mothers supplement their infants' diet with formula, the breast is not entirely emptied and the remaining milk contains higher levels of the virus.

- Breast milk naturally contains several substances that can inhibit virus growth. Although more breast milk will present more virus, the effects may be countered because the infant also ingests more of the substances that inhibit virus growth.

In "Infant Feeding and HIV: Avoiding Transmission Is Not Enough" (*British Medical Journal*, vol. 334, no. 7592, March 10, 2007), Nigel C. Rollins of the Nelson R. Mandela School of Medicine in South Africa states that, in view of the results of this research, the WHO changed its recommendations in 2007. The new recommendations suggest that decision making be based on individual circumstances and acknowledge that infant survival, as opposed to simply preventing HIV transmission, should be the goal of infant feeding practices.

The WHO has revised its recommendations several times in response to new research findings. In *Guidelines on HIV and Infant Feeding 2010: Principles and Recommendations for Infant Feeding in the Context of HIV and a Summary of Evidence* (2010, http://whqlibdoc.who.int/publications/2010/9789241599535_eng.pdf), the WHO recommends that HIV-infected women either breast-feed exclusively or avoid breast-feeding altogether, as opposed to doing some breast-feeding and some formula or soft foods. If they do breast-feed exclusively, women are recommended to take ART to reduce transmission. In countries where ART is available, the WHO advises breast-feeding until infants are 12 months old.

Louise Kuhn et al. find in "HIV-1 Concentrations in Human Breast Milk before and after Weaning" (*Science Translational Medicine*, vol. 5, no. 181, April 2013) that HIV-infected mothers are less likely to transmit the virus to their newborns if they breast-feed their child exclusively for more than four months. Because even slight changes in breast-feeding patterns appear to increase HIV in the mother's breast milk, mothers are discouraged from supplementing their infants' diets with formula. Kuhn et al. also observe that when HIV-infected mothers adhere to ART during breast-feeding, the risk of transmission is very low.

Nonetheless, in the United States and other resource-rich countries, HIV-infected women, including those receiving ART, are advised against breast-feeding because safe infant formula is readily available. The HHS reports in *Recommendations for Use of Antiretroviral Drugs in Pregnant HIV-1-Infected Women for Maternal Health and Interventions to Reduce Perinatal HIV Transmission in the United States* (August 6, 2015, https://aidsinfo.nih.gov/contentfiles/lvguidelines/Perinatal GL.pdf) that avoidance of breast-feeding, routine HIV counseling and testing, ART, rapid HIV testing in labor and delivery, and scheduled cesarean delivery have reduced the rate of HIV transmission from mother to child in the United States and Europe to 2%.

TREATMENTS FOR CHILDREN

Prescribing drug therapy for children is often more difficult than prescribing for adults because children respond to drugs differently at different ages and because oral medication must have an acceptable taste to ensure that children will take it as prescribed.

In "Approved Antiretroviral Drugs for Pediatric Treatment of HIV Infection" (January 1, 2014, http://www.fda.gov/forpatients/illness/hivaids/treatment/ucm118951.htm), the U.S. Food and Drug Administration

(FDA) lists 35 drugs that are approved to treat pediatric HIV patients. Nine of these were protease inhibitors (PIs). PI compounds act by preventing the reproduction of HIV that is already in the host cells. However, safety and effectiveness in children had not been established for two of the PIs: Indinavir and Saquinavir. The seven PIs approved for use and deemed safe and effective by the FDA were:

- Aptivus
- Kaletra
- Lexiva
- Norvir
- Prezista
- Reyataz
- Viracept

Another group of drugs used in treating HIV are known as nucleoside reverse transcriptase inhibitors (NRTIs). NRTIs, which are structurally similar to a nucleoside constituent of deoxyribonucleic acid (DNA), limit HIV replication by incorporating themselves into a strand of DNA and causing the chain to end. Although 12 NRTIs are approved for pediatric use, one of these drugs, Trizivr, had not been determined safe and effective in pediatric patients. The other drugs were:

- Combivir
- Emtriva
- Epivir
- Epzicom
- Truvada
- Videx
- Videx EC
- Viread
- Zerit
- Ziagen
- Zidovudine

Another group of antiretroviral drugs are known as nonnucleoside reverse transcriptase inhibitors (NNRTIs). NNRTIs slow down the functioning of the enzyme that allows the virus to become a part of the infected cell's nucleus. Six NNRTIs were approved for pediatric use as of January 2014, but one, Edurant, had not had its safety and efficacy in pediatric patients established. Another, Rescriptor, had not had its safety and efficacy established in patients aged 15 years and younger infected with HIV-1. The other four NNRTIs were:

- Intelence
- Sustiva

- Viramune
- Viramune XR

HIV integrase strand inhibitors (INSTI) block an enzyme HIV uses to insert its viral DNA into the DNA of the host CD4 cell. Blocking the enzyme prevents HIV replication. Figure 5.1 shows how the two FDA-approved INSTIs, Isentress and Tivicay, act to keep HIV from replicating.

Fuzeon is a fusion inhibitor. The only drug in this class in 2014, it is approved for use in children aged six years and older. It acts by inhibiting the fusion of HIV to the host cell membrane. Entry inhibitors work by blocking a receptor, CCR5, that some strains of HIV use to enter white blood cells. Selzentry was the only entry inhibitor approved for pediatric use in 2014; it has not had its safety and efficacy in these patients established.

The FDA has approved three other drugs for pediatric use called Atripla, Complera, and Stribild. Each of these drugs combines several of the previously listed medications into a single pill to provide a complete regimen of HIV treatment in an easy-to-take form. However, of the three drugs, as of 2014 only Atripla had its safety and efficacy established in pediatric patients, and even that drug was recommended only for children aged 12 years and older.

2015 Treatment Guidelines for Children and Adolescents

The NIH Panel updated the *Guidelines for the Use of Antiretroviral Agents in Pediatric HIV Infection* in March 2015. Table 5.3 summarizes the NIH Panel's treatment recommendations for HIV-infected infants and children. Depending on the age of the child and the severity of his or her symptoms, drug treatment may be recommended. In these cases, the NIH Panel calls for combination antiretroviral therapy (cART) regimens that feature at least three drugs drawn from two or more drug classes because these drug regimens "have been associated with enhanced survival, reduction in opportunistic infections and other complications of HIV infection, improved growth and neurocognitive function, and improved quality of life in children."

The NIH Panel also notes specific issues that arise when treating HIV-infected adolescents including:

- The need for regular discussions about reproductive health, contraception methods and safer sex techniques to prevent HIV transmission
- Ensuring that adolescents considering a planned pregnancy receive a maximally suppressive ART therapy regimen to reduce the risk of transmission to offspring
- The potential for combination antiretroviral therapy to reduce the effectiveness of hormonal contraceptives

FIGURE 5.1

How integrase-inhibitors prevent HIV replication

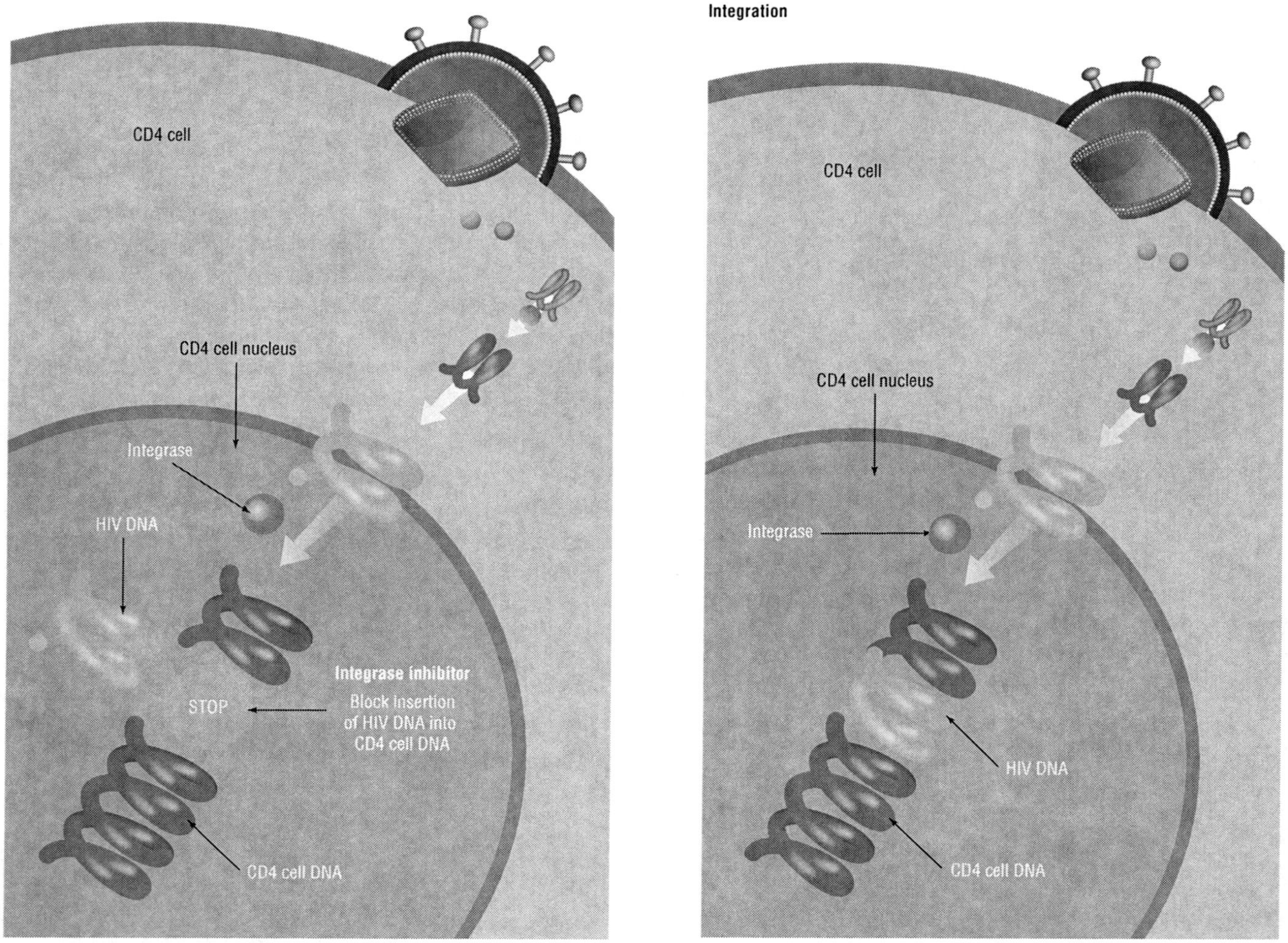

SOURCE: "Integrase Strand Transfer Inhibitor (INSTI)," in *Glossary*, AIDSinfo, U.S. Department of Health and Human Services, July 26, 2015, https://aidsinfo.nih.gov/education-materials/glossary/380/integrase-strand-transfer-inhibitor (accessed July 27, 2015)

• Continuing emphasis on the importance of adherence to treatment and consideration of a once-daily drug regimen to improve adherence. Table 5.4 enumerates strategies to improve adherence to ART.

Monitoring Treatment

In order to monitor disease progression and the effectiveness of treatment the NIH Panel recommends that absolute CD4 T lymphocyte (CD4) cell count should be used for monitoring immune status in children of all ages. After initiation of cART or following a change in cART regimen, children should be evaluated for clinical side effects of treatment within one to two weeks, and should have laboratory testing for toxicity and viral load response two to four weeks after treatment begins. Children and adolescents should be routinely assessed every three to four months for adherence to treatment, effectiveness

(by CD4 cell count/percentage and plasma viral load), and toxicities (by history, physical, and selected laboratory tests).

CHILDREN ARE AT HIGHER RISK OF DRUG RESISTANCE

In "Risk of Triple-Class Virological Failure in Children with HIV: A Retrospective Cohort Study" (*Lancet*, vol. 377, no. 9777, May 7, 2011), the project team for the Collaboration of Observational HIV Epidemiological Research Europe looked at more than 1,000 children who had been infected with HIV perinatally and became resistant to the three major classes of drugs that are used to treat HIV: NRTIs, NNRTIs, and PIs. The team aimed to estimate the number of children who will need new classes of drugs as they age. It finds that 12% of the

TABLE 5.3

Treatment recommendations for HIV-infected infants and children

	Panel recommendations

Recommend urgent treatment[a]	Combination Antiretroviral Therapy (cART) should be initiated urgently in all HIV-infected children with any of the following:
	Age <12 months:
	• AI for infants age <12 weeks
	• AII for infants 12 weeks–12 months
	Age ≥1 year:
	• CDC Stage 3-defining opportunistic illnesses
	• CDC Stage 3 immunodeficiency:
	    • Aged 1 to <6 years, CD4 count[c] <500 cells/mm
	    • Aged ≥6 years, CD4 count[c] <200 cells/mm

Recommend treatment[b]	cART should be initiated in HIV-infected children aged ≥1 year with any of the following: • Moderate HIV-related symptoms • Plasma HIV RNA >100,000 copies/mL[d] CDC stage 2: • Age 1 to <6 years, CD4 count[c] 500–999 cells/mm • Age ≥6 years, CD4 count[c] 200–499 cells/mm
Consider treatment[b]	cART should be considered for HIV-infected children aged ≥1 year with: • Mild HIV-related symptoms or asymptomatic and CDC stage 1: • Ages 1 to <6 years, CD4 count[c] ≥1,000 cells/mm • Age ≥6 years, CD4 count[c] ≥500 cells/mm

[a]Within 1–2 weeks, including an expedited discussion on adherence.
[b]More time can be taken to fully assess and address issues associated with adherence with the caregivers and the child prior to initiating therapy. Patients/caregivers may choose to postpone therapy, and on a case-by-case basis, providers may elect to defer therapy based on clinical and/or psychosocial factors.
[c]CD4 counts should be confirmed with a second test to meet the treatment criteria before initiation of cART.
[d]To avoid overinterpretation of temporary blips in viral load (which can occur, for example, during intercurrent illnesses), plasma HIV RNA level >100,000 copies/mLshould be confirmed by a second level before initiating cART.
Note: Adherence should be assessed and discussed with HIV-infected children and their caregivers before initiation of therapy.

SOURCE: Adapted from Panel on Antiretroviral Therapy and Medical Management of HIV-Infected Children, "Treatment Recommendations for Initiation of Therapy in Antiretroviral-Naive, HIV-Infected Infants and Children," in *Guidelines for the Use of Antiretroviral Agents in Pediatric HIV Infection*, AIDSinfo, U.S. Department of Health and Human Services, July 26, 2015, https://aidsinfo.nih.gov/guidelines/html/2/pediatric-arv-guidelines/55/diagnosis-of-hiv-infection-in-infants-and-children (accessed July 27, 2015)

children developed resistance to all three drugs within five years of starting ART. The team also notes that the children who started ART at older ages were more likely to suffer drug resistance.

The NIH Panel observes that drug treatment of pediatric HIV infection has improved since the introduction of potent combination drug regimens that effectively suppress viral replication in most patients, resulting in a lower risk of treatment failure due to development of drug resistance. Despite this progress, the NIH Panel notes that poor adherence to treatment increases the risk of drug resistance and recommends that drug resistance testing be used to choose effective initial and subsequent drug regimens.

HOW MANY CHILDREN ARE INFECTED?

In 2013 an estimated 187 children under the age of 13 years contracted an HIV infection in the United States. (See Table 3.2 in Chapter 3.) Of the estimated new 26,688 AIDS cases in 2013, just 8 were in children aged 12 years and under. (See Table 3.1 in Chapter 3 and Table 5.5.)

In 2013 African American children accounted for a disproportionate share of HIV infections among children. That year African Americans made up 14% of all children in the United States, but the estimated 108 new HIV infections in that group constituted 65.2% of new HIV infections among children. (See Table 5.6.)

Global Outlook

The HHS reports in "Global Statistics" (November 13, 2014, https://www.aids.gov/hiv-aids-basics/hiv-aids-101/global-statistics) that in 2013 there were 3.2 million children living with HIV worldwide. Most were infected during pregnancy, at birth, or via breast-feeding by their HIV-infected mothers.

In *HIV/AIDS and Children: Analysis of Achievements and Challenges* (September 8, 2014, http://www.unicef.org/publicpartnerships/files/FA3_HIV_thematic_briefing_presentation_2014.pdf), UNICEF reports that between 2001 and 2009 effective prevention of mother-to-child transmission resulted in a 26% decline in the annual number of new HIV infections in children worldwide. Between 2009 and 2012 there was a further reduction of 35%. During this same period AIDS deaths in children aged zero to four years fell by more than 50%. However, deaths among children 10 to 19 years of age more than doubled.

Gene Mutation in Some Babies May Help

A gene mutation that slows the progress of HIV in adults was shown during the late 1990s to help HIV-infected

TABLE 5.4

Strategies to improve adherence to antiretroviral treatment

Initial intervention strategies

- Establish trust and identify mutually acceptable goals for care.
- Obtain explicit agreement on the need for treatment and adherence.
- Identify depression, low self-esteem, substance abuse, or other mental health issues for the child/adolescent and/or caregiver that may decrease adherence. Treat mental health issues before starting ARV drugs, if possible.
- Identify family, friends, health team members, and others who can support adherence.
- Educate patient and family about the critical role of adherence in therapy outcome.
- Specify the adherence target: ≥95% of prescribed doses.
- Educate patient and family about the relationship between partial adherence and resistance.
- Educate patient and family about resistance and constraint in later choices of ARV drug (i.e., explain that although a failure of adherence may be temporary, the effects on treatment choice may be permanent).
- Develop a treatment plan that the patient and family understand and to which they feel committed.
- Establish readiness to take medication through practice sessions or other means.
- Consider a brief period of hospitalization at start of therapy in selected circumstances for patient education and to assess tolerability of medications chosen.

Medication strategies

- Choose the simplest regimen possible, reducing dosing frequency and number of pills.
- Choose a regimen with dosing requirements that best conform to the daily and weekly routines and variations in patient and family activities.
- Choose the most palatable medicine possible (pharmacists may be able to add syrups or flavoring agents to increase palatability).
- Choose drugs with the fewest adverse effects; provide anticipatory guidance for management of adverse effects.
- Simplify food requirements for medication administration.
- Prescribe drugs carefully to avoid adverse drug-drug interactions.
- Assess pill-swallowing capacity and offer pill-swallowing training.

Follow-up intervention strategies

- Monitor adherence at each visit and in between visits by telephone, email, text, and social media, as needed.
- Provide ongoing support, encouragement, and understanding of the difficulties associated with demands to attain 95% adherence with medication doses.
- Use patient education aids including pictures, calendars, and stickers.
- Encourage use of pill boxes, reminders, alarms, pagers, and timers.
- Provide follow-up clinic visits, telephone calls, and text messages to support and assess adherence.
- Provide access to support groups, peer groups, or one-on-one counseling for caregivers and patients, especially for those with known depression or drug use issues that are known to decrease adherence.
- Provide pharmacist-based adherence support, such as medication education and counseling, blister packs, refill reminders, automatic refills, and home delivery of medications.
- Consider directly observed therapy at home, in the clinic, or in selected circumstances, during a brief inpatient hospitalization.
- Consider gastrostomy tube use in selected circumstances.

SOURCE: Panel on Antiretroviral Therapy and Medical Management of HIV-Infected Children, "Table 12. Strategies to Improve Adherence to Antiretroviral Medications," in *Guidelines for the Use of Antiretroviral Agents in Pediatric HIV Infection,* AIDSinfo, U.S. Department of Health and Human Services, July 26, 2015, https://aidsinfo.nih.gov/guidelines/html/2/pediatric-arv-guidelines/55/diagnosis-of-hiv-infection-in-infants-and-children (accessed July 27, 2015)

newborns avoid serious AIDS-associated illnesses longer than those who do not have the mutation. Michael Fischer-eder et al. report in "CC Chemokine Receptor 5 and Renal-Transplant Survival" (*Lancet*, vol. 357, no. 9270, June 2, 2001) that the gene CC chemokine receptor 5 (CCR5) is present in 10% to 15% of whites but is not found in Asian Americans or African Americans.

The gene codes for a protein called CCR5. This protein and another one called CXCR4 are located on the surface of a number of human cells. In "Analysis of the Mechanism by Which the Small-Molecule CCR5 Antagonists SCH-351125 and SCH-350581 Inhibit Human Immunodeficiency Virus Type 1 Entry" (*Journal of Virology*, vol. 77, no. 9, May 2003), Fotini Tsamis et al. demonstrate that CCR5 and CXCR4 can be used as receptors by HIV-1 to enter and infect CD4+ T cells, dendritic cells, and macrophages. Furthermore, CCR5 has been shown to be essential for viral transmission and replication during the early phase of the disease, even before symptoms of infection appear. Researchers expect that further investigation of the CCR5 gene will eventually help them develop drugs to prevent or destroy HIV in newborns.

Some researchers, such as Michael Marmor et al., in "Resistance to HIV Infection" (*Journal of Urban Health*, vol. 83, no. 1, January 2006), speculate that because several of the same genetic mutations have been found in both exposed uninfected populations and in long-term nonprogressor populations (people who become infected but do not develop AIDS), a single theory may explain both phenomena—that the genetic traits prevent or hinder HIV-1 entry into cells, which reduces the likelihood of infection and, should infection occur, slows or entirely eliminates the development of serious disease.

HIV TESTING RECOMMENDED FOR ALL PREGNANT WOMEN

When HIV-infected pregnant women know their HIV infection status, they are better able to make informed decisions about ART to reduce perinatal transmission of HIV to their infants. In September 2008 the American College of Obstetrics and Gynecology's (ACOG) Committee on Obstetric Practice expanded its recommendations about prenatal and perinatal HIV testing in "ACOG Committee Opinion No. 418: Prenatal and Perinatal Human Immunodeficiency Virus Testing: Expanded

TABLE 5.5

AIDS diagnoses in children aged 13 and under, 2009–13 and cumulative

Race/ethnicity	2009			2010			2011			2012			2013			Cumulative[b]	
		Estimated[a]			Estimated[a]			Estimated[a]			Estimated[a]			Estimated[a]			
	No.	No.	Rate	No.	No.	Rate	No.	No.	Rate	No.	No.	Rate	No.	No.	Rate	No.	Est. No.[a]
American Indian/Alaska Native	0	0	0.0	0	0	0.0	0	0	0.0	0	0	0.0	0	0	0.0	26	26
Asian[c]	1	1	0.0	1	1	0.0	0	0	0.0	0	0	0.0	0	0	0.0	46	46
Black/African American	8	8	0.1	15	15	0.2	11	12	0.2	8	8	0.1	3	3	0.0	5,601	5,615
Hispanic/Latino[d]	4	4	0.0	4	4	0.0	2	2	0.0	1	1	0.0	2	2	0.0	1,955	1,960
Native Hawaiian/other Pacific Islander	0	0	0.0	0	0	0.0	0	0	0.0	0	0	0.0	0	0	0.0	6	6
White	1	1	0.0	3	3	0.0	2	2	0.0	1	1	0.0	0	0	0.0	1,540	1,542
Multiple races	0	0	0.0	0	0	0.0	0	0	0.0	0	0	0.0	2	2	0.1	225	226
Total[e]	**14**	**14**	**0.0**	**23**	**24**	**0.0**	**15**	**16**	**0.0**	**10**	**10**	**0.0**	**7**	**8**	**0.0**	**9,399**	**9,421**

[a]Estimated numbers resulted from statistical adjustment that accounted for reporting delays, but not for incomplete reporting. Rates are per 100,000 population.
[b]From the beginning of the epidemic through 2013.
[c]Includes Asian/Pacific Islander legacy cases.
[d]Hispanics/Latinos can be of any race.
[e]Because column totals for estimated numbers were calculated independently of the values for the subpopulations, the values in each column may not sum to the column total.
Note: Reported numbers less than 12, as well as estimated numbers (and accompanying rates and trends) based on these numbers, should be interpreted with caution.

SOURCE: "Table 6a. Stage 3 (AIDS) among Children Aged <13 Years, by Race/Ethnicity, 2009–2013 and Cumulative—United States," in HIV Surveillance Report: Diagnoses of HIV Infection in the United States and Dependent Areas, 2013, vol. 25, Centers for Disease Control and Prevention, National Center for HIV/AIDS, Viral Hepatitis, Sexual Transmitted Diseases, and Tuberculosis Prevention, Division of HIV/AIDS Prevention, February 2015. http://www.cdc.gov/hiv/pdf/g-l/hiv_surveillance_report_vol_25.pdf#Page=56f (accessed July 22, 2015)

TABLE 5.6

HIV infection in children aged 13 and under, by race/ethnicity, 2009–13

Race/ethnicity	2009 No.	2009 Est. No.[a]	2010 No.	2010 Est. No.[a]	2011 No.	2011 Est. No.[a]	2012 No.	2012 Est. No.[a]	2013 No.	2013 Est. No.[a]
American Indian/Alaska Native	0	0	0	0	1	1	0	0	0	0
Asian	8	8	2	2	6	6	12	13	14	15
Black/African American	152	156	148	152	118	124	164	177	108	122
Hispanic/Latino[b]	33	34	37	39	25	26	15	17	11	13
Native Hawaiian/other Pacific Islander	0	0	0	0	1	1	1	1	0	0
White	17	17	31	32	30	31	31	33	23	26
Multiple races	9	9	11	11	9	9	9	10	8	10
Total[c]	**219**	**224**	**229**	**236**	**190**	**199**	**232**	**250**	**164**	**187**

[a]Estimated numbers resulted from statistical adjustment that accounted for reporting delays, but not for incomplete reporting.
[b]Hispanics/Latinos can be of any race.
[c]Because column totals for estimated numbers were calculated independently of the values for the subpopulations, the values in each column may not sum to the column total.
Note: Data include persons with a diagnosis of HIV infection regardless of stage of disease at diagnosis. Reported numbers less than 12, as well as estimated numbers (and accompanying rates and trends) based on these numbers, should be interpreted with caution.

SOURCE: "Table 5b. Diagnoses of HIV Infection among Children Aged <13 Years, by Race/Ethnicity, 2009–2013—United States and 6 Dependent Areas," in *HIV Surveillance Report: Diagnoses of HIV Infection in the United States and Dependent Areas, 2013*, vol. 25, Centers for Disease Control and Prevention, National Center for HIV/AIDS, Viral Hepatitis, Sexual Transmitted Diseases, and Tuberculosis Prevention, Division of HIV/AIDS Prevention, February 2015, http://www.cdc.gov/hiv/pdf/g-l/hiv_surveillance_report_vol_25.pdf#Page=56f (accessed July 22, 2015)

Recommendations" (*Obstetrics and Gynecology*, vol. 112, no. 3). The committee recommended that all pregnant women be screened for HIV infection as early as possible during each pregnancy and informed that they will receive an HIV test as part of routine prenatal testing unless they decline or opt-out of HIV screening. Repeat conventional or rapid HIV testing during the third trimester of pregnancy is recommended for:

- Women living in areas with high HIV prevalence rates
- Women known to be at high risk for acquiring HIV
- Women who declined testing earlier in the pregnancy

In 2012 Roger Chou et al. conducted a review of the medical literature on the prevention of HIV transmission during pregnancy on behalf of the U.S. Preventive Services Task Force. In "Screening for HIV in Pregnant Women: Evidence Summary" (November 2012, http://www.uspreventiveservicestaskforce.org/Page/Document/screening-for-hiv-in-pregnant-women-evidence-summary/human-immunodeficiency-virus-hiv-infection-screening#figure-analytic-framework-and-key-questions-for-screening-for-hiv-in-pregnant-women), they conclude that HIV screening is accurate and can lead to interventions that reduce the risk of mother-to-child transmission.

SURVIVING INTO ADOLESCENCE AND ADULTHOOD

In "HIV Infection in Infants and Children," the NIAID distinguishes three distinct patterns of disease progression among HIV-infected children. The first group consists of those who display symptoms within their first 18 months following infection. Even with treatment, progression to AIDS in this group is rapid and most children die by age four. Children in the second group experience a less aggressive progression and often have milder or less prolonged symptomatic periods. These children tend to live longer. The third group are children who grown up with few, if any, symptoms. Researchers are eager to determine precisely why and how these children remain asymptomatic in spite of their infections.

Research indicates that some of the difference in response to HIV is attributable to polymorphisms (common genetic variations). Kumud K. Singh and Stephen Spector find in "Host Genetic Determinants of HIV Infection and Disease Progression in Children" (*Pediatric Research*, vol. 65, May 2009) that HIV-infected children with a specific polymorphism called CCR5-delta32 had half the rate of disease progression compared with children with normal CCR5. They also observe that the most rapid progression of HIV symptoms occurred in children with normal CCR5 plus a polymorphism called 59029-A/A. This particular polymorphism was identified in about 25% of the HIV-infected children studied, representing the genotype that most often accelerated the rate of disease progression in children with normal CCR5. Furthermore, Singh and Spector find that there were some polymorphisms that had an impact in adults but not in children and some that seemed to have an important impact in children but only a modest impact in adults.

In "Host and Viral Genetic Correlates of Clinical Definitions of HIV-1 Disease Progression" (*PLoS One*, vol. 5, no. 6, June 11, 2010), Concepción Casado et al. describe patterns of HIV disease progression that are based on host genetic markers and viral factors. The researchers attempt to better define long-term nonprogressor elite controllers (HIV-infected people who show no signs of disease progression for over 12 years and remain asymptomatic), viremic controllers (HIV-infected people who progress to AIDS very slowly, after a long period, or in some instances do not progress to AIDS), viremic noncontrollers (HIV-infected people who have high levels of viral load), chronic progressors (HIV-infected people who progress to AIDS within 10 years of diagnosis), and rapid progressors (HIV-infected people who progress to AIDS within four years of diagnosis).

In "HLA Correlates of Long-Term Survival in Vertically Infected HIV-1-Positive Adolescents in Harare, Zimbabwe" (*AIDS Research and Human Retroviruses*, vol. 31, no. 5, May 1, 2015), Brittany L. Shepherd et al. report that HIV typically progresses rapidly among infected infants in Africa, with only 50% surviving past the age of two if not treated. Despite this fact, some untreated older children reach adolescence with no symptoms and normal CD4+ counts. Shepard et al. performed genetic analyses of these long-term slow-progressors and found that slow progression was associated with specific subtypes of the polymorphic human leukocyte antigen (HLA) gene network. HLA-C*08:02 and C*08:04 were significantly enriched in the HIV-1 long-term survivor group, and may confer the observed survival advantage.

Some children who were born with HIV infection were in their 30s as of 2015. If they continue to receive treatment, it may be that they will have life spans comparable to people without HIV. No one, however, can say for sure since the epidemic and its treatments have been underway and studied for only a few decades and thus the effects of 40 or more years of infection are unknown.

Dealing with Physical and Emotional Problems

When HIV-infected children died during the early years of the HIV/AIDS epidemic, they were generally unaware of what was happening to them. In the 21st century, at the Children's Evaluation and Rehabilitation Center of the Albert Einstein College of Medicine of Yeshiva University, school-aged children meet with social workers in a support group to handle the physical and emotional ordeals of growing up with HIV/AIDS. These children are part of the increasing number born with HIV who have survived long enough to realize what it means. They must learn to cope with the physical, psychological, and emotional consequences of HIV/AIDS.

Claude A. Mellins and Kathleen M. Malee review in "Understanding the Mental Health of Youth Living with Perinatal HIV Infection: Lessons Learned and Current Challenges" (*Journal of the International AIDS Society*, vol. 16, June 18, 2013) studies that examine the mental health problems of children aged 10 years and older living with perinatal HIV infection. The researchers find that although many of these youth fare well in terms of mental health, a substantial proportion experience emotional and behavioral problems, including psychiatric

disorders, at higher than expected rates. Adolescents coping with lifelong HIV infection must contend with medical treatment, hospitalizations, and physical pain as well as the psychosocial impact of HIV, a stigmatized and sexually transmittable illness that may make their teen years especially challenging. Mellins and Malee cite building resilience—positive development despite exposure to significant adversity—as a preventive measure that can be used to promote mental health and emotional well-being.

Lisa Henry-Reid, Lori Wiener, and Ana Garcia observe in "Caring for Youth with HIV" (*Achieve*, Winter 2009) that adolescents with HIV require significant psychological and emotional support because they face unique challenges, including:

- Experiencing stigma and fear of rejection

- Dealing with the side effects of HIV drugs

- Coping with a potentially life-threatening illness and an uncertain life span

- Dealing with disclosure and transmission

- Enduring the impact of loss

- Navigating the health care system

Henry-Reid, Wiener, and Garcia report that adolescents who share their HIV diagnosis with others fare better psychologically and socially than those who do not disclose their HIV status. They assert that HIV-infected adolescents must deal with the normal challenges of adolescence and illness as well as with additional stressors such as poverty, barriers to care and social services, violence, racism, homophobia, broken families, homelessness, and child abuse.

Global HIV Infection in Young People

In *Fact Sheet: 2014 Statistics* (2015, http://www.unaids.org/en/resources/campaigns/HowAIDSchangedeverything/factsheet), the Joint United Nations Programme on HIV/AIDS (UNAIDS) notes that most parts of the world have seen a reduction in new HIV infections among young people. By 2014, an estimated 32% of children had access to antiretroviral therapy, up from 14% in 2010. However there was still a considerable treatment gap for children.

According to UNAIDS, in 2014, 220,000 children were newly infected with HIV, down from 520,000 in 2000. Most of this decrease was attributable to PMTCT. Nearly three-quarters (73%) of pregnant women living with HIV had access to antiretroviral medicines to prevent transmission of HIV in 2014.

Almost none of the children who acquired HIV in 2014 lived in high-income countries, and more than 91% lived in sub-Saharan Africa. Regardless, the situation is improving globally. Between 2009 and 2014 there was a 48% decline in new HIV cases among children in the 21

African countries targeted as priorities in the Global Plan to Eliminate New HIV Infections among Children and Keeping Their Mothers Alive.

WHO WILL CARE FOR THEM?

The HIV/AIDS epidemic has created many tragedies, including millions of orphans. AVERT, an international HIV and AIDS charity, based in the United Kingdom, reports that worldwide there were an estimated 25 million orphans due to AIDS in 2015. In "Children Orphaned by HIV and AIDS" (2015, http://www.avert.org/children-orphaned-hiv-and-aids.htm), AVERT observes that about 85% of these orphaned children live in sub-Saharan Africa. AIDS is responsible for about three-quarters of all orphaned children in Zimbabwe and 63% of such children in South Africa.

It is not always possible to find someone to care for an orphan of parents who died of AIDS, particularly if the child also has HIV or AIDS. Some family members may be hesitant to take in the child for fear he or she may spread the infection. In a growing number of cases, however, grandparents (in most cases, grandmothers) are taking these orphans into their home. This may be a burden on older people who have lost their own children and may feel too old, tired, or impoverished to rear another family. They may also fear that they will die before their grandchildren do, leaving no one to care for them. It is no less difficult for the children who have lost their parents and fear they will probably miss the advantages they would have had with younger parents, such as being able to play more active childhood games.

Older orphans struggle with the rage, shame, and isolation of losing a parent to AIDS. Observers are finding that the HIV/AIDS epidemic is creating a class of particularly troubled youth. All children who lose a parent suffer to some degree, but for those whose parents die from AIDS, embarrassment and secrecy often compound the trauma. Teens whose parents became infected as a result of injecting drugs or practicing unsafe sex are often torn between feeling sorry for their parents and blaming them for their illness.

ADOLESCENTS, YOUNG ADULTS, AND HIV/AIDS
Patterns of Infection

The transmission and course of AIDS among adolescents aged 13 to 19 years and young adults aged 20 to 24 years follow similar patterns to those over the age of 25 years. The CDC reports in *HIV Surveillance in Men Who Have Sex with Men* (June 5, 2015, http://www.cdc.gov/hiv/pdf/statistics_surveillance_msm.pdf) that between 2009 and 2013 HIV infections in males aged 13 to 24 years attributed to MSM increased about 18%. (See Figure 5.2.) In 2013, 8,777 males aged 13 to 24 years were diagnosed with HIV in the United States. (See Table 5.7.) Almost all (91.8%) were infected via MSM contact. By contrast, 1,299

FIGURE 5.2

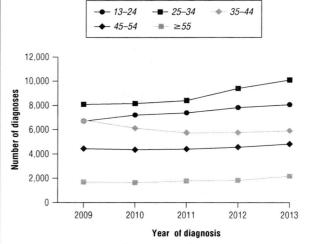

HIV infection among men who have sex with men by age group, 2009–13

[United States and 6 dependent areas]

Note: Data include persons with a diagnosis of HIV infection regardless of stage of disease at diagnosis. All displayed data have been statistically adjusted to account for reporting delays and missing transmission category, but not for incomplete reporting. Data on men who have sex with men do not include men with HIV infection attributed to male-to-male sexual contact *and* injection drug use.

SOURCE: "Diagnosis of HIV Infection among Men Who Have Sex with Men, by Age Group, 2009–2013—United States and 6 U.S. Dependent Areas," in *HIV Surveillance—Men Who Have Sex with Men (MSM)*, Centers for Disease Control and Prevention, National Center for HIV/AIDS, Viral Hepatitis, Sexual Transmitted Diseases, and Tuberculosis Prevention, Division of HIV/AIDS Prevention, June 2015, http://www.cdc.gov/hiv/pdf/statistics_surveillance_msm.pdf (accessed July 28, 2015)

TABLE 5.7

Diagnosed HIV infection among adolescent and young adult males by transmission category, 2013

Transmission category	13–19 years		20–24 years	
	No.	%	No.	%
Male-to-male sexual contact	1,441	92.6	6,620	91.7
Injection drug use (IDU)	21	1.4	117	1.6
Male-to-male sexual contact and IDU	28	1.8	218	3.0
Heterosexual contact[a]	51	3.3	251	3.5
Other[b]	15	0.9	16	0.2
Total	**1,556**	**100**	**7,221**	**100**

[a]Heterosexual contact with a person known to have, or to be at high risk for, HIV infection.
[b]Includes hemophilia, blood transfusion, perinatal exposure, and risk factor not reported or not identified.
Note: Data include persons with a diagnosis of HIV infection regardless of stage of disease at diagnosis. All displayed data have been statistically adjusted to account for reporting delays and missing transmission category, but not for incomplete reporting.

SOURCE: "Diagnosis of HIV Infection among Adolescent and Young Adult Males, by Age Group and Transmission Category, 2013—United States and 6 U.S. Dependent Areas," in *HIV Surveillance—Adolescents and Young Adults*, Centers for Disease Control and Prevention, National Center for HIV/AIDS, Viral Hepatitis, Sexual Transmitted Diseases, and Tuberculosis Prevention, Division of HIV/AIDS Prevention, June 2015, http://www.cdc.gov/hiv/pdf/statistics_surveillance_Adolescents.pdf (accessed July 28, 2015)

female adolescents and young adults aged 13 to 24 years became infected with HIV in 2013, most of them through heterosexual contact (86.67%) or injection drug use (8.6%). (See Table 5.8.)

The characteristics of adolescence—a time of development, uncertainty, and a misleading sense of bravado and immortality, often combined with pushing the boundaries of good sense—create the potential for some young people to become particularly vulnerable to HIV infection. For many, this is a time of experimentation and risk taking, often in terms of sexual behavior or use of alcohol and illicit drugs.

Many Adolescents Are Sexually Active

More than one-third of adolescents are sexually active. In "The Youth Risk Behavior Surveillance—United States, 2013" (*Morbidity and Mortality Weekly Report*, vol. 63, no. 4, June 13, 2012), Laura Kann et al. indicate that in 2013 nearly half (46.8%) of high school students said they had ever had sexual intercourse. The fact that only 59.1% of high school students said they had used a condom during their last sexual intercourse indicates that many were at risk of contracting HIV. (See Table 5.9.)

In 2013 the overwhelming majority (85.3%) of teens said they had been taught in school about HIV/AIDS. (See Table 5.10.) A small percentage of students (12.9%) reported that they had ever been tested for HIV. Females were more likely to have been tested than males, and African Americans were more likely to have been tested than other racial and ethnic groups.

SEXUALLY TRANSMITTED DISEASES. Teenagers engaging in sexual activity before becoming sufficiently mature, with inadequate regard for contraceptive methods or safe sex practices, have led to high rates of sexually transmitted infections (STDs) among adolescents and young adults. According to the CDC, in the fact sheet "Reported STDs in the United States: 2013 National Data for Chlamydia, Gonorrhea, and Syphilis" (December 2014, http://stacks.cdc.gov/view/cdc/26427/cdc_26427_DS1.pdf), approximately 20 million new STDs occur every year in the United States, and half of these occur among people aged 15 to 24 years. Figure 5.3 shows that most chlamydia and gonorrhea infections occur among this age group.

Overall rates of infection for some STDs, such as gonorrhea, declined during the 1990s and leveled off during the first decade of the 21st century. The CDC notes in "STDs in Adolescents and Young Adults" (December 16, 2014, http://www.cdc.gov/std/stats13/adol.htm) that between 2012 and 2013 gonorrhea rates decreased 11.6% for people aged 15 to 19 years and decreased 1.9% among people aged 20 to 24 years. The chlamydia rate for people aged 15 to 19 years decreased 8.7%, but for people aged 20 to 24 years the rate remained the same.

The rates of syphilis infection show a different trend. The rate among 15- to 19-year-old females decreased from 2.9 cases per 100,000 population in 2010 to 1.9 cases in 2013. Among women aged 20 to 24 years there were 3.9 cases in 2013. Among 15- to 19-year-old males the rate rose from 1.3 cases in 2009 to 6.4 cases in 2013. Men aged 20 to 24 years had the highest rate of any age group, 28 cases per 100,000 people in 2013. This is driven largely by

TABLE 5.8

Diagnosed HIV infection among adolescent and young adult females by transmission category, 2013

Transmission category	13–19 years		20–24 years	
	No.	%	No.	%
Injection drug use	23	6.1	90	9.8
Heterosexual contact[a]	316	84.0	810	87.7
Other[b]	37	9.9	23	2.5
Total	**376**	**100**	**923**	**100**

[a]Heterosexual contact with a person known to have, or to be at high risk for, HIV infection.
[b]Includes blood transfusion, perinatal exposure, and risk factor not reported or not identified.
Note: Data include persons with a diagnosis of HIV infection regardless of stage of disease at diagnosis. All displayed data have been statistically adjusted to account for reporting delays and missing transmission category, but not for incomplete reporting.

SOURCE: "Diagnosis of HIV Infection among Adolescent and Young Adult Females, by Age Group and Transmission Category, 2013—United States and 6 U.S. Dependent Areas," in *HIV Surveillance—Adolescents and Young Adults*, Centers for Disease Control and Prevention, National Center for HIV/AIDS, Viral Hepatitis, Sexual Transmitted Diseases, and Tuberculosis Prevention, Division of HIV/AIDS Prevention, June 2015, http://www.cdc.gov/hiv/pdf/statistics_surveillance_Adolescents.pdf (accessed July 28, 2015)

TABLE 5.9

Percentage of high school students that used a condom during last sexual intercourse, 2013

	Condom use		
	Female	Male	Total
Category	%	%	%
Race/ethnicity			
White*	53.2	61.8	57.1
Black*	55.3	73.0	64.7
Hispanic	50.7	66.5	58.3
Grade			
9	56.5	69.5	62.7
10	55.5	69.3	61.7
11	54.8	70.6	62.3
12	48.4	58.0	53.0
Total	**53.1**	**65.8**	**59.1**

*Non-Hispanic.
Notes: Among the 34.0% of students nationwide who were currently sexually active.

SOURCE: Adapted from Laura Kann et al., "Table 67. Percentage of High School Students Who Used a Condom during Last Sexual Intercourse and Who Used Birth Control Pills before Last Sexual Intercourse, by Sex, Race/Ethnicity, and Grade—United States, Youth Risk Behavior Survey, 2013," in "Youth Risk Behavior Surveillance—United States, 2013," *MMWR*, vol. 63, no. 4, June 13, 2014, http://www.cdc.gov/mmwr/pdf/ss/ss6304.pdf (accessed July 28, 2015)

TABLE 5.10

Percentage of high school students taught in school about HIV/AIDS by sex, 2013

	Taught in school about AIDS or HIV infection			Tested for HIV		
	Female	Male	Total	Female	Male	Total
Category	%	%	%	%	%	%
Race/ethnicity						
White*	86.8	86.3	86.6	12.7	8.7	10.7
Black*	83.0	80.6	81.9	20.9	18.7	19.8
Hispanic	84.9	83.9	84.4	13.4	12.2	12.8
Grade						
9	80.1	82.4	81.3	7.8	10.4	9.1
10	86.2	84.5	85.3	12.6	8.5	10.6
11	88.2	86.7	87.4	17.3	13.2	15.3
12	89.3	86.6	88.0	21.3	13.1	17.2
Total	**85.8**	**85.0**	**85.3**	**14.6**	**11.2**	**12.9**

*Non-Hispanic.
Note: HIV tests do not include tests done when donating blood.

SOURCE: Laura Kann et al., "Table 75. Percentage of High School Students Who Were Ever Taught in School about Acquired Immunodeficiency Syndrome (AIDS) or Human Immunodeficiency Virus (HIV) Infection and Who Were Ever Tested for HIV, by Sex, Race/Ethnicity, and Grade—United States, Youth Risk Behavior Survey, 2013," in "Youth Risk Behavior Surveillance—United States, 2013," *MMWR*, vol. 63, no. 4, June 13, 2014, http://www.cdc.gov/mmwr/pdf/ss/ss6304.pdf (accessed July 28, 2015)

FIGURE 5.3

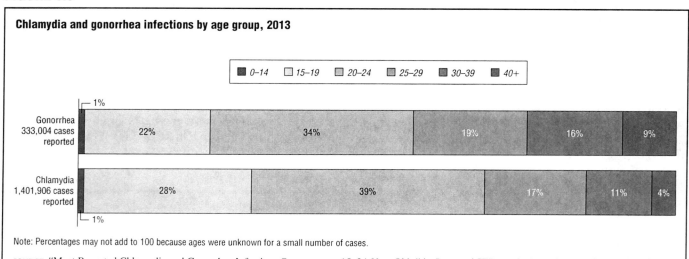

Chlamydia and gonorrhea infections by age group, 2013

Legend: 0–14 | 15–19 | 20–24 | 25–29 | 30–39 | 40+

Gonorrhea 333,004 cases reported: 1%, 22%, 34%, 19%, 16%, 9%

Chlamydia 1,401,906 cases reported: 28%, 39%, 17%, 11%, 4%, 1%

Note: Percentages may not add to 100 because ages were unknown for a small number of cases.

SOURCE: "Most Reported Chlamydia and Gonorrhea Infections Occur among 15–24-Year-Olds," in *Reported STDs in the United States: 2013 National Data for Chlamydia, Gonorrhea, and Syphilis*, Centers for Disease Control and Prevention, National Center for HIV/AIDS, Viral Hepatitis, Sexual Transmitted Diseases, and Tuberculosis Prevention, Division of HIV/AIDS Prevention, December 2014, http://stacks.cdc.gov/26427/cdc_26427_DS1.pdf (accessed July 28, 2015)

MSM. "Adolescents and Young Adults" notes that MSM account for 75% of all cases of primary and secondary syphilis, and that the number of infected people in this category has been increasing. (See Figure 5.4.) It goes on to state that being infected with syphilis increases the risk of someone acquiring or transmitting HIV.

LEADING THE WAY: YOUNG PEOPLE AS AIDS ACTIVISTS AND ORGANIZATIONS THAT HELP YOUNG PATIENTS

Almost since the beginning of the HIV/AIDS epidemic, children and teenagers have been among the activists campaigning for HIV/AIDS reforms and awareness of the disease. Their role has been a profoundly personal one. For example, until his death from AIDS in April 1990, Ryan White—an Indiana teenager—brought worldwide attention to the disease and, in particular, to the stigmas and misconceptions surrounding it. White, who contracted the virus during treatment for his hemophilia, was a white, middle-class, heterosexual boy, which ran counter to the public's perception at the time of AIDS as a disease of gay men.

Being expelled from school because of the supposed health risk to other students galvanized White to educate others on the nature of HIV/AIDS. His legacy includes

FIGURE 5.4

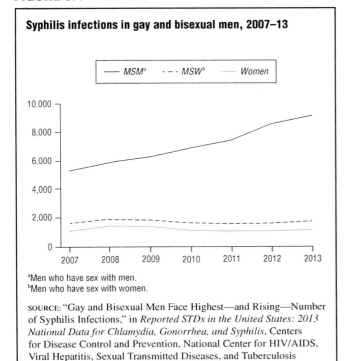

Syphilis infections in gay and bisexual men, 2007–13

aMen who have sex with men.
bMen who have sex with women.

SOURCE: "Gay and Bisexual Men Face Highest—and Rising—Number of Syphilis Infections," in *Reported STDs in the United States: 2013 National Data for Chlamydia, Gonorrhea, and Syphilis,* Centers for Disease Control and Prevention, National Center for HIV/AIDS, Viral Hepatitis, Sexual Transmitted Diseases, and Tuberculosis Prevention, Division of HIV/AIDS Prevention, December 2014, http://stacks.cdc.gov/26427/cdc_26427_DS1.pdf (accessed July 28, 2015)

the Ryan White Comprehensive AIDS Resources Emergency Act, the multibillion-dollar program that funds programs to help provide primary health care and support to those living with HIV/AIDS.

The National Association of People with AIDS, founded in 1983, advocates for people, including children, who live with HIV/AIDS. The nonprofit organization—the oldest national AIDS organization in the United States—is a strong advocate for HIV/AIDS social programs and research funding.

The AIDS Alliance for Children, Youth, and Families was established in 1994 to publicize the concerns of women, children, young people, and families who are affected by HIV/AIDS. The nonprofit organization is also a clearinghouse for relevant information and advocates for public policy changes in the areas of HIV/AIDS social welfare and disease prevention.

Metro TeenAIDS focuses on prevention, education, and treatment needs of teenagers. Through its website (http://www.metroteenaids.org) and in-person contact at schools, nightclubs, youth centers, shelters, and on the street, Metro TeenAIDS connects with teenagers in a language that is relevant to them. The intent is to help teenagers protect themselves from the risks of HIV exposure and contamination and in securing medical care for HIV infection and AIDS.

Metro TeenAIDS has been working in conjunction with other youth and AIDS activist groups since 1994 to host annual conferences around the country that focus on educating young people about HIV/AIDS. In 1995 the conference became known as the Ryan White National Youth Conference on HIV and AIDS (RWNYC). In 2001 the first Positive Youth Institute—a one-day gathering specifically focusing on the needs of HIV-positive young people—was held before and in conjunction with the RWNYC. Each year several hundred young people, health care workers, and AIDS activists attend the conference.

Many other organizations work to provide HIV/AIDS prevention, treatment, and support programs, including:

- Save the Children (2015, http://www.savethechildren.org), which supports children and youth at risk for, and affected by, HIV. Save the Children focuses on orphans and others who are at risk and supports PMTCT efforts.

- Keep a Child Alive (http://keepachildalive.org) supports innovative, community-based initiatives to improve access to HIV treatment and care and support for children and families living with and affected by HIV in Kenya, Rwanda, South Africa, Uganda, and India.

- The Elizabeth Glaser Pediatric AIDS Foundation (http://www.pedaids.org) is dedicated to preventing pediatric HIV infection and eliminating HIV/AIDS in children through research, advocacy, and prevention. It operates care and treatment programs in 14 countries around the world.

CHAPTER 6
HIV/AIDS COSTS AND TREATMENT

FINANCING HEALTH CARE DELIVERY

Care for HIV/AIDS patients is expensive. Drug treatments, most prominently antiretroviral therapy (ART), have high per-unit costs. Nonetheless, their introduction in 1996 reduced total health care spending on AIDS by decreasing the rate of hospitalization and outpatient care. According to Samuel A. Bozzette et al., in "Expenditures for the Care of HIV-Infected Patients in the Era of Highly Active Antiretroviral Therapy" (*New England Journal of Medicine*, vol. 344, no. 11, March 15, 2001), the average HIV patient incurred costs of approximately $1,410 per month in 1998 (about $2,047 in 2015 dollars). For a full year, a patient's drug treatment for HIV could cost as much as $18,300 ($26,561 in 2015 dollars). People with AIDS could spend up to $77,000 ($111,761 in 2015 dollars) per year on treatment. By the second decade of the 21st century, the costs of treating AIDS increased more than sixfold. Jessica Camille Aguirre reports in "Cost of Treatment Still a Challenge for HIV Patients in U.S." (NPR.org, July 27, 2012) that in 2012 the average drug treatment cost was between $2,000 and $5,000 per month, and the lifetime cost was estimated at more than $500,000.

Longer survival following infection with HIV leads to even greater costs for care and treatment. The lifetime costs of care for HIV-infected people depend on the disease stage at which people are diagnosed and when ART is started. For example, Paul G. Farnham et al. note in "Updates of Lifetime Costs of Care and Quality-of-Life Estimates for HIV-Infected Persons in the United States: Late versus Early Diagnosis and Entry into Care" (*Journal of Acquired Immune Deficiency Syndromes*, vol. 64, no. 2, October 1, 2013) that average lifetime costs vary from $253,000 to $402,000 (in 2011 dollars). HIV-infected patients who enter care early incur greater lifetime costs, improved quality of life, and reduced transmissions compared with patients who enter care late. Farnham et al.

conclude that early ART initiation and early entry into care increases the costs of care, in large part because it extends patients' years of life and treatment.

Some HIV/AIDS patients rely on health insurance to help pay these costs. Many patients, however, are not insured. Also, until enactment of the Patient Protection and Affordable Care Act of 2010 (ACA), which prohibits preexisting condition exclusions and lifetime limits, many policies excluded or denied coverage to people with preexisting conditions, and, as a result, many HIV-positive people were denied private health insurance.

The ACA also provides financial assistance for people with low and middle incomes in the form of tax credits that offset the cost of their monthly premiums and reduce their out-of-pocket costs. These tax credits depend on a family's household size and income.

According to AIDS.gov, in "The Affordable Care Act and HIV/AIDS" (March 6, 2015, https://www.aids.gov/federal-resources/policies/health-care-reform), many people living with HIV/AIDS in the United States have the costs of their treatment paid for by Medicaid and Medicare. Medicaid is an entitlement program that is run by the federal and state governments to provide health care insurance to patients under the age of 65 years who cannot afford to pay for private health insurance. It is the largest payer for HIV care, and under the ACA states were able to expand Medicaid to include those with incomes at or below 138% of the federal poverty line (FPL; $16,105 for an individual and $32,913 for a family of four in 2015), including single adults without children who were previously not generally eligible for Medicaid. In states that expanded Medicaid enrollment (29 of the 50 states), people with HIV no longer have to wait until they are diagnosed with AIDS to become eligible for Medicaid. As a result, they can gain access to life-extending care and treatment before the disease has significantly harmed their immune system.

Medicare is the federal health insurance program for adults aged 65 years and older and younger adults with permanent disabilities. The ACA improved prescription drug benefits for Medicare enrollees. Under the ACA, AIDS drug assistance program (ADAP) benefits count toward Medicare Part D out-of-pocket spending limit, which means that ADAP clients will more quickly qualify for prescription drug benefits. The Ryan White HIV/AIDS Program is another key source of funding for health and social services for this population.

The toll of HIV/AIDS on Medicaid and Medicare is huge. The Kaiser Family Foundation estimates in the fact sheet "U.S. Federal Funding for HIV/AIDS: The President's FY 2016 Budget Request" (April 13, 2015, http://kff.org/global-health-policy/fact-sheet/u-s-federal-funding-for-hivaids-the-presidents-fy-2016-budget-request) that the federal contribution to Medicaid for HIV/AIDS care rose to $7 billion in fiscal year (FY) 2016 from $4.7 billion in FY 2010. The Kaiser Family Foundation projects that Medicare spending for HIV/AIDS will grow to $7.5 billion in FY 2016 from $5.1 billion in FY 2010.

AIDS Drug Assistance Programs

During the late 1980s state-administered programs were established to help AIDS patients pay for zidovudine, the most effective drug at the time. ADAPs provide free drugs to low-income AIDS patients who are not poor enough to qualify for Medicaid coverage but who do not have private health insurance coverage or who have used up their prescription drug coverage. The federal government provides two-thirds of the funding for the state programs, and the balance comes mostly from the states. These programs financed most of the cost of medication for low-income patients until 2006, when the Medicare prescription drug benefit Part D took effect. People eligible for both Medicaid and Medicare have the cost of their drugs covered by Part D.

During the late 1990s, however, the development of more effective antiretroviral drugs prompted additional patients to take advantage of the ADAPs. This growing demand put a financial strain on the ADAPs, and many states began rationing HIV/AIDS drugs or turning patients away to remain solvent. Some states made it harder for people to qualify for the programs, and some charged patients a small copayment (a percentage of the total cost that the patient is responsible for paying) to offset the cost of the drugs. Other state programs attempted to obtain larger price discounts or rebates on HIV/AIDS drugs in an effort to reduce their costs so they could continue to provide the drugs to an expanding population of patients.

The National Alliance of State and Territorial AIDS Directors reports in *National ADAP Monitoring Project 2015 Annual Report* (May 2015, http://www.nastad.org/ sites/default/files/NASTAD-ADAP-Monitoring-Project-Annual-Report-May-2015.pdf) that as of June 2014 the ADAPs provided medications to more than 146,000 clients, a 4% decrease from June 2013. Most clients (71%) were male, 56% were below 138% of the FPL and more than half were African American (35%) or Hispanic (28%). ADAP spending on prescription drugs was more than $159 million in 2014.

According to the National Alliance of State and Territorial AIDS Directors, aspects of health care reform, such as whether states expanded Medicaid and the types of state health insurance marketplaces (online sites where eligible individuals could shop for health insurance coverage) they established, affected ADAP. For example, ADAP enrollment decreased slightly in states that expanded Medicaid enrollment because enrollees no longer needed ADAP. However, because some private insurance plans offered at the marketplaces do not cover specific antiretroviral drugs, ADAP remains the primary payer for many clients with private insurance.

Changes to the Health Care System

Since the 1960s U.S. government spending on health services has consistently increased. The Centers for Medicare and Medicaid Services' Office of the Actuary projects in *National Health Expenditure Projections 2014–2024* (July 28, 2015, https://www.cms.gov/Research-Statistics-Data-and-Systems/Statistics-Trends-and-Reports/NationalHealthExpendData/Downloads/proj2014.pdf) that health care spending will grow at an average annual rate of 5.8% between 2014 and 2024. By 2024 government spending for health care is projected to reach nearly 47% of total national health expenditures, with the federal government accounting for about two-thirds.

Along with Medicaid and Medicare, managed-care plans (also known as managed-care organizations [MCOs]), which control the use of and reimbursement for services in an effort to contain costs, rely heavily on primary care practitioners (general and family physicians). These plans have become the health care providers for increasing numbers of HIV/AIDS patients. Since 2000 many HIV-infected people have enrolled in managed-care plans. This is partly because more companies are offering employees only managed-care plans and partly because government insurance programs are directing Medicaid recipients to such programs.

A MANAGED-CARE PLAN FOR HIV/AIDS PATIENTS: THE TENNESSEE "CENTERS OF EXCELLENCE" PROGRAM. On January 1, 1994, Tennessee withdrew from the federal Medicaid program and began implementing a state health care reform plan called Tennessee Medicaid (TennCare). One of the oldest Medicaid managed-care programs in the country, in 1998 TennCare introduced a managed-care plan for its members with HIV or AIDS. The model plan features "Centers of Excellence" providers—practitioners with expertise in the care of HIV/AIDS patients. The providers must agree to adopt and adhere to a clinical protocol (practice and care guidelines) developed by a committee composed of providers, consumers, MCOs, and public health officials. The committee meets periodically to evaluate and recommend new drug therapies as they become available and to inform participating providers about new treatments.

Providers may be individual practitioners with access to needed services or full-service clinics composed of a group of practitioners. There are no financial incentives to participate in the program. However, providers who meet the Centers of Excellence criteria do not have to obtain prior authorization when they prescribe drugs or treatments that fall under the clinical protocols.

The Centers of Excellence program frees MCOs from the clinical and administrative responsibility of keeping close tabs on HIV/AIDS care. It also allows MCOs to remain confident that providers are capable and have access to a wide range of services needed by members. MCO members know that participating providers meet high standards of HIV/AIDS clinical care. Other managed-care plans are developing comparable programs to meet the unique health and social service needs of people living with HIV/AIDS.

With an annual budget of about $10 billion, TennCare (2015, http://www.tennessee.gov/tenncare) provides health care to 1.3 million people per year. Many industry observers cite TennCare as an early exemplar and model for the kind of Medicaid expansion many states implemented in response to the ACA. Darin Gordon, Wendy Long, and Casey Dungan report in *Health Care Finance and Administration FY 2016 Budget Presentation* (March 2015, https://www.tn.gov/assets/entities/tenncare/attachments/HCFAbudgetFY16.pdf) that in 2014 TennCare exceeded its goal of achieving member satisfaction above 90% for the sixth consecutive year.

Nonetheless, TennCare has faced some serious operational challenges. In "TennCare Timeline: Major Events and Milestones from 1992 to 2014" (October 2014, http://csl.iismemphis.org/mlche/pdfs/tenncare/tenncare_bulleted_timeline.pdf), Cyril F. Chang and Stephanie C. Steinberg of the University of Memphis report that in June 2014 the director of the federal Medicaid program put Tennessee on notice for "failing to provide services as required by the Affordable Care Act, a problem TennCare has blamed on a faulty $35 million computer system." Tennessee officials attributed delays in signing up enrollees to problems with the federally run health care insurance exchange, HealthCare.gov. In September 2014 a U.S. district court ordered Tennessee's Medicaid program to assume responsibility for the delayed applications, which kept people waiting months to find out whether they would receive coverage.

In July 2015 TennCare contracted with a new vendor to provide call-center services for state residents checking on their Medicaid eligibility. In "TennCare Scraps Another Multimillion-Dollar Contract" (Tennessean.com, July 6, 2015), Tom Wilemon reports that the state also canceled a $35.7 million contact for a computer system to determine Medicaid eligibility according to new income guidelines. Wilemon observes, "Tennessee's government has a history of dealing with failed computer systems across state agencies."

CHALLENGES FOR THE DELIVERY SYSTEM

HIV/AIDS poses a major challenge to health care institutions, health care professionals, and others who provide direct health care services. Since its emergence and identification, HIV infection has undergone a dramatic transformation; it has gone from being an infectious disease that was an almost certain death sentence to a chronic disease that for many can be managed for decades. Furthermore, unlike most chronic diseases that afflict older Americans, HIV/AIDS affects people of all ages, and young adults are disproportionately affected. The health care system also plans to deliver services to the tens of thousands of people in the United States who are HIV positive and will require specialized health care services during the coming years, even though only a small proportion will need intensive medical care at any one time.

The number of indigent people in need of HIV/AIDS care, particularly those who bring the added complications of drug addiction, homelessness, and other socioeconomic problems, has strained public hospitals in particular. Patients in public hospitals are often different from those in private hospitals. They generally seek care later in the course of the disease's progression and are, therefore, sicker and require more intensive services.

Health Care Reform Legislation Improves Access to Care

In 2010 President Barack Obama (1961–) signed the ACA into law. It is considered the most comprehensive and important health care reform legislation since the 1965 passage of Medicaid and Medicare. Certain provisions of the legislation were intended to improve access to care for people with HIV/AIDS. These include:

- Eliminating the Medicaid disability requirement (people with HIV no longer must wait for an AIDS diagnosis to be eligible for Medicaid coverage) and extending access to Medicaid to people with an income 133% of the FPL

- Closing the Medicare Part D donut hole (a gap in Medicare that stops paying for prescriptions, so the beneficiary must pay the entire cost) by 2020, and allowing the ADAP to be used to meet the Medicare Part D True Out of Pocket Spending Limit

- Requiring pharmaceutical companies to offer a 50% discount on brand-name drugs in the donut hole

- Increasing access to private health insurance by prohibiting discrimination or higher premiums based on health status or gender and banning preexisting condition exclusions and lifetime limits on coverage

- Expanding the scope of coverage by mandating benefits that include prescription drugs, mental health and substance abuse treatment, preventive care, and chronic disease management

- Increasing affordability of insurance coverage by providing subsidies for people with incomes up to 400% of the FPL

Thousands of people with HIV, some of whom did not have insurance previously, obtained health care coverage under the ACA. In "Nearly 50,000 HIV Patients Will Gain Coverage under Obamacare, Medicaid" (Healthline.com, February 10, 2014), David Heitz reports that about 23,000 people with HIV gained private health insurance coverage as a direct result of the ACA and an additional 26,000 gained coverage through the states' Medicaid expansions. Prior to ACA implementation, many of these people had been cared for by the federal Ryan White HIV/AIDS Program.

In "Health Insurance Coverage for People with HIV under the Affordable Care Act: Experiences in Five States" (December 2014, http://kff.org/hivaids/issue-brief/health-insurance-coverage-for-people-with-hiv-under-the-affordable-care-act-experiences-in-five-states), Jennifer Kates et al. of the Kaiser Family Foundation report the results of focus group interviews conducted in five states (California, Florida, Georgia, New York, and Texas) to learn how the ACA affected people with HIV. The researchers find that people living with HIV who enrolled in private coverage sold on the marketplaces had access to more comprehensive health services than they had before the ACA was enacted. Some were able to find much more affordable coverage through the marketplace compared with pre-ACA insurance costs. Interviewees in states that opted not to expand their Medicaid programs continued to receive care through the Ryan White program but worried about how to meet other health needs. Kates et al. note that these interviewees "were frustrated by their state's decision not to expand and continued to be worried about health and economic insecurity that accompanied being uninsured."

Preventing HIV Is Cost Effective

Although HIV treatment increases health care costs, prevention efforts are cost effective. In "The Cost and Impact of Scaling Up Pre-exposure Prophylaxis for HIV Prevention: A Systematic Review of Cost-Effectiveness Modelling Studies" (*PLoS Medicine*, vol. 10, no. 3, March 2013), Gabriela B. Gomez et al. evaluate the anticipated health gains and costs of HIV pre-exposure prevention efforts—giving people at high risk for HIV exposure ART to reduce their risk of becoming infected. The researchers find that pre-exposure prophylaxis has "the potential to be a cost-effective addition to HIV prevention programmes in some settings."

In "The Lifetime Medical Cost Savings from Preventing HIV in the United States" (*Medical Care*, vol. 53, no. 4, April 2015), Bruce Schackman et al. estimated lifetime medical costs in people with and without HIV to determine the cost saved by preventing a single HIV infection. The researchers calculated that the average patient with HIV spends $230,000 more than a person without HIV in lifetime medical costs. Patients who receive the best possible treatment spend more than $338,000 more than someone without HIV. More than half (60%) of costs are for antiretroviral medications, one-quarter (25%) for nonmedication costs, and 15% for chronic disease medications and treating/preventing opportunistic infections. Preventing just one case of HIV infection would save between $229,800 and $338,400.

Hospital Care

Most HIV/AIDS patients are cared for in inner-city public hospitals that are already overburdened with inadequate revenues, staff shortages, lack of referral facilities, and emergency departments that are used by many poor neighborhood residents as sources of primary medical care. Many health care professionals praise a model of hospital care that was pioneered in San Francisco, California. The city was hit hard during the early days of the HIV/AIDS epidemic and developed a range of innovative, effective programs in response to acute need. This model of care relies on extensive outpatient services and volunteer social support services that are provided by the well-established and well-organized gay and lesbian community.

In "HIV Care: The San Francisco Model" (July 18, 2012, http://www.coe.ucsf.edu/coe/patient/ucsf_hiv_care.html), Susan Davis of the University of California, San Francisco, School of Medicine reports that "Within a few short years, the San Francisco model became the global standard for HIV patient care, inspiring and educating communities around the world to emulate the city's practices and policies. Thirty years later, that model is still alive and well, but it has evolved in ways that reflect the changing nature of both the epidemic and the field of HIV research." Davis explains that the current challenge is to encourage people to be tested and to keep them engaged in care. Modern HIV care also must be culturally sensitive and customized for specific populations such as non-English-speaking patients, incarcerated patients, veterans, women, and patients over age 50.

Changes in Health Care Delivery

Although fewer people are acquiring HIV/AIDS, the evolution of HIV care is altering the ways in which health care is delivered. In the late stages of AIDS, most patients require intermittent hospitalization and home health care. Those who are not as severely affected and have symptoms or conditions that once required intravenous therapy (which had to be administered in a hospital or by home health professionals) are now able to self-medicate at home. Most drugs are now available for oral administration in pill or liquid form. These home care and community-based measures lessen the burden on the health care delivery system and make it easier for HIV/AIDS patients to care for themselves.

People with AIDS who receive informal home health care (such as care from friends and family) often use fewer hospital services, perhaps reflecting a greater desire to remain at home. People with AIDS who have strong social support systems and who prefer to remain at home may also be less likely to demand an aggressive approach to treating their illness. Those who receive formal home health care (visits from physicians, nurses, therapists, social workers, case managers, and other paid caregivers) often use more hospital services. This may reflect a greater use of all types of health services by people with AIDS with weaker social support systems and/or an aggressive approach to treatment by medical professionals.

An AIDS Care Alternative

In an effort to offer uninsured AIDS patients in Atlanta, Georgia, treatment equal to that available to patients with private insurance, in 1986 Grady Memorial Hospital (2015, http://www.gradyhealth.org/specialty/ponce-de-leon-center.html) opened the Ponce De Leon Center, one of the largest centers that is dedicated to the treatment of advanced HIV/AIDS. The center provides internal medicine and infectious disease care, mental health counseling, social and support services, HIV research and education, and case management. It also works closely with many local AIDS service organizations, some housed on-site, to meet the complex needs of people living with HIV/AIDS. The Ponce De Leon Center is the largest publicly funded program of its kind in the eastern United States and is consistently named as one of the top-three HIV/AIDS outpatient clinics in the country.

Hospice Care

The AIDS epidemic has had a significant impact on hospices. Hospice care, both in the home and in specialized centers, offers care that is aimed at comfort rather than cure. This includes expert pain relief, along with emotional, psychological, and spiritual support for patients, their families, and friends. Most hospice patients are older adults who suffer from terminal diseases such as cancer and face imminent death.

At the beginning of the AIDS epidemic, patients did not fit well into the hospices of the era. AIDS patients were typically younger than traditional hospice patients, and the progression of their disease was less predictable than many cancers. In the 21st century, however, home-based hospice programs were designed to meet the needs of AIDS patients, their partners, and families and gained acceptance in the medical community as well as among HIV-infected people and the voluntary social service agencies that are organized to support them.

HEALTH CARE PROVIDERS
Physicians

Physicians from many medical specialties—primary care physicians such as family practitioners, internists, and specialists in infectious diseases, pulmonary medicine, and cancer medicine— care for people with HIV/AIDS. Many are also AIDS activists and may be involved in developing policies, planning for care needs, and dealing with the media.

One challenge in preparing physicians to treat AIDS patients is that AIDS care requires skills and training in the multitude of conditions that are known to be part of HIV/AIDS. However, the amount of experience (rather than the kind of training) may be a better predictor of the quality of care the physician is able to deliver.

In parts of the world such as sub-Saharan Africa a shortage of health care workers has impeded the provision of HIV treatment. Connor A. Emdin, Nicholas J. Chong, and Peggy E. Millson analyze in "Non-physician Clinician Provided HIV Treatment Results in Equivalent Outcomes as Physician-Provided Care: A Meta-analysis" (*Journal of International AIDS Society*, vol. 16, July 3, 2013) the results of nine studies that examined how patients with HIV infection fare when treated by nonphysicians (nurses and others). The researchers find that nonphysician-provided care produced comparable outcomes to physician-provided treatment and also decreased the number of patients who did not return for follow-up care.

Nurses

Nurses often have a different view from that of physicians regarding their professional obligations to patients with HIV/AIDS. As hospital employees, nurses seldom have the option of choosing whether to treat a particular patient (nor do patients have much choice of nurses). Nurses, however, report that caring for HIV/AIDS patients can take an enormous emotional toll because they often provide the primary source of continuous physical and emotional care for these patients, who generally require more intensive care and services than other patients.

Nurses face a wide range of emotional issues when caring for these patients, from feelings of failure when treatment is unsuccessful to grief when witnessing the deaths of patients. In "How Caring for Persons with HIV/AIDS Affects Rural Nurses" (*Issues in Mental Health Nursing*, vol. 30, no. 5, May 2009), Iris L. Mullins of New Mexico State University explains that caring for patients with HIV/AIDS affects nurses in three distinct areas of their personal and professional lives: their personal sense of self as a nurse in practice; their interactions with their family members, friends, and colleagues; and their interactions with patients with HIV/AIDS. Nurses caring for HIV/AIDS patients in rural areas expressed additional concerns including the need for ongoing continued education about the care of people with HIV/AIDS.

Irish Patrick Williams and Lorona Searcy examine in "Study: Is Bedside Nursing Still Affected by HIV Stigma?" (*HIV Clinician*, vol. 24, no. 4, Fall 2012) nurses' feelings about HIV/AIDS and whether stigma associated with the disease influences the care nurses deliver. The researchers find that some nurses remain reluctant to care for patients with HIV/AIDS because of fear of contracting the disease and that stigmatization continues to challenge efforts to optimize treatment of this vulnerable patient population. Williams and Searcy assert that improved HIV/AIDS education for nursing students and professional development for nurses is needed.

Centers for Disease Control and Prevention Guidelines

In response to an incident in which five patients acquired HIV from David J. Acer (1949–1990), a Florida dentist, the Centers for Disease Control and Prevention (CDC) addressed occupational exposure to blood-borne pathogens in "Recommendations for Preventing Transmission of Human Immunodeficiency Virus and Hepatitis B Virus to Patients during Exposure-Prone Invasive Procedures" (*Morbidity and Mortality Weekly Report*, vol. 40, no. RR-8, July 12, 1991). The updated guidelines were intended to prevent the accidental spread of the infection from health care providers to patients and from patients to health care workers. The recommendations stressed the careful and consistent use, with all patients, of standard infection control procedures for blood-borne agents (the so-called universal precautions) that were published by the CDC in 1987.

The CDC guidelines recommended that HIV-infected health care workers stop performing exposure-prone invasive procedures and that professional medical and dental groups draw up lists of exposure-prone procedures for their disciplines. The CDC recommended that HIV-infected health care workers consult with a panel of experts to determine which, if any, limits should be placed on their medical practices and further advised practitioners to inform patients of their HIV-infection status before performing medical procedures.

The CDC guidelines resulted in some unforeseen consequences. Professional groups, hospital attorneys, state courts, legislatures, and Congress reacted with alarm to a perception of dangers to patients posed by HIV-infected health care professionals totally out of proportion to the largely theoretical risk. Adelisa L. Panlilio et al. of the CDC note in "Updated U.S. Public Health Service Guidelines for the Management of Occupational Exposures to HIV and Recommendations for Postexposure Prophylaxis" (*Morbidity and Mortality Weekly Report*, vol. 54, no. RR-9, September 30, 2005) that the average risk of HIV infection after skin contact with HIV-infected blood is estimated to be about 0.3%, and the risk for transmission is even lower from contact with bodily fluids or tissues other than blood. In "Surveillance of Occupationally Acquired HIV/AIDS in Healthcare Personnel, as of December 2010" (May 2011, http://www.cdc.gov/HAI/organisms/hiv/Surveillance-Occupationally-Acquired-HIV-AIDS.html), the CDC indicates that 57 documented cases had been reported between 1981 and 2010 (although no documented cases were reported between 2000 and 2010), and it was possible that 143 additional cases of HIV infection were linked to occupational exposures.

HEALTH CARE WORKERS AND INFECTION
Updated Guidelines for Occupational Exposure to HIV

In "Updated U.S. Public Health Service Guidelines for the Management of Occupational Exposures to HIV and Recommendations for Postexposure Prophylaxis" (September 25, 2013, http://stacks.cdc.gov/view/cdc/20711), the U.S. Public Health Service Working Group updated the guidelines for treatment to prevent health care workers with occupational exposure to HIV from becoming infected with the virus. Known as postexposure prophylaxis (PEP), the recommendation was that affected workers be given a four-week regimen of two antiretroviral drugs such as zidovudine and lamivudine, with the addition of a third drug for HIV exposures that pose an increased risk of transmission. The new guidelines advise, "To ensure timely postexposure management and administration of HIV PEP, clinicians should consider occupational exposures as urgent medical concerns, and institutions should take steps to ensure that staff are aware of both the importance of, and the institutional mechanisms available for, reporting and seeking care for such exposures." Although the best strategy to protect health care workers is to avoid exposure to HIV and other blood-borne pathogens, PEP has, as of 2015, proven generally effective in preventing HIV infection in workers who have been exposed.

Risks to Patients

Health care officials are not the only ones worried about HIV transmission in the health care setting. Patients also fear that infected health care workers can transmit the virus to them. In the landmark study "HIV Transmission from Health Care Worker to Patient: What Is the Risk?" (*Annals of Internal Medicine*, vol. 116, no. 10, May 15, 1992), Mary E. Chamberland and David M. Bell of the CDC develop a model of the risk of HIV transmission to patients and estimate that the risk of a patient becoming infected by an HIV-positive surgeon during a single operation is anywhere from 1 out of 42,000 to 1 out of 420,000. This risk is considerably less than the risks that are associated with many other medical procedures.

The CDC indicates in "HIV and Its Transmission" (July 1999, http://www.hivlawandpolicy.org/sites/www .hivlawandpolicy.org/files/CDC%2C%20HIV%20and%20 its%20transmission.pdf) that of more than 22,000 patients of 63 HIV-infected health care workers, no documented evidence had been found that links HIV infection to medical or dental care, except for the five patients of Acer in 1990. Medical researchers have tried without success to determine how Acer infected his patients and whether the exposure was accidental or deliberate. One theory is that he did not properly sterilize his dental tools; another is that he accidentally cut his finger or jabbed himself with a hypodermic needle, did not notice it, and bled into the patients' mouths. Before his death in 1990, Acer denied intentionally exposing his patients.

Although HIV transmission through transplanted organs occurs very rarely, in November 2007 the national media reported the first known cases in 20 years of HIV transmission from a high-risk donor. The most likely explanation for this transmission is that the donor, who was deceased when the organs were harvested, had tested HIV negative because the infection was recent and antibodies had not yet formed to the virus.

As described in Chapter 2, another instance of HIV transmission from a kidney transplant (the first documented case of this kind) was reported in March 2011 Also described in Chapter 2 is the Department of Health and Human Services (HHS) 2015 ruling that enables HIV-infected donors to give organs to HIV-infected recipients.

WHAT DOES IT COST TO TREAT HIV/AIDS PATIENTS?

The Kaiser Family Foundation notes in "U.S. Federal Funding for HIV/AIDS: The President's FY 2016 Budget Request" that President Obama's federal budget request for FY 2016 included an estimated $31.7 billion—$25.3 billion for domestic programs and $6.3 billion for global initiatives and activities. Federal funding has increased significantly throughout the course of the epidemic, and the FY 2016 federal budget for domestic programs and research represented a 3.1% increase over FY 2015. Much of the federal funding for HIV/AIDS care, as opposed to other assistance such as housing, was for Medicaid and

Medicare, which were budgeted for 11.3% and 13.8% increases, respectively, in funding.

HIV/AIDS-related costs are expected to increase in response to the rising costs of hospitalization, home care, insurance premiums and co-payments, physician services, and pharmaceutical drugs. Growing concern about rising drug prices led to a self-imposed price freeze by some pharmaceutical companies in 2002. However, price increases were eventually instituted. In "Using Drugs to Discriminate—Adverse Selection in the Insurance Marketplace" (*New England Journal of Medicine*, vol. 372, no. 5, January 29, 2015), Douglas B. Jacobs and Benjamin D. Sommers scrutinized 48 health plans in 12 states and found that one-quarter of the plans used "adverse tiering"—placing all HIV drugs in a specialty drug tier that requires consumers to pay at least 30% of the cost of the drug. The financial impact of this kind of pricing is significant. For example, a patient taking Atripla (a common HIV medication), would pay $3,000 more per year in a plan using adverse tiering compared with a patient in a plan that did not use adverse tiering. Although insurance companies are prohibited from discriminating against people with specific medical conditions under the ACA, industry observers say that some appear to be circumventing the spirit of the law by restricting access to all drugs that treat certain conditions.

Other HIV/AIDS care–related expenses have actually been reduced by relocating services from the hospital to outpatient settings. Examples of cost-saving services include outpatient transfusions and outpatient treatment for opportunistic infections such as *Pneumocystis carinii* pneumonia and cryptococcal meningitis. Increased volunteer-based social service programs that enable patients to be cared for at home can also prevent expensive hospital stays.

The Ryan White Comprehensive AIDS Resources Emergency Act

As of 2015 the Ryan White Comprehensive AIDS Resources Emergency (CARE) Act was the only federal program that exclusively funded medical and supportive services for people with HIV/AIDS. The act was named after Ryan White (1971–1990), who died of AIDS. White was an Indiana teenager with hemophilia who was infected through a blood transfusion. Shunned by his community because many people feared becoming infected through any kind of contact with him, White fought to attend school and attain rights for those infected with HIV/AIDS. White's efforts helped change the way the world treated those with the disease.

The Ryan White HIV/AIDS Program meets the needs of people living with HIV/AIDS who are not covered by other resources or payers and serves as payer of last resort. According to the HHS, in *FY 2016 Congressional*

Justification for the Health Resources and Services Administration (April 2013, http://www.hrsa.gov/about/budget/budgetjustification2014.pdf), every year the program serves over 500,000 low-income people with HIV/AIDS. More than one-quarter (28%) are uninsured, and 59% are underinsured. Funding priority is given to urban areas with the highest number of people living with AIDS, while helping eligible metropolitan areas (EMAs) and midsized cities with emerging needs, which are called transitional grant areas.

The funds from the Ryan White HIV/AIDS Treatment Extension Act are appropriated using five formulas. Part A funds eligible EMAs that are disproportionately affected by HIV/AIDS and transitional grant areas. Part B funds states to improve the quality, availability, and organization of HIV/AIDS health care and support services. Part C funds early intervention services and ambulatory care. Part D funds do not have to be used for primary care; instead, they may be used to help improve access to clinical trials and research. Part F funds encompass Special Projects of National Significance, which support the demonstration and evaluation of innovative models of HIV/AIDS care delivery for hard-to-reach populations as well as for AIDS Education and Training Centers, dental programs, and the Minority AIDS Initiative.

To qualify for Part A funds, EMAs must have more than 2,000 cumulative AIDS cases reported during the preceding five years and a population of at least 500,000. (The population provision does not apply to any EMA that was named and funded before FY 1997.) Table 6.1 is an overview of funding by the Ryan White HIV/AIDS Treatment Extension Act for FYs 2014, 2015, and 2016.

THE ACA AND THE RYAN WHITE HIV/AIDS PROGRAM. The ACA has enrolled previously uninsured people living with HIV/AIDS in private health insurance and in many states, covered others under expanded Medicaid, slightly reducing the number of people in need of services funded by the "payer of last resort." The Ryan White programs continue to fill gaps in coverage for people with HIV/AIDS. For example, ADAP, which provides HIV-related prescription medications, helps people with limited or no drug coverage. Also, depending on the state, ADAP may help privately insured or Medicaid enrollees pay for antiretroviral drugs that are not included in their health insurance plan's formulary (list of prescription drugs covered by a health insurance plan).

The scope of coverage for Ryan White HIV/AIDS services under expanded Medicaid programs is determined by the states. Coverage for the Ryan White service categories is included in the benefits package in many states' Medicaid programs and in the health plans offered through the exchanges. Nonetheless, Medicaid and subsidies for insurance obtained through the exchanges are unlikely to be sufficient for people living with HIV/AIDS because of limitations in the scope of coverage. Services that may not be covered by Medicaid or plans offered by the exchanges include dental care, counseling, and psychosocial support services.

Until 2014 Ryan White clinics were funded through grants. Under the ACA, they contract directly with Medicaid programs and insurance plans. Because reimbursement rates may not always be sufficient to operate their programs, some Ryan White clinics are seeking to become federally qualified health centers, which enables them to continue to receive grant funding.

TABLE 6.1

Ryan White Act, fiscal years 2014–16

	Fiscal year 2014 final	Fiscal year 2015 enacted	Fiscal year 2016 president's budget	Fiscal year 2016 +/− Fiscal year 2015
BA	$2,288,024,000	$2,318,781,000	$2,322,781,000	+$4,000,000
ADAP (non add)	$900,313,000	$900,313,000	$900,313,000	—
MAI (non add)	$168,587,435	$169,077,000	$169,077,000	—
PHS evaluation fund appropriation	$25,000,000	—	—	—
Total funding	**$2,313,024,000**	**$2,318,781,000**	**$2,322,781,000**	**+$4,000,000**
FTE	171	176	176	—

BA = Budget Authorization.
ADAP = AIDS Drug Assistance Program.
MAI = Minority AIDS Initiative.
PHS = Public Health Service.
SPNS = Special Projects of National Significance.
FTE = Full-Time Equivalents.
Note: The amounts include funding for Special Projects of National Significance (SPNS) funded from Department PHS Act evaluation set-asides in fiscal year 2014. SPNS included in budget authority in fiscal year 2015 and fiscal year 2016.

SOURCE: "Ryan White HIV/AIDS Treatment Extension Act of 2009 Overview," in *FY 2016 Congressional Justification for the Health Resources and Services Administration (HRSA)*, Health Resources and Services Administration, 2015, http://www.hrsa.gov/about/budget/budgetjustification2016.pdf (accessed July 30, 2015)

Some people living with HIV are unable to purchase coverage on the exchanges and are not eligible for Medicaid. Persons who continue to rely on Ryan White clinics include:

- Low-income residents of states that have not expanded Medicaid and who cannot afford health insurance

- Undocumented immigrants, who are not eligible to buy health insurance through exchanges

- Documented immigrants who are subject to a five-year waiting period for Medicaid eligibility

Private Insurance and Medicaid

The financing of HIV/AIDS care has increasingly become the responsibility of Medicaid. The greater reliance on Medicaid funding is due in large part to the increase in the number of HIV/AIDS cases among injection drug users and poor people who are unlikely to be covered by private health insurance. In addition, some patients who once had private insurance through their workplace lost their coverage when the illness made them too sick to work, or they lost their job and job-related health benefits during the so-called Great Recession (which lasted from late 2007 to mid-2009), and turned to Medicaid and other public programs.

Added to this list are those whose employment or economic status would normally ensure them insurance coverage, but who were virtually ineligible for private health insurance coverage once they tested positive for HIV before the ACA (which prohibits denying people coverage because they have preexisting conditions). Even insurance companies that do cover HIV treatment often impose caps, limiting coverage to relatively small dollar amounts.

Death Benefits

Since 1988 an industry has developed that offers dying AIDS patients the opportunity to collect a portion of their life insurance benefits before they die, either to pay for their treatment or to spend as they wish during their remaining time. These viatical (money for necessities given to a person dying or in danger of death) settlements are reached when an insured person sells his or her life insurance policy to an independent insurance company at a reduced or discounted price. This enables the patient to have some cash from the policy while he or she is still alive. After the patient dies, the company that bought the policy is paid the full death benefits. Regulators with the U.S. Securities and Exchange Commission are scrutinizing some practices they believe may victimize AIDS patients.

Some larger companies, such as Prudential, offer policyholders more than 90% of their policy payouts, but only with a physician's certification that they have

less than six months to live. Smaller companies usually pay 50% to 80% of the benefit payable at death, although they will pay benefits to people who still have up to five years to live. The longer the policyholders are expected to live, the less the cash disbursement they receive.

Most insurers will not write new life insurance policies for people known to have AIDS. Those that do offer life insurance policies to people infected with HIV or people with AIDS often have stringent requirements and limited benefits. For example, some policies for AIDS patients stipulate that should death occur due to illness during the first two or three years of coverage, then the benefits paid are simply a return of premiums paid plus an annual interest rate. Others offer an initial two- or three-year incremental period; after that initial period full benefits are paid whether death occurs due to accident or to illness.

TREATMENT RESEARCH

Medical and pharmaceutical research to develop and conduct clinical trials of antiretroviral drugs is expensive. According to the National Institutes of Health (NIH), nearly $3.1 billion was allocated for AIDS research in FY 2016. Table 6.2 shows budget allocations by the type of activity funded between FY 2012 and FY 2016.

Decisions about how much is spent to research a particular disease are not based solely on how many people develop the disease or die from it. Rightly or wrongly, economists base the societal value of an individual on his or her earning potential and productivity (the ability to contribute to society as a worker). The bulk of the people who die from heart disease, stroke, and cancer are older adults. Many have retired from the workforce, and their potential economic productivity is often minimal. This economic measure of present and future financial productivity should not be misinterpreted as a casting-off of older adults; instead, it is simply an economic measure of present and future financial productivity.

In contrast, AIDS patients are usually much younger and, until recently, often died young—in their 20s, 30s, and 40s. Until they develop AIDS, the potential productivity of these people, measured in economic terms, is high. The number of work years lost when they die is considerable. Using this economic equation to determine how disease research should be funded, it may be considered economically wise to invest more money to research AIDS because the losses, measured in potential work years rather than in lives, are so much greater.

The primary goals of HIV/AIDS therapy are to prolong life and improve its quality. Even though during the early days of AIDS research a cure for the disease was envisioned, few researchers at the turn of the 21st century realistically expected any one drug to cure HIV infection

TABLE 6.2

Office of AIDS Research budget allocation by activity, fiscal years 2012–16

Area of emphasis	Fiscal year 2012 actual	Fiscal year 2013 actual	Fiscal year 2014 actual	Fiscal 2015 enacted	Fiscal year 2016 president's budget	Fiscal year 2016 +/− Fiscal year 2015
Vaccines	$556,613	$518,170	$532,671	$537,402	$567,947	$30,545
HIV microbicides	129,919	111,240	107,843	108,349	113,072	4,723
Behavioral and social science	420,084	397,377	411,723	414,873	423,038	8,165
Etiology and pathogenesis	668,244	625,027	666,569	670,527	698,310	27,783
Therapeutics						
Therapeutics as prevention	*56,561*	*69,375*	*75,638*	*73,696*	*74,472*	*776*
Drug discovery, development, and treatment	*650,059*	*632,123*	*660,194*	*671,857*	*685,653*	*13,796*
Total, therapeutics	**706,620**	**701,498**	**735,832**	**745,553**	**760,125**	**14,572**
Natural history and epidemiology	257,973	243,454	228,830	230,437	236,868	6,431
Training, infrastructure, and capacity building	280,775	261,921	259,866	257,591	264,978	7,387
Information dissemination	54,567	39,178	34,245	35,329	35,723	394
Total	**$3,074,795**	**$2,897,865**	**$2,977,579**	**$3,000,061**	**$3,100,061**	**$100,000**

SOURCE: "National Institutes of Health Office of AIDS Research Budget Authority by Activity," in *Office of AIDS Research Trans-NIH AIDS Research Budget*, U.S. Department of Health and Human Services, National Institutes of Health, 2015, http://www.oar.nih.gov/budget/pdf/2016_OARTransNIHAIDSResearchBudget.pdf (accessed July 30, 2015)

in all people. The bottom-line objective became making the virus less deadly by foiling its efforts to reproduce within the body.

A major obstacle to the discovery of such treatments is the cost of drug research and development (R&D). Pharmaceutical manufacturers spend millions of dollars researching and developing new medicines. According to the Pharmaceutical Research and Manufacturers of America (PhRMA), since 1992 U.S. pharmaceutical companies have consistently spent more money each year on R&D activities than the NIH has spent on its annual budget. For example, PhRMA reports in *2015 Profile Biopharmaceutical Industry* (2015, http://www.phrma.org/sites/default/files/pdf/2015_phrma_profile.pdf) that in 2014 the estimated total pharmaceutical R&D budget was $51.2 billion. By contrast, the HHS states in *Fiscal Year 2014 Budget in Brief: Strengthening Health and Opportunity for All Americans* (2013, https://wayback.archive-it.org/3920/20150326110529/http://www.hhs.gov/budget/fy2014/fy-2014-budget-in-brief.pdf) that the NIH budget for research was $31.3 billion in 2014. Furthermore, private-sector spending has been outpacing government spending since 1995.

PhRMA explains that pharmaceutical manufacturers must cover the cost not only of R&D for the approximately two out of 10 drugs that succeed but also for many of the drugs (eight out of 10) that fail to make it to the marketplace. Because of this cost, once a new drug receives U.S. Food and Drug Administration (FDA) approval, its manufacturer ordinarily holds a patent or gains exclusivity rights, which guarantee that it will be the sole marketer for a specified time (usually from three to 20 years) to recoup its investment. During this time the drug is priced much higher than if other manufacturers

were allowed to compete by producing generic versions of the same drug. In contrast to the original manufacturer, the generic manufacturer does not have to pay for the successes and failures that occurred in the drug development pathway or pursue the complicated, time-consuming process of seeking FDA approval. The producer of generic drugs has the formula and must simply manufacture the drugs properly. Because of the lower cost of the generic drug after the original patent or exclusivity period has expired, competition among pharmaceutical manufacturers generally lowers the price. HIV/AIDS drugs are granted seven years of exclusivity under legislation that is aimed at encouraging research and promoting development of new treatments.

The issue of patent protection for HIV/AIDS drugs is understandably contentious. Pharmaceutical manufacturers and others argue that patent protection is necessary to allow for the financial investments necessary to breed innovation. However, to those directly affected by HIV/AIDS and those governments or health care systems that provide care, the enormous costs can be infuriating, especially with the knowledge that generic drugs carrying a lower price tag are possible. The need for less expensive HIV/AIDS drugs is especially urgent in the developing world.

In light of this need, the Medicines Patent Pool (2015, http://www.medicinespatentpool.org), a United Nations–backed organization, was established in 2010 with the intent to foster generic competition by reducing the price of drugs and stimulating development of new formulations. It negotiates for licenses from key HIV medicines patent holders (pharmaceutical companies, research institutes, governments, and universities) and then makes sublicenses available to generic companies, enabling them to produce low-cost HIV drugs for use in developing countries before the patent terms expire.

FDA-APPROVED DRUGS

The first drug thought to delay symptoms was zidovudine. Although initially promising, zidovudine's effects were found to be temporary at best. Several other drugs worked using the same mechanism of action as zidovudine—exclusion of HIV from the host chromosome. Another class of drugs called protease inhibitors (PIs) prevents HIV already in the host cells from reproducing. PIs block the ability of HIV to mature and infect new cells by suppressing a protein enzyme of the virus, called protease, which is crucial to the progression of HIV. Roy M. Gulick et al. indicate in the landmark study "Treatment with Indinavir, Zidovudine, and Lamivudine in Adults with Human Immunodeficiency Virus Infection and Prior Antiretroviral Therapy" (*New England Journal of Medicine*, vol. 337, no. 11, September 11, 1997) that a combination of indinavir, zidovudine, and lamivudine reduces the viral load and raises CD4 cell counts. In the researchers' study, impacts on the viral load and the CD4 cell count lasted for as long as 52 weeks, and the drugs were generally well tolerated.

Even when the effectiveness of PIs proves to be transient, they improve patients' prospects simply by creating more roadblocks for HIV, which mutates so rapidly that it becomes resistant to most drugs when the drugs are used alone. These drugs, when used in various combinations, have helped transform HIV infection from a certain death sentence to a chronic but manageable disease, much like diabetes.

Types of Antiretroviral Agents

The FDA notes in "Antiretroviral Drugs Used in the Treatment of HIV Infection" (October 8, 2015, http://www.fda.gov/forpatients/illness/hivaids/ucm118915.htm) that it approves seven classes of antiretroviral agents for the treatment of HIV/AIDS.

PROTEASE INHIBITORS. As of October 2015 the FDA had approved the following PIs:

- Amprenavir (no longer marketed)
- Atazanavir sulfate
- Darunavir
- Fosamprenavir calcium
- Indinavir
- Lopinavir and ritonavir
- Nelfinavir mesylate
- Saquinavir (no longer marketed)
- Saquinavir mesylate
- Tipranavir

NUCLEOSIDE REVERSE TRANSCRIPTASE INHIBITORS. Nucleoside reverse transcriptase inhibitors (NRTIs) were among the first compounds shown to be effective against viral infections. Research during the 1970s led to the development of the drug acyclovir, which is still being used to treat herpes infections. The first four anti-HIV drugs to be approved—zidovudine, didanosine, dideoxycytosine, and stavudine—were nucleoside analogs.

As their name implies, NRTIs exert their action based on their three-dimensional structure, which mimics the structure of the nucleoside building blocks of deoxyribonucleic acid (DNA). By becoming incorporated into the DNA as the molecule is replicated, the analogs can preserve the structure of DNA but make it impossible for the HIV to use its reverse transcriptase to hijack the host replication machinery to make new viral copies.

As of October 2015 the following NRTIs had received FDA approval for use with HIV/AIDS:

- Abacavir and lamivudine
- Abacavir sulfate
- Abacavir, zidovudine, and lamivudine
- Didanosine and dideoxyinosine
- Emtricitabine
- Enteric coated didanosine
- Lamivudine
- Lamivudine and zidovudine
- Stavudine
- Tenofovir disoproxil fumarate
- Tenofovir disoproxil fumarate and emtricitabine
- Zalcitabine and dideoxycytidine (no longer marketed)
- Zidovudine and azidothymidine

NONNUCLEOSIDE REVERSE TRANSCRIPTASE INHIBITORS. Another class of antiretroviral drugs that were approved during the late 1990s is nonnucleoside reverse transcriptase inhibitors (NNRTIs). NNRTI compounds slow down the process of the reverse transcriptase enzyme that allows the virus to become part of the infected cell's nucleus. The compounds accomplish this by binding to the viral enzyme, which blocks the ability of the enzyme to function.

As of October 2015 there were six NNRTIs approved for use by the FDA:

- Delavirdine
- Efavirenz
- Etravirine

- Nevirapine (extended release)
- Nevirapine (immediate release)
- Rilpivirine

MULTICLASS COMBINATION PRODUCTS. The FDA approves another class of HIV medications that consist of combinations of specific drugs. As of October 2015 there were three combinations approved for use:

- Efavirenz, emtricitabine, and tenofovir disoproxil fumarate
- Elvitegravir, cobicistat, emtricitabine, tenofovir disoproxil fumarate
- Emtricitabine, rilpivirine, and tenofovir disoproxil fumarate

OTHER APPROVED DRUGS. As of October 2015 the FDA also approved the fusion inhibitor drug enfuvirtide, which interferes with the fusion of HIV with the host cell membrane; the entry inhibitor drug maraviroc, which binds CC chemokine receptor 5 (CCR5), an essential co-receptor for most HIV strains, and blocks HIV from entering T cells; and the HIV integrase strand inhibitor drugs raltegravir, which acts against an enzyme that HIV uses to integrate its viral material into the host's chromosomes, and dolutegravir, which is a once-daily integrase inhibitor that prevents HIV replication and reduces the amount of HIV in the blood.

Aggressive Treatment

With new drugs in the anti-HIV/AIDS arsenal, many people with HIV/AIDS who had given up hope of effective treatment returned to clinics and doctors' offices. Although treatment guidelines previously promoted early intervention with zidovudine, recommended treatment now combines PIs with other antiretroviral drugs. Treatment recommendations change rapidly in response to the development of new drugs and clinical trials indicating the effectiveness of different combinations of antiretroviral drugs. Because HIV mutates to resist any drug it faces, including all PIs, researchers find that varying the combination of drugs prescribed can "fool" the virus before it has time to mutate.

Patients undergoing therapy with new drugs or drug combinations must be highly disciplined. For example, indinavir must be taken on an empty stomach, every eight hours, not less than two hours before or after a meal, and with large amounts of water to prevent the development of kidney stones. Patients must also be careful to never skip doses of indinavir, otherwise the virus will quickly grow immune to the drug. (Indinavir has been found to generate cross-resistance, meaning it makes patients resistant to other PIs.) Saquinavir mesylate must be taken in large doses. Ritonavir must be carefully prescribed and administered because it interacts negatively with some

antifungals and antibiotics used by AIDS patients. Because there are many minor and serious risks that are associated with use of these drugs, patients must be closely monitored.

When effective AIDS drugs were introduced, patients sometimes had to wake up during the middle of the night to take pills, and some treatment regimens consisted of as many as 50 or 60 pills administered several times a day. Even with intense pressure to simplify treatment regimens, pharmaceutical companies remained skeptical about an effective once-a-day pill despite the consensus opinion that it would help more people start, and stick with, treatment. Even as recently as 2005, many combined HIV/AIDS medication regimens were administered two to three times per day. Once-a-day regimens were not available until 2006.

Early Treatment Is Better

The results of a clinical trial, the Strategic Timing of Antiretroviral Treatment (START) confirm that immediate treatment with antiretrovirals (as soon as the diagnosis is made) reduced the risk of developing AIDS or other serious illnesses by half. In "Initiation of Antiretroviral Therapy in Early Asymptomatic HIV Infection" (*New England Journal of Medicine*, July 20, 2015), the INSIGHT START Study Group reported the results of a study involving 4,685 patients in 35 countries that found a large difference between patients who received treatment early and those who received treatment when their CD4+ cell count dropped below 350 cells per cubic millimeter.

As soon as the results of the study were published, the Joint United Nations Programme on HIV/AIDS (UNAIDS) called for all people with HIV to get immediate access to antiretroviral therapy. In "Breakthrough HIV Study Could Change Course of Treatment for Millions" (WashingtonPost.com, May 28, 2015), Ariana Eunjung Cha quotes Anthony S. Fauci, the director of the National Institute of Allergy and Infectious Diseases (one of the NIH institutes), who declared, "We now have clear-cut proof that it is of significantly greater health benefit to an HIV-infected person to start antiretroviral therapy sooner rather than later."

Once-a-Day AIDS Treatment

In 2006 the FDA approved the first once-a-day AIDS treatment, a combination of efavirenz, emtricitabine, and tenofovir disoproxil fumarate. Although this once-a-day drug combination reduces the number of pills a patient must take and as a result improves adherence to treatment, it is probably not the sole drug an AIDS patient needs. Many patients also require additional prescription medications to support their immune system and help them resist infection. In 2010 the FDA approved a second once-a-day AIDS treatment, a combination of emtricitabine, rilpivirine, and tenofovir disoproxil fumarate. A third once-a-day treatment became available in 2012, a combination of elvitegravir, cobicistat, emtricitabine, and tenofovir disoproxil fumarate. In 2014 a fourth once-a-day treatment was approved, a combination of dolutegravir (integrase strand transfer inhibitor), abacavir sulfate and lamivudine (both nucleoside analog reverse transcriptase inhibitors).

THE DISCOVERY OF AN HIV-RESISTANT GENE

In 1996 scientists working independently at the Aaron Diamond AIDS Research Center in New York City and the Free University of Brussels, Belgium, announced that some white (Caucasian) people have genes that may protect them from HIV, regardless of how many times they are exposed to the virus. The researchers hoped that their findings would lead to new HIV/AIDS therapies or to the development of drugs or vaccines to prevent HIV infection.

The researchers discovered that a gene called CCR5 is associated with HIV resistance. The gene codes for a protein called CC chemokine receptor 5 (CCR5) that is located on the surface of host cells including macrophages, monocytes, and T cells. HIV exploits this protein by using it as a receptor to bind to, and subsequently infect, cells such as T cells. The CCR5 mutation blocks the manufacture of CCR5. Thus, HIV loses its surface target and cannot invade the immune system.

Subsequent studies conducted in the United States found that one out of 100 people inherits two copies of this gene (one from each parent) and is completely immune to HIV infection. One out of five people with only one copy of the CCR5 gene can become infected, but will remain healthy two to three years longer than those without the altered gene. This may be because these people have half as many CCR5 receptors as normal, which limits or slows the spread of the virus.

According to Michael Fischereder et al., in "CC Chemokine Receptor 5 and Renal-Transplant Survival" (*Lancet*, vol. 357, no. 9270, June 2, 2001), the gene is most common in white Americans (10% to 15% of the population). It is rarely found in African Americans and almost never in Asian Americans, perhaps reflecting the origins of the mutation.

Certain populations appear to be resistant to HIV because they lack or have a mutated form of the CCR5 receptor. Most populations that carry the mutant CCR5 gene come from Europe, and there are indications that the mutation arose only about 700 years ago. For a mutation to be sustained in a population at a rate of 10%, there must be some benefit bestowed by the mutation. It is likely nothing to do with HIV, because HIV did not appear until the late 20th century.

The exact nature of the selective pressure that caused the appearance of the CCR5 mutation is the subject of considerable debate. The prevailing theory has been that the selective pressure was the bubonic plague; however, new research suggests that smallpox may have been the trigger. Which of these, if either, is true remains to be determined.

Research is also under way to learn more about other genes such as CCR2 that, when expressed dominantly, appears to slow the progression of AIDS. Vijay Kumar et al. confirm in "Genetic Basis of HIV-1 Resistance and Susceptibility: An Approach to Understand Correlation between Human Genes and HIV-1 Infection" (*Indian Journal of Experimental Biology*, vol. 44, no. 9, September 2006) that site-specific mutations in these genes determine the susceptibility or resistance to HIV-1 infection and AIDS. Researchers hope that the study of host genes in relation to HIV-1 infection may speed the development of drug therapies to prevent or cure HIV-1 infection effectively.

Although the impact of genetic variation on HIV susceptibility is clear, in "The Impact of Host Genetic Variation on Infection with HIV-1" (*Nature Immunology*, vol. 16, May 19, 2015), Paul J. McLaren and Mary Carrington explain that the extent to which genetic variation influences the progression of HIV is not yet known, nor have all of the genetic variants associated with susceptibility and gene progression been identified.

ENGINEERING AN HIV-RESISTANT GENE

In 2013 researchers announced that they had found a way to engineer key cells of the immune system so they remain resistant to HIV infection. In "Generation of an HIV Resistant T-cell Line by Targeted 'Stacking' of Restriction Factors" (*Molecular Therapy*, vol. 21, no. 4, April 2013), Richard A. Voit et al. describe the use of a kind of molecular scissors to insert a series of HIV-resistant genes into T cells. By inactivating a receptor gene and inserting additional anti-HIV genes, the virus was completely blocked from entering the cells, effectively preventing it from harming the immune system.

RESEARCH LOOKS FOR PROTECTION AGAINST HIV INFECTION
Natural Barriers to HIV

Olivier Schwartz of the Pasteur Institute identifies in "Langerhans Cells Lap Up HIV-1" (*Nature Medicine*, vol. 13, no. 3, March 2007) a protein that acts as a natural barrier to HIV infection. The protein is called langerin because it is produced by Langerhans cells, which form a network in the skin and mucosa (the membrane lining the vagina) and were previously thought to promote the spread of HIV. Instead, the Langerhans cells contain a protein that eats viruses. Langerin scavenges for viruses in the surrounding environment and thereby helps prevent infection. Langerhans cells do not become infected by HIV-1 because they have langerin on their surfaces. It appears that HIV infection occurs when levels of invading HIV are high, or if langerin activity is especially weak. In either of these instances, Langerhans cells can become overwhelmed by the virus and infected.

In "Elevated Elafin/Trappin-2 in the Female Genital Tract Is Associated with Protection against HIV Acquisition" (*AIDS*, vol. 23, no. 13, August 24, 2009), Shehzad M. Iqbal et al. identify the protein elafin/trappin-2 as a novel innate immune factor that is strongly associated with HIV resistance. This innate immune factor was found in the mucosal secretions from the genital tracts of HIV-resistant women who are sex workers. Discovery of this factor enhances understanding of natural immunity to HIV infection.

Researchers are also looking at so-called elite suppressors, a small fraction (0.5%) of people who are infected with HIV that appear able to control infection without antiretroviral drugs. Robert W. Buckheit, Robert F. Siliciano, and Joel N. Blankson of the Johns Hopkins University School of Medicine find in "Primary CD8+ T Cells from Elite Suppressors Effectively Eliminate Nonproductively HIV-1 Infected Resting and Activated CD4+ T Cells" (*Retrovirology*, vol. 10, July 2013) that elite suppressors have much lower levels of HIV integrated into their immune cells than do HIV-infected people treated with antiretroviral drugs. This finding is believed to reflect the fact that elite suppressors mount a more effective immune response to HIV (meaning that their T cells more effectively combat the virus). Elite suppressors are able to efficiently eliminate CD4+ T cells shortly after viral entry and before they produce infection. Buckheit, Siliciano, and Blankson note that elite suppressors are significantly more effective at eliminating these cells than are chronic progressors. The researchers posit that a vaccine that helps generate killer T cells comparable to those in active elite suppressors might help others to more effectively combat infection.

Morning-After Treatment

Drugs that are used to treat established infections as "morning after" also may prevent the transmission of HIV after risky sexual encounters. Because some forms of HIV are halted by prompt use of the drugs, many believe it is a worthwhile approach. To be effective, PEP must begin as soon as possible (always within 72 hours of exposure). Jonathan E. Kaplan et al. describe the evidence supporting the use of PEP and World Health Organization (WHO) guidelines in "Postexposure Prophylaxis against Human Immunodeficiency Virus (HIV): New Guidelines from the WHO: A Perspective" (*Clinical Infectious Diseases*, vol. 1, no. 60, Suppl., June 1, 2015). Kaplan et al. observe that although "the evidence supporting the use of PEP for the prevention of HIV infection is limited, PEP has come to be accepted as a standard of care in the medical community for the prevention of HIV infection after isolated exposures." The WHO guidelines recommend the use of a two- or three-drug regimen—tenofovir and lamivudine (or emtricitabine) with lopinavir/ritonavir (LPV/r) or atazanavir/ritonavir as the third drug.

The use of PEP in an attempt to prevent the spread of HIV is not without risks and side effects, some of which may be potentially life threatening. PIs may cause high blood sugar and diabetes, lipodytrophy (problems with fat metabolism that can result in dangerously high cholesterol levels), and liver problems. Furthermore, some researchers fear that if people believe morning-after treatment will prevent HIV infection, they may stop taking precautions, such as using condoms, to prevent exposure to HIV.

Finally, postexposure treatment is expensive. The costs of two or three drugs taken for a month, plus laboratory tests and visits to the doctor, may cost more than $1,000. Of course, this is a fraction of the cost for lifetime treatment of HIV infection and certainly money well spent if it prevents a person from acquiring the virus.

Pre-exposure Prevention

In "Antiretroviral Therapy for Prevention of HIV Transmission in HIV-Discordant Couples" (*Cochrane Database of Systemic Review*, vol. 5, May 11, 2011), a meta-analysis of seven studies, Andrew Anglemyer et al. find that antiretroviral drugs may prevent the transmission of HIV from an infected person to an uninfected sexual partner by suppressing viral replication. In couples in which the infected partner was taking antiretroviral drugs, the uninfected partner had more than five times lower the risk of becoming infected than in couples where the infected partner was not receiving antiretroviral treatment.

In "PrEP Implementation: Moving from Trials to Policy and Practice" (*Journal of the International AIDS Society*, vol. 18, Suppl. 3, July 20, 2015), Carlos F. Cáceres et al. observe that the safety and efficacy of pre-exposure prophylaxis (PrEP; the daily use of tenofovir/emtricitabine to prevent HIV infection) has been demonstrated, but that its use is not yet widespread or optimal. The researchers note that a 2014 WHO recommendation to include PrEP as a prevention choice for men who have sex with men has been controversial. Some observers are concerned about low rates of adherence to treatment leading to low effectiveness and drug resistance, or that people will engage in risky behaviors because they believe they are completely protected.

Topical Drugs to Block HIV Infection

In recent years there have been many efforts to develop topical microbicides (preparations to prevent HIV infection). In "Barrier Methods for Human Immunodeficiency Virus Prevention" (*Infectious Disease Clinics*, vol. 28, no. 4, December 2014), Ellen F. Eaton and Craig J. Hoesley state that microbicides, which may be formulated as gels, creams, films, or suppositories, are a promising barrier against vaginal and rectal HIV transmission. Although more than 50 topical microbicides have been tested during the past decade there are no FDA-approved topical drugs and only intravaginal gel containing tenofovir has demonstrated efficacy in preventing sexual transmission of HIV.

THE PROMISE OF GENE THERAPY

In 2011 researchers reported progress using genetic engineering techniques to create HIV-resistant blood cells. This effort was inspired by the apparent cure of Timothy Ray Brown (1966–) after he received a transplant of blood stem cells in 2007 to treat the leukemia (cancer of the blood cells) he had in addition to his AIDS diagnosis. Brown's physician, Gero Huetter, thought that the best chance of curing the leukemia was with a blood stem-cell transplant, so he searched for a donor who was not only a tissue match for Brown but was also among the 1% of people with gene mutations that confer resistance to HIV. In preparation for the transplant, Brown was given chemotherapy and radiation treatment to destroy his immune system so that he would not reject the donor blood stem cells. Remarkably, four years after the procedure Brown was still disease free—there was no evidence of HIV in his body, and he no longer required antiretroviral drug treatment. Although this treatment is physically grueling, involves considerable risk, and is prohibitively expensive, it offers tantalizing clues about new approaches for HIV/AIDS treatment.

In 2013 two HIV-infected men who were taking ART prior to bone marrow transplants to treat cancer appeared to be cured of HIV as well. The mechanism of the apparent cure is different from the cure affected in Brown because neither of the two patients received bone marrow from donors with mutations that confer immunity to HIV infection. As described in Chapter 1, in both men the virus rebounded after they stopped ART at 12 and 32 weeks, respectively.

Researchers remain optimistic about the use of novel technologies such as gene therapies. In "Gene Therapy: A Possible Future Standard for HIV Care" (*Science & Society*, vol. 33, no. 7, July 2015), Mohamed Abou-El-Enein, Gerhard Bauer, and Petra Reinke write, "We believe that sufficiently universal gene therapy coverage would eventually pay for itself by suppressing HIV spread, improving survival and quality of life, and preventing the future need for HIV care, particularly the lifelong use of ART."

IN SEARCH OF A VACCINE

Some vaccines use a weakened and medically safe version of viruses as a delivery vehicle to carry various HIV genes into the human participants. The hope is that antibody production of the HIV-critical proteins encoded by these genes will occur and that this production will offer protection from HIV infection. Other vaccines use a DNA plasmid to ferry HIV genes into the human participants; the aim again is to stimulate antibody production.

Unsurprisingly, there are experimental design challenges and ethical considerations involved in vaccine trials using human volunteers. Vaccines may be made using recombinant DNA technology—DNA that has been altered by joining genetic material from two different sources. Figure 6.1 shows how recombinant DNA is used to develop vaccines. Although some recombinant technology uses live attenuated viruses (viruses that are genetically altered so they are less virulent), this is not feasible with HIV because it would be unwise to create any risk of infection. The challenges are to elicit cell-mediated immune responses against HIV and the need for a balanced immune response consisting of not only cellular immunity but also a broad and strong antibody response that can prevent infection with HIV. Concerning ethical considerations, most volunteers for a vaccine have behaviors that put them at risk for contracting HIV. Some may mistakenly believe that participating in the clinical trial of an experimental vaccine—which may be a vaccine or a placebo (which contains no active drug)—protects them and, with a false sense of security, they may resume high-risk behaviors.

Despite optimistic projections during the early 1990s that a vaccine would be found in a few years, a considerable number of promising experimental HIV vaccines have proven ineffective against strains of HIV taken from

FIGURE 6.1

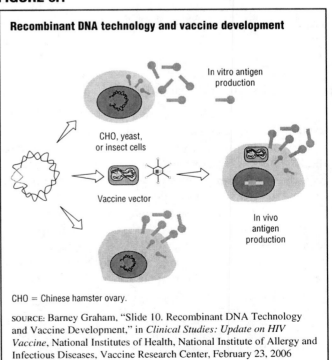

Recombinant DNA technology and vaccine development

In vitro antigen production

CHO, yeast, or insect cells

Vaccine vector

In vivo antigen production

CHO = Chinese hamster ovary.

SOURCE: Barney Graham, "Slide 10. Recombinant DNA Technology and Vaccine Development," in *Clinical Studies: Update on HIV Vaccine*, National Institutes of Health, National Institute of Allergy and Infectious Diseases, Vaccine Research Center, February 23, 2006

infected people. Researchers reported developing antibodies that worked successfully against HIV grown in test tubes, but in every case they failed when used against HIV in human beings. The progress and setbacks in vaccine development as well as the results of recent clinical trials of vaccines are described in Chapter 1. As of October 2015 none of the candidate vaccines had shown sufficient promise in clinical trials to warrant approval, manufacture, and widespread use.

History of Human Vaccine Trials

In "F.D.A. Authorizes First Full Testing for H.I.V. Vaccine" (NYTimes.com, June 4, 1998), Lawrence K. Altman reports that in 1998 the FDA granted permission to VaxGen to conduct the first full-scale test of a vaccine to prevent HIV infection. The VaxGen vaccine (a genetically engineered molecule called AIDSvax) had been found "safe in tests involving 1,200 uninfected volunteers beginning in March 1992 and induced production of antibodies in more than 99 percent of the vaccinated participants." The 1998 test involved 5,000 volunteers in 40 clinics throughout the United States and Canada and 2,500 volunteers in 16 clinics in Thailand.

AIDSvax was made from part of HIV's outer coat, specifically a molecule called gp120, which functions in the attachment of the virus to host cells. The vaccine did not contain the intact virus, only the gp120 protein from two strains of HIV. The two strains of the vaccine that were tested in North America were made with strains common in North America. The vaccine used in Thailand contained strains common to that part of the world. Participants in the North American study were men who have sex with men and uninfected partners of HIV-positive people. In Thailand, volunteers were uninfected injection drug users. Two-thirds of the North American volunteers were given the vaccine, and the rest received a placebo. In Thailand, half the group received the vaccine, and half were given a placebo. The four-year trial ended in 2002.

The trial results were reported in 2003. David R. Baker explains in "Vaccine Has No Impact, AIDSVAX's Failure a Blow to Treatment" (SFGate.com, November 13, 2003) that AIDSvax was a failure, as the comparison of those who received the vaccine versus those who received a placebo demonstrated a slight reduction in new HIV infections in the vaccine population. Surprisingly, Asian Americans and African Americans who received the vaccine displayed a lower rate of infection than their racial counterparts who received the placebo. Considerable debate has arisen concerning these latter observations. Was this a statistical fluke? Or did AIDSvax display demographically specific protection, and if so, why?

One potential problem with AIDSvax, and perhaps a partial explanation of the poor overall results, is that previous tests indicated that it boosted only one part of the immune system—the component of the immune system that is responsible for antibody production. It is generally believed that a truly effective anti-HIV vaccine must boost another part of the immune system: the killer T cells that destroy virus-infected cells. Some experts consider the vaccine a long shot, but others point out that a failed vaccine does not mean that the experiment failed. Negative results can teach researchers what not to do in the future.

In 2011 another vaccine trial reported disappointing results. According to Glenda E. Gray et al., in "Safety and Efficacy of the HVTN 503/Phambili Study of a Clade-B-Based HIV-1 Vaccine in South Africa: A Double-Blind, Randomised, Placebo-Controlled Test-of-Concept Phase 2b Study" (Lancet Infectious Diseases, vol. 11, no. 7, July 2011), researchers conducted a clinical trial in South Africa with a vaccine that was designed to elicit T cell–mediated immune responses capable of providing complete or partial protection from HIV-1 infection or a decrease in viral load after acquisition. When the researchers compiled the results following the completion of the trial, they determined that the vaccine failed to accomplish either of these objectives. Gray et al. opine that there are lessons to be learned from such trials, noting that "this is now the third study in human beings that has failed after initial successful data from studies in non-human primates, highlighting once again that human HIV-1 vaccines should not be based simply on non-human primate models. We should still strive for innovative strategies that prevent HIV, despite the success of antiretroviral drugs in those for whom they are available. It would not be surprising if further prophylactic studies yielded new mechanistic and therapeutic insights outside the remit of the initial endpoints, ultimately enabling the eradication of HIV."

As detailed in Chapter 1, two vaccine trials were halted in 2013 when it was found that HIV infections occurred as often among the vaccine recipients as they did in subjects who received the placebo vaccine and that the vaccine failed to reduce viral load among volunteers who acquired HIV infection.

Vaccine Research Center

In 2000 the Dale and Betty Bumpers Vaccine Research Center (VRC) opened on the NIH campus in Bethesda, Maryland. The facility brings together private companies and federal agencies to research, develop, and produce vaccines. The VRC is not exclusively devoted to HIV research and works to develop vaccines for other diseases.

In 2011 a study that was directed by researchers from NIAID uncovered another genetic mechanism of protection that may be helpful in the design of an HIV vaccine for humans. The researchers administered to monkeys a vaccine made from DNA that encodes immunodeficiency virus proteins, followed by a booster vaccine containing an inactivated cold virus (adenovirus) and immunodeficiency virus proteins to help protect monkeys from simian immunodeficiency virus (SIV; the monkey analog of HIV). Norman L. Letvin et al. find in "Immune and Genetic Correlates of Vaccine Protection against Mucosal Infection by SIV in Monkeys" (*Science Translational Medicine*, vol. 3, no. 81, May 4, 2011) that neutralizing antibodies are a key component of the immune response needed to prevent HIV infection. This finding may help future vaccine development efforts.

Most researchers are optimistic that an effective vaccine will be developed, but many believe that perfecting a vaccine will take years. VRC researchers believe that more than one vaccine formulation, or a vaccine that works two ways—by boosting immunity provided by T cells and by producing antibodies to attach to HIV and mark it for destruction—may be necessary to provide complete protection.

In "Co-evolution of a Broadly Neutralizing HIV-1 Antibody and Founder Virus" (*Nature*, vol. 496, no. 7446, April 25, 2013), Hua-Xin Liao et al. report increased understanding of how HIV and a strong antibody response develop in an HIV-infected person who naturally develops antibodies to the virus after several years of infection. This understanding is helping researchers create a vaccine that mimics the virus and results in the body generating neutralizing HIV antibodies.

Arik Cooper et al. note in "HIV-1 Causes CD4 Cell Death through DNA-Dependent Protein Kinase during Viral Integration" (*Nature*, vol. 498, no. 7454, June 20, 2013) the discovery of how HIV triggers a signal that tells infected immune cells (the very cells that mobilize to fight the infection) to die. These findings suggest that treating HIV-infected individuals with drugs that block the first steps of viral replication can not only prevent viral replication but

may also improve CD4+ T-cell survival and immune function. This discovery may also help researchers figure out how to eliminate reservoirs of the resting virus.

Renewed Optimism

Reports of the stem-cell therapy cure of Timothy Ray Brown and the two patients with no detectable virus after receiving bone marrow transplants lead many to believe that a cure is close at hand. According to the article "Cure for AIDS 'Possible' Says Nobel Prize–Winning Scientist Who Helped Discover HIV" (Telegraph.co.uk, March 5, 2013), Françoise Barré-Sinoussi (1947–), who along with Luc Montagnier (1932–) and Harald zur Hausen (1936–) was awarded the 2008 Nobel Prize in Physiology or Medicine for pinpointing the cause of AIDS, expresses optimism about the possibility of a cure. Barré-Sinoussi suggests, "We are now in a position that we have evidence suggesting a cure might be possible. We have to stimulate funding for research into cures. It's ongoing, and it will take time, but more and more data [are] indicating that we have to move forward and work on a cure."

Other researchers are optimistic as well. In "HIV Infection en Route to Endogenization: Two Cases" (*Clinical Microbiology and Infection*, vol. 20, no. 12, December 2014), Philippe Colson et al. report that they have uncovered the genetic path by which two men were spontaneously cured of HIV infection. the virus was inactivated due to an altered HIV gene coding integrated into human cells. Colson et al. believe that the inactivation occurred in response to stimulation of an enzyme, which could be targeted by drug treatment to produce the same response. The researchers, "propose a new vision of HIV cure through integration, inactivation and potential endogenization of a viral genome into the human genome."

CHAPTER 7
PEOPLE WITH HIV/AIDS

Large numbers of people are afflicted with HIV/AIDS in the United States. An increasing proportion of the population lives with HIV infection. In the second decade of the 21st century more Americans than ever before are likely to know someone who is affected by HIV or AIDS. Even people who live in remote geographic areas and do not believe they are personally at risk of acquiring HIV are aware of the epidemic from public health education campaigns, reports in the media, school health programs, and health and social service agencies, all of which work to improve community awareness of HIV/AIDS.

PUBLIC FIGURES WITH HIV/AIDS

Perhaps one of the most famous HIV-infected people in the world is Magic Johnson (1959–), an internationally known former basketball player for the Los Angeles Lakers. When Johnson announced his HIV infection in November 1991, the world was shocked. He had no idea he was infected until he received the results of a routine physical examination for life insurance. He freely admitted that before his marriage he had unprotected sexual contact with many women.

Following this announcement, Johnson became an HIV/AIDS spokesperson and began working in prevention programs. In 1991 he started the Magic Johnson Foundation, which seeks to fund and establish community-based education and social and health programs (including HIV/AIDS awareness) in inner-city communities, and briefly served on the President's Commission on AIDS. Although he officially retired from professional basketball in 1996, he continues to play on the Magic Johnson All-Stars Team and is an active spokesperson for HIV/AIDS.

In 1992 the former tennis star Arthur Ashe (1943–1993) announced that he had become infected with HIV from a blood transfusion in the mid-1980s during a heart bypass operation. His was not a voluntary announcement, but one made necessary when the news media discovered his HIV infection and threatened to announce it before he did. Ashe was reluctant to make his condition public, fearing the effect on his five-year-old daughter. He maintained that because he did not have a public responsibility, he should have been allowed to maintain his privacy. He died of pneumonia, a complication of AIDS, in 1993.

The diver Greg Louganis (1960–), who competed in the 1976, 1984, and 1988 Olympic games, was diagnosed with HIV infection in 1988, before his competition in the 1988 games. During the games, Louganis hit his head on the diving board while competing. Although his injury was not serious, it did result in an open wound—making Louganis concerned that his blood might have entered the pool. Nevertheless, Louganis did not reveal his HIV status at the time. The Olympic gold medalist announced that he had HIV in 1995. Louganis now competes in dog agility competitions with his dogs, is a published author of two books, and coaches athletes in diving. He advocates safe sexual practices, because he attributes his HIV infection to unsafe sexual behavior.

Another sports celebrity who succumbed to AIDS was the National Association for Stock Car Auto Racing (NASCAR) racecar driver Tim Richmond (1955–1989). During his heyday on the NASCAR race circuit in the 1980s, Richmond was one of the circuit's premier drivers. He was also well known for his expensive tastes and playboy lifestyle. Whether his lifestyle contributed to his illness is conjecture. Nonetheless, by the end of the 1986 racing season Richmond had become noticeably ill. He was diagnosed with AIDS that same year. He was able to race again in 1987, but soon thereafter his health deteriorated precipitously. During another attempted comeback in 1988, when his illness was still unpublicized, Richmond faced the hostility and innuendo of his fellow drivers, who, guessing the nature of the illness, speculated about his sexual orientation and the possibility of drug abuse. In response, Richmond filed a defamation of character lawsuit against NASCAR. He subsequently withdrew the lawsuit to avoid making his condition public. Richmond ultimately retired from competitive racing and lived in seclusion with his mother until his death. After his death, as news of his illness and the treatment he received from his fellow drivers and NASCAR became public, many people were outraged at the NASCAR organization.

Other sports figures diagnosed with HIV infection include Rudy Galindo (1969–), an American figure skater who earned a bronze medal at the 1996 world championships, and Roy Simmons (1956–2014), an American athlete who played for the National Football League.

Mary Fisher (1948–), a heterosexual and nondrug user who contracted HIV from her husband, stood before her peers during the 1992 Republican National Convention and announced that she was infected with HIV. A former television producer and assistant to President Gerald R. Ford (1913–2006), she said she considered her announcement part of her contribution to the fight against HIV/AIDS. The wealthy and well-educated Fisher was among the first women to publicly dispel the image that still comes to mind when many people think of HIV/AIDS: homosexual, poor, drug addicted, and lacking access to support systems or adequate medical care and housing.

Fisher established the Mary Fisher Clinical AIDS Research and Education Fund at the University of Alabama, Birmingham, in 2000. She is an accomplished artist, public speaker, and author of four books. In 2006 Peter Piot (1949–), the under-secretary-general of the United Nations, appointed Fisher to a two-year term as a special representative of the Joint United Nations Programme on HIV/AIDS, which Piot directed.

The actor Anthony Perkins (1932–1992), who is best known for his role as Norman Bates in the classic Alfred Hitchcock (1899–1980) film *Psycho* (1960), also died of AIDS. Forever typecast by that performance, Perkins was in fact an accomplished film and stage actor. He was bisexual and had relationships with a number of men. Shortly before his death in 1992, Perkins commented in a press release about a *National Enquirer* article that revealed his AIDS-positive status by saying, "I have learned more about love, selflessness, and human understanding from the people I have met in this great adventure in the world of AIDS than I ever did in the cutthroat, competitive world in which I spent my life."

Another movie star who succumbed to AIDS was Rock Hudson (1925–1985). Indeed, Hudson was the first major U.S. celebrity known to have died from AIDS. His death was especially noteworthy, given his status during the 1950s as the quintessential rugged, all-American male. Despite his many movie roles as a leading man opposite many beautiful actresses, Hudson was homosexual, a fact that was covered up by movie studios. His 1955 marriage to the studio employee Phyllis Gates (1925–2006), which ended in divorce in 1958, is thought to have been a studio-orchestrated attempt to cover up his sexual orientation. Hudson died at the age of 59.

The African American rap star Eazy-E (c. 1963–1995) rose to fame as one of the members of the group N.W.A. (Niggaz with Attitude), based in Compton, California. Using money obtained from illegal drug sales, Eazy-E founded Ruthless Records. Soon after, he recruited Ice Cube (1969–), Dr. Dre (1965?–), MC Ren (1969–), DJ Yella (1967–), and Arabian Prince (1965–) to form N.W.A. Following the dissolution of N.W.A., Eazy-E went on to have a successful solo career. In 1995 he entered the hospital for treatment of what he thought was asthma. However, he was diagnosed with AIDS and died soon after. Eazy-E is now regarded as one of the influential founders of the style of music known as gangsta rap. Every year, the city of Compton celebrates his life by observing Eazy-E Day.

Another music icon who died of AIDS was Freddie Mercury (1946–1991), the lead vocalist of the British rock band Queen. His more than three-octave vocal range and operatic compositional approach to rock resulted in classic hits such as "Bohemian Rhapsody," "Somebody to Love," and "We Are the Champions." The video made for the 1975 release of "Bohemian Rhapsody" is considered by some music insiders to be one of the decisive influences that spurred the popularity of music videos. Mercury was well known for his extravagance and bisexuality. His diagnosis and deteriorating physical condition were kept private. Indeed, his eventual announcement that he had AIDS was made only one day before his death in 1991.

Rudolf Nureyev (1938–1993) was a Soviet-born ballet and modern dancer who defected to the West in 1961. He was one of the most celebrated dancers of the 20th century. Nureyev tested positive for HIV in 1984 and died of AIDS at the age of 54. The British actor and Oscar-winning director Tony Richardson (1928–1991), the former husband of Vanessa Redgrave (1937–), died of AIDS at the age of 63.

Elizabeth Glaser (1947–1994), the wife of the actor Paul Michael Glaser (1943–), was motivated to cofound the Pediatric AIDS Foundation in 1988 (now called the Elizabeth Glaser Pediatric AIDS Foundation), following the discovery that she and her children, Ariel (1981–1988) and Jake (1984–), were all infected with HIV. She originally contracted the virus from contaminated blood that was administered during pregnancy, but she was unaware of her illness until much later, already having passed it to her children. In the ensuing years she became a vocal AIDS activist. The foundation that is her legacy contributes more than $1 million annually to pediatric AIDS research. Ariel died at the age of seven, and Elizabeth died in 1994. Because Jake has a mutation of the CCR5 gene that delays onset by restricting the virus's ability to enter white blood cells, he remains symptom free and no longer takes HIV medication. He and Paul continue to raise money and AIDS awareness through Elizabeth's foundation.

Although he did not confirm his HIV status when he was alive, an autopsy performed on the flamboyant entertainer Liberace (1919–1987) confirmed that he was HIV infected. The award-winning playwright and lyricist Howard Ashman (1950–1991) also died of AIDS. Ashman wrote the lyrics for several Disney films, including *The Little Mermaid*, *Aladdin*, and *Beauty and the Beast*, which was dedicated to him.

The artist and photographer Robert Mapplethorpe (1946–1989) was 42 when he died of AIDS complications. The artist Keith Haring (1958–1990), who was known for his striking murals and political themes, also died of AIDS-related complications.

In November 2015 the actor Charlie Sheen (1965–) revealed that he is HIV positive and has known of his status for four years. Sheen has a well-publicized history of drug use and sex with prostitutes. However, in a November 17, 2015, interview on the *Today* show, Sheen asserted that he did not know how he had become infected.

Finally, in a list of examples that is by no means complete, the prolific and influential science-fiction author Isaac Asimov (1920–1992) contracted HIV from infected blood that was given to him in a transfusion during heart bypass surgery in 1983. He died in 1992 of heart and renal failure that were complications of AIDS.

OLDER ADULTS WITH HIV/AIDS

In "AIDS among Persons Aged Greater Than or Equal to 50 Years—United States, 1991–1996" (*Morbidity and Mortality Weekly Report*, vol. 47, no. 2, January 23, 1998), the U.S. Centers for Disease Control and Prevention (CDC) reports that older people infected with HIV early in the epidemic were typically infected through contaminated blood or blood products. Through 1989 only 1% of HIV/AIDS cases among people aged 13 to 49 years were due to contaminated blood. However, during this same period 6% of cases among people aged 50 to 59 years, 28% of cases among people aged 60 to 69 years, and 64% of cases among people aged 70 years and older resulted from contaminated blood or blood products.

Improved safety of the nation's blood supply, including routine screening of blood donations for HIV, sharply reduced the risk of contracting the virus from contaminated blood or blood products. Subsequently, the proportion of people aged 50 years and older who acquired HIV from other types of exposure increased. Although male-to-male sexual contact and injection drug use remain the primary means by which HIV is transmitted among all age groups in the United States, heterosexual transmission of HIV is steadily increasing in people aged 50 years and older.

HIV/AIDS Cases among Older Adults

As described in Chapter 4, adults aged 50 years and older accounted for 18% of new HIV diagnoses and 27% of AIDS diagnoses in 2013. The proportion of adults over the age of 50 years with HIV/AIDS is expected to increase as HIV-infected people of all ages live longer thanks to effective drug therapy and other advances in medical treatment.

HIV Testing for Those over the Age of 50 Years

Many older adults do not seek routine screening for HIV infection because they do not believe they are at risk of acquiring the disease. Figure 7.1 shows that in 2014 the lowest rates of testing among adults over the age of 18 years were among people aged 65 years and older—just 16.9% of this group had ever been tested for HIV. By comparison, 59.1% of those aged 25 to 34 years, 53.3% of those aged 35 to 44 years, and 36.5% of those aged 45 to 64 years had ever been tested. Among women over the age of 50 years, the absence of the risk of pregnancy may lead to a false sense of security and the mistaken belief that they are at less risk for sexually transmitted infections, including HIV.

The failure to test or the late testing of older patients may be occurring because physicians are less apt to look for HIV in people of this age group. Another factor is that some AIDS-related illnesses that occur in older people, such as encephalopathy (any of various diseases of the brain) and wasting disease, have symptoms that are similar to other diseases that are associated with aging.

It is vitally important to overcome older adults' reluctance to seek testing and other delays to diagnosis because research shows that age speeds the progression of HIV to AIDS and blunts CD4 response to highly active antiretroviral therapy.

YOUNG ADULTS WITH HIV/AIDS

The CDC estimates that about one-quarter of new HIV infections occur in youth and young adults aged 13 to 24 years. The majority of new infections among this age group occur in men who have sex with men (MSM). In 2009, 72% of all new diagnoses among people aged 13 to 24 years in the United States were attributed to MSM; in 2013 this percentage stood at 80%. (See Figure 7.2.) By contrast, HIV infections attributed to heterosexual contact decreased from 20% to 14% during the same period and diagnosed HIV infections attributed to injection drug use also decreased slightly, from 4% to 3%.

FIGURE 7.1

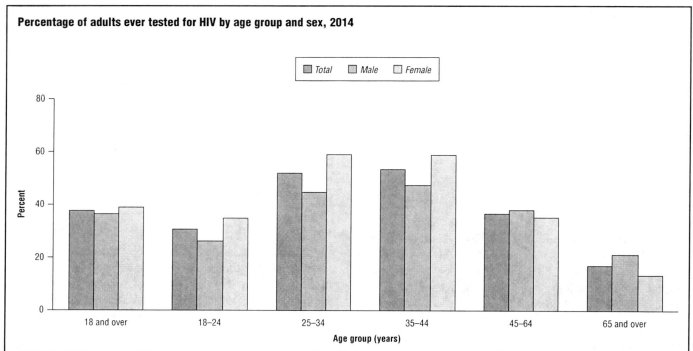

Percentage of adults ever tested for HIV by age group and sex, 2014

Notes: Data are based on household interviews of a sample of the civilian noninstitutionalized population. Individuals who received HIV testing solely as a result of blood donation were considered not to have been tested for HIV. The AIDS Knowledge and Attitudes section of the National Health Interview Survey (NHIS) was dropped in 2011; only the HIV testing question was retained, and it was moved to the Adult Access to Health Care and Utilization section of the Sample Adult questionnaire. In 2013, the HIV testing question was moved to the Adult Selected Items section of the Sample Adult questionnaire and is not comparable to the years 2011–2012. Differences observed in estimates based on the 2010 and earlier NHIS and the 2011 and later NHIS may be partially or fully attributable to these changes in placement of the HIV testing question on the NHIS questionnaire. The analyses excluded the 4.3% of adults with unknown HIV test status.

SOURCE: "Figure 10.2. Percentage of Adults Aged 18 and over Who Had Ever Been Tested for Human Immunodeficiency Virus (HIV), by Age Group and Sex: United States, 2014," in *Early Release of Selected Estimates Based on Data from the 2014 National Health Interview Survey, January—June 2014*, Centers for Disease Control and Prevention, December 2014, http://www.cdc.gov/nchs/data/nhis/earlyrelease/earlyrelease201412_10.pdf (accessed August 1, 2014)

In *HIV among Youth* (June 30, 2015, http://www.cdc.gov/hiv/group/age/youth/index.html), the CDC notes that youth aged 13 to 24 years account for a disproportionate share of new HIV diagnoses. The CDC cites the following as some of the reasons why this is the case:

- Underestimation of risk—Surveys reveal that teens and young adults are generally not very concerned about becoming infected with HIV, which means they may fail to take actions to prevent infection.

- Lack of HIV/AIDS education—The prevalence of HIV education in school fell from 92% in 1997 to 85% in 2013. In addition, some sex education programs do not present information that is relevant to gay and bisexual young men.

- Low levels of awareness—The CDC estimates that as of 2010, half of all infected youth did not know they had HIV, a much lower percentage than the overall population. In 2013, just 13% of high school students (22% of those who had ever had sexual intercourse) had been tested for HIV.

- Low rates of condom use—A substantial percentage (41%) of high school students who had sexual intercourse in 2013 report that they did not use a condom.

- High rates of sexually transmitted diseases (STDs)— Other STDs are relatively common among people aged 20 to 24 years. People infected with an STD have a greater likelihood of catching and transmitting HIV.

- Substance use—Alcohol and illicit drug use increase the likelihood of high-risk behaviors. Of the 34% of high school students who were sexually active in 2013, 22% had used alcohol or drugs before engaging in sexual intercourse.

- Homelessness—Runaways and homeless youth are at high risk for HIV infection if they trade sex for drugs, money, or shelter.

LIVING WITH HIV/AIDS

To gain a more complete view of the impact of HIV/ AIDS, it is important to understand the psychosocial and emotional consequences of diagnosis with a potentially fatal disease.

FIGURE 7.2

HIV diagnoses in persons aged 13–24, by transmission category, 2009–13

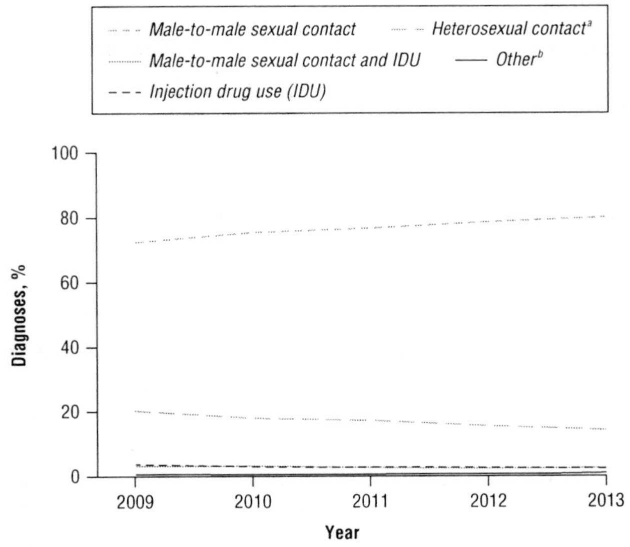

- - - Male-to-male sexual contact .... Heterosexual contact[a]
.... Male-to-male sexual contact and IDU ——— Other[b]
- - - Injection drug use (IDU)

[a]Heterosexual contact with a person known to have, or to be at high risk for, HIV infection.
[b]Includes hemophilia, blood transfusion, perinatal exposure, and risk factor not reported or not identified.
Note: Data include persons with a diagnosis of HIV infection regardless of stage of disease at diagnosis. All displayed data have been statistically adjusted to account for reporting delays and missing transmission category, but not for incomplete reporting.

SOURCE: "Diagnoses of HIV Infection among Adolescents and Young Adults Aged 13–24 Years, by Transmission Category, 2009–2013, United States and 6 Dependent Areas," in *HIV Surveillance— Adolescents and Young Adults*, Centers for Disease Control and Prevention, National Center for HIV/AIDS, Viral Hepatitis, Sexual Transmitted Diseases, and Tuberculosis Prevention, Division of HIV/AIDS Prevention, June 2015, http://www.cdc.gov/hiv/pdf/statistics_surveillance_Adolescents.pdf (accessed July 28, 2015)

Still a Worrisome Diagnosis

By the dawn of the 21st century, a diagnosis of HIV infection was no longer a certain death sentence, but it was still likely to elicit feelings of fear, confusion, depression, and anger. Researchers have identified another reason that people who are diagnosed with HIV infection require additional emotional support: there is an association between psychosocial stress and HIV disease progression. Gail Ironson et al. explain in "Psychosocial and Neurohormonal Predictors of HIV Disease Progression (CD4 Cells and Viral Load): A 4 Year Prospective Study" (*AIDS and Behavior*, September 19, 2014) that psychosocial factors such as depression, hopelessness, coping, and life event stress predict HIV disease progression. Specifically, the researchers find a strong relationship between adverse psychosocial factors, such as difficulty coping with stress, and HIV disease progression.

Coping with Discrimination

Unlike people who are diagnosed with other terminal or catastrophic illnesses such as cancer or multiple sclerosis, people with HIV/AIDS often confront the social isolation and discrimination that accompany a stigmatized status. Many people continue to think of HIV/AIDS as a disease that people bring on themselves through risky or inappropriate behavior, and they may condemn HIV-infected people for inflicting themselves with the condition. Some still believe that AIDS is divine retribution for an "immoral lifestyle." The fear of unfavorable judgment keeps many infected individuals from disclosing their HIV infection to others, even friends and family. Others simply do not want the pity that is often extended to people with potentially fatal conditions. Still others worry that friends and family, fearing infection, will abandon them.

Under the Americans with Disabilities Act (ADA) of 1990, people infected with HIV and those diagnosed with AIDS are considered disabled and as such are subject to the antidiscrimination provisions of this landmark legislation. As a result, employers may not ask job applicants if they are HIV infected or have AIDS, nor can they require an HIV test of prospective employees. The only exceptions to this provision are those employers who can demonstrate that such questions or testing are job-related and absolutely necessary for the employer to conduct business.

More important, the ADA requires employers to make "reasonable accommodations" for disabled employees. Reasonable accommodation is an adjustment to a job or modification of the responsibilities or work environment that will enable the worker with a disability to gain equal employment opportunity. Examples include flexible work schedules to allow for medical appointments, treatments, and counseling and the provision of additional unpaid leave.

The Stigma of AIDS

In "A Comparison of HIV Stigma and Discrimination in Five International Sites: The Influence of Care and Treatment Resources in High Prevalence Settings" (*Social Science and Medicine*, vol. 68, no. 12, June 2009), a study designed to examine HIV stigma and discrimination in five high prevalence settings, Suzanne Maman et al. observe that the factors that contribute to HIV stigma and discrimination include the fear of transmission, the fear of suffering and death, and the burden of caring for people with AIDS.

According to Maman et al., the family, access to antiretroviral drugs, and other resources offered some protection against HIV stigma and discrimination. Variation in the availability of health and social services designed to lessen the impact of HIV/AIDS helps explain differences in HIV stigma and discrimination across the settings. The researchers opine that "increasing access to treatment and care resources may function to lower HIV stigma, however, providing services is not enough." They also assert that it is necessary to develop "effective strategies to reduce HIV stigma as treatment and care resources are scaled up in the settings that are most heavily impacted by the HIV epidemic."

More than three decades after the first diagnosis of AIDS and widespread public health and community education efforts to inform people about HIV infection and prevent the spread of HIV, ignorance and misunderstanding of HIV/AIDS persist. Health educators and HIV/AIDS activists stress the importance of intensified, ongoing education to destigmatize people who are affected by HIV/AIDS and prevent discrimination. Reducing the stigma that is associated with HIV/AIDS may also encourage individuals to get tested and, for those who are infected, begin treatment as soon as possible.

Because stigma, even among personnel who work with people with HIV/AIDS, persists, efforts to reduce it continue. The HIV/AIDS Stigma Program, which is funded by the Health Resources and Services Administration's HIV/AIDS Bureau, offers training programs that explore the stigma associated with HIV/AIDS. The programs, which are made available to staff employed by agencies and organizations funded by the Ryan White Comprehensive AIDS Resources Emergency Act of 1990, focus on:

- Defining stigma and its origins in society

- The impact of stigma on an individual's decision-making process and how it deters him or her from seeking HIV testing and counseling services

- How stigma affects access to care and disclosure of HIV-positive status

Dealing with Emotions

Not unexpectedly, anger and depression are natural and common reactions to discovering that one is infected with HIV. Experts stress the importance of recognizing and expressing anger and depression; however, if these feelings become all consuming, they can prevent health- and life-improving actions. Many people with HIV/AIDS say that sharing feelings with friends and family members and participating in support groups ease anguish and help generate more positive attitudes and actions.

Many HIV/AIDS sufferers report that the most difficult thing they had to do after being diagnosed with HIV was to inform people in their present or recent past whom they might have exposed to the virus. If the patient is unable to do this, a physician or public health official can notify present or former sexual partners without revealing the infected person's name.

ONLINE SUPPORT AND RESOURCES HELP WITH DISCLOSURE. There are many agencies and organizations that offer support services for people with HIV/AIDS who are concerned about sharing their status with friends, family and colleagues. For example, "Do You Have to Tell?" at the AIDS.gov website and "Telling Others You Are HIV Positive," (July 23, 2014, AIDS InfoNet, http://www.aidsinfonet.org/fact_sheets/view/204) offer advice about disclosing HIV status to partners, coworkers and health care providers.

Early Medication Improves Outlook and Protects against Spread of HIV

The earlier people learn of their infection, the earlier they can begin medical treatment to suppress the virus's destructive growth, delay the onset of AIDS symptoms, and extend life. Along with antiretroviral drugs there are medications that fight the life-threatening opportunistic infections that eventually may afflict people who are HIV infected. Although these drugs do not eliminate HIV infection, they have been shown to keep HIV/AIDS patients healthy and symptom free for increasingly longer periods.

In 2011 the results of an international study definitively concluded that prompt treatment of HIV infection, before a person develops symptoms, dramatically reduces the risk that the person with HIV will transmit the virus to a sexual partner. According to the article "Early HIV Therapy Protects against Virus Spread" (Associated Press, May 12, 2011), the study followed 1,763 couples in which one partner was HIV infected and the other was not. The study participants were from Botswana, Brazil, India, Kenya, Malawi, South Africa, Thailand, the United States, and Zimbabwe. Half of the couples received early treatment of the infected partner and the other half waited until the infected partner's CD4 cell count fell below 250 per cubic millimeter of blood or until symptoms appeared. Among the untreated couples, 28 previously uninfected partners were infected. Among the treated couples, just one previously uninfected person became infected. Anthony S. Fauci (1940–), the head of the National Institute of Allergy and Infectious Diseases, said the study's finding "promises to change practice worldwide."

Practicing Good Health Habits

Experts advise HIV-infected people to exercise and maintain a balanced diet with sufficient lean protein. Not only does exercise improve overall fitness and generate a sense of well-being, it releases endorphins, which are natural substances produced by the brain that boost immunity, reduce stress, and elevate mood. People with HIV/AIDS are advised to avoid smoking, excessive alcohol consumption, and using illegal drugs, all of which can act to depress the immune system.

HOUSING PROBLEMS

The difficulty of finding affordable and appropriate housing can be an acute crisis for people living with HIV/AIDS. HIV-infected people need more than just a safe shelter that provides protection and comfort; they may also require a base from which to receive services, care, and support. Adherence to complicated medical regimens is challenging for many HIV-infected people, but for some homeless people it is nearly impossible.

Some individuals are homeless when they acquire the HIV infection, whereas others lose their homes when they are no longer able to hold jobs or cannot afford to pay for health care and housing costs. The National AIDS Housing Coalition (NAHC) indicates in the fact sheet "Breaking the Link between Homelessness and HIV" (February 2011, http://www.nationalaidshousing.org/PDF/Factsheets-Homelessness.pdf) that:

- Housing status is a key factor affecting access to care and health behaviors among people with HIV/AIDS. Housing assistance reduces HIV health risk behaviors, improves health outcomes, and reduces use of costly emergency and inpatient hospital services.

- Housing remains one of the greatest unmet needs of Americans with HIV/AIDS. At least half of all people with HIV/AIDS experience housing instability or homelessness.

- Although about 500,000 households affected by HIV/AIDS will require some form of housing assistance during the course of their illness, the federal program Housing Opportunities for Persons with AIDS (HOPWA) serves less than 60,000 households per year.

In the fact sheet "Housing Is HIV Prevention & Care" (2013, http://nationalaidshousing.org/PDF/FactSheet.pdf), the NAHC describes the relationship between HIV risk and housing instability and homelessness. More than 145,000 households living with HIV/AIDS had unmet housing needs in 2013 and less than 60,000 were being served by HOPWA. The NAHC asserts that "improved housing status also prevents new HIV infections by reducing HIV risk behaviors by as much as half and by facilitating effective [antiretroviral therapy] that lowers viral load to an undetectable level, virtually eliminating ongoing HIV transmission."

According to the NAHC, in the fact sheet "Housing Is Cost-Effective HIV Prevention and Care" (February 2011, http://nationalaidshousing.org/PDF/Factsheets-Cost%20Effective.pdf), housing for people with HIV/AIDS not only saves lives but also saves money. The NAHC observes that housing assistance improves health outcomes, reduces utilization of emergency and other costly health services such as hospitalization by 57%, and reduces involvement with the criminal justice system.

Each new HIV infection that is prevented saves an estimated $300,000 in lifetime health care costs.

SUICIDE

Depression is a common psychiatric problem among patients who are seriously ill with HIV/AIDS. Although this is a normal grief response, the combination of alienation, hopelessness, guilt, and lack of self-esteem can lead some to contemplate and plan for suicide in search of lost dignity and control. Others counter that the real dignity is in seeing the disease to the end. Those who encourage people with HIV/AIDS to "stick it out" often see the disease as becoming increasingly manageable with drugs and improved treatment techniques.

Several factors make HIV/AIDS patients more likely to commit suicide. They may feel they are certain to die sooner than they expected and worry that their death will be prolonged and emotionally and physically painful. They may also be despondent about the prospects of losing their jobs, insurance, or their homes. Furthermore, they may be ostracized from society. Researchers find that factors that have a considerable impact on the quality of life include security, family, love, pleasurable activity, and freedom from pain, suffering, and debilitating disease. AIDS patients may lose all of these, or they may be consumed by the fear of losing vital capacities and freedoms. For some, suicide seems like a reasonable alternative; it offers an end to pain and suffering, insecurity, self-pity, dependency, and hopelessness.

According to Pablo Aldaz et al., in "Mortality by Causes in HIV-Infected Adults: Comparison with the General Population" (*BMC Public Health*, May 11, 2011), people with HIV infection have higher mortality (deaths) than uninfected people of the same age and sex for many causes of death, including suicide. The researchers analyzed deaths among HIV-infected people aged 20 to 59 years between 1999 and 2006 and compared mortality from the same causes in the general population. Aldaz et al. conclude that "in agreement with other studies, we found a high mortality from suicide among HIV-infected persons."

Susane Müller Klug Passos, Luciano Dias de Mattos Souza, and Bárbara Coiro Spessato evaluated 211 HIV/AIDS patients in Brazil for suicide risk and report their findings in "High Prevalence of Suicide Risk in People Living with HIV: Who Is at Higher Risk?" (*AIDS Care*, vol. 26, no. 11, 2014). The researchers found that about one-third (34.1%) were at risk for suicide. Characteristics associated with suicide risk included being female, less than age 47, unemployed, suffering from anxiety and/or depression, and abuse of alcohol and/or illicit drugs.

The Physician's Role

During the 1990s there were heated debates, voter initiatives, and court decisions about the legalization of physician-assisted suicide. As of September 2015, four states had legalized physician-assisted suicide: Oregon (in 1994), Washington (in 2008), and Vermont (in 2013) through legislation, and Montana (in 2009) through court order. Voters in Oregon, Washington, and Vermont determined that the right to end one's own life is intensely personal and should not be forbidden by law. (Although attempts and acts of suicide are no longer subject to criminal prosecution in the United States, aiding a suicide is considered a criminal offense.)

Both the public and physicians themselves are divided about the issue of physician-assisted suicide. People who support the practice believe that doctors should make their skills available to patients to end anguish and suffering. Those who oppose physician-assisted suicide argue that better end-of-life care—effective pain management, emotional and spiritual support, and widespread education to reduce anxiety about dying—may reduce the frequency of requests for physician-assisted suicide. Opponents also fear that the legal right to assist suicide can be misused or abused and that such abuses might victimize already vulnerable populations.

In 2015 a Gallup survey found that 68% of Americans supported allowing physicians to help patients end their own lives under certain circumstances. (See Table 7.1.) According to Andrew Dugan of the Gallup Organization, in *In U.S., Support up for Doctor-Assisted Suicide* (May 27, 2015, http://www.gallup.com/poll/183425/support-doctor-

TABLE 7.1

Public opinion on the acceptability of physician-assisted suicide, 2014 and 2015

WHEN A PERSON HAS A DISEASE THAT CANNOT BE CURED AND IS LIVING IN SEVERE PAIN, DO YOU THINK DOCTORS SHOULD OR SHOULD NOT BE ALLOWED BY LAW TO ASSIST THE PATIENT TO COMMIT SUICIDE IF THE PATIENT REQUESTS IT?

[% Yes, should be allowed]

	May 2014	May 2015	Change
	%	%	pct. pts.
18 to 34 years old	62	81	+19
35 to 54 years old	57	65	+8
55 and older	56	61	+5
Republicans	51	61	+10
Independents	64	80	+16
Democrats	59	72	+13

SOURCE: Andrew Dugan, "Support for Doctor-Assisted 'Suicide,' by Year," in *In U.S., Support up for Doctor-Assisted Suicide*, The Gallup Organization, May 27, 2015, http://www.gallup.com/poll/183425/support-doctor-assisted-suicide.aspx?utm_source=physician%20assisted%20suicide&utm_medium=search&utm_campaign=tiles (accessed August 3, 2015). Copyright © 2015 Gallup, Inc. All rights reserved. The content is used with permission; however, Gallup retains all rights of republication.

assisted-suicide.aspx), support had increased sharply among young adults aged 18 to 34 years, rising from 62% in 2014 to 81% in 2015. This increase of support was probably due in part to the widely publicized story of Brittany Maynard, a 29-year-old woman suffering from terminal brain cancer who traveled to Oregon in 2014 to end her life.

CHAPTER 8
TESTING, PREVENTION, AND EDUCATION

HIV TESTING
Voluntary, Not Mandatory

Few issues about the HIV/AIDS epidemic prompted more controversy than the use of antibody tests to identify people who are infected with HIV. When the enzyme-linked immunosorbent assay test was developed and licensed in 1985, many public health officials supported testing in an attempt to change "undesirable" behaviors that were determining the course of the epidemic (such as unsafe male-to-male sexual contact and injection drug use). Those who favored testing claimed that if a person knew he or she was HIV positive, the infected person would change his or her behavior. Others argued that aggressive public health education and thoughtful counseling would be more productive strategies to achieve the desired results, even if people did not know their HIV status.

During the early years of the epidemic, health care officials in the public and private sectors refrained from advocating mandatory testing; instead, they focused on HIV testing that would be performed by physicians for patients they considered to be at risk for infection. In 1990 the House of Delegates of the American Medical Association voted to declare HIV/AIDS a sexually transmitted disease (STD; also known as sexually transmitted infection, or STI). This designation allowed physicians more freedom to decide the conditions under which HIV testing should take place.

During the late 1980s, when the research community announced that HIV-infected, symptom-free people could receive early intervention with azidothymidine (now called zidovudine) to slow the effects of the illness and delay the onset of *Pneumocystis carinii* pneumonia, the debate took another turn. Gay rights advocates, such as the Gay Men's Health Crisis in New York, began encouraging those who were at risk for HIV infection to get tested rather than discouraging testing, as they had previously done. In June

1997 the Gay Men's Health Crisis Center opened its own testing facility. This service was still available in 2015 as part of the range of care and support services offered by the Michael Palm Center (http://www.gmhc .org). The center also offered a "harm reduction program" that was designed to curb risky behaviors such as substance abuse and unprotected sex. The intent of the program was to encourage people to change their risky behavior in a supportive atmosphere of care.

Another controversy surrounding testing concerns reporting HIV-positive patients by name. Every state is required to report AIDS cases. Since 2011 all 50 states and six dependent areas (American Samoa, Guam, the Northern Mariana Islands, Palau, Puerto Rico, and the U.S. Virgin Islands) have implemented HIV case surveillance using the same confidential system for name-based case reporting for both HIV infection and AIDS.

Critics, including the American Civil Liberties Union, assailed name reporting as an invasion of privacy that carries social and economic risks. They claimed that any benefit that would result from reporting names could not override the negative consequences (such as ostracism and the potential loss of jobs and insurance) of being classified as infected. They added that name reporting discourages those at risk for HIV from coming forward to seek testing and timely treatment.

Name-based reporting became the norm in 2013 because the Ryan White HIV/AIDS Treatment Extension Act of 2009 required grantees to convert to name-based reporting by fiscal year (FY) 2013 or risk the loss of funding. The name-reporting debate subsided in 2013, with the states acquiescing to federal requirements.

Previous HIV Testing among Adults and Adolescents Newly Diagnosed with HIV Infection

In 2006 the Centers for Disease Control and Prevention (CDC) recommended HIV testing for adults, adolescents, and pregnant women in health care settings and HIV testing at least annually for people who were at high risk for HIV infection. The three populations at highest risk for HIV in the United States are men who have sex with men (MSM), injection drug users (IDUs), and high-risk heterosexuals (e.g., sex workers). The CDC collects information from all these groups.

The most recent data that have been analyzed are from 18 jurisdictions participating in the CDC National HIV Surveillance System. In "Previous HIV Testing among Adults and Adolescents Newly Diagnosed with HIV Infection—National HIV Surveillance System, 18 Jurisdictions, United States, 2006–2009" (*Morbidity and Mortality Weekly Report*, vol. 61, no. 24, June 22, 2012), the CDC observes that many people diagnosed with HIV infection have never been tested previously. Between 2006 and 2009, 40.8% were diagnosed with HIV infection at their first HIV test, and 59.2% had a negative test at some point before HIV diagnosis. The highest percentage of people testing HIV negative less than 12 months before HIV diagnosis were those aged 13 to 29 years (33%), males with HIV transmission attributed to MSM (29%), and whites (28%).

Contact Tracing/Partner Notification

A by-product of testing is contact tracing, or partner notification. When individuals test positive for HIV, health officials ask them to provide, with the promise of anonymity, the names of those with whom they have had sexual contact or shared needles. The CDC asks counselors to inform contacts if the patient is reluctant to do so and strongly endorses contact-tracing programs, but results vary. States struggling under the strain of many HIV/AIDS cases continue to support programs that encourage the infected people to notify partners on their own. Contact-tracing programs in states with fewer HIV/AIDS cases are more likely to contact partners. Many patients who are HIV infected or have AIDS fear that promises of confidentiality will be broken; others fear retribution from those they may have infected.

Binwei Song et al. explain in "Partner Referral by HIV-Infected Persons to Partner Counseling and Referral Services (PCRS)—Results from a Demonstration Project" (*Open AIDS Journal*, vol. 6, 2012) that "the success of partner notification depends on whether [patients] are willing to provide information about their partners, the content of the information that they provide (i.e., whether they provide names and locating information of their partners), and how they choose to inform their partners that they have been exposed to HIV." The researchers report on their research to determine factors associated with refusal and agreement to provide partner information. They find that clients who were aged 25 years and older, male, or reported MSM or injection drug use in the past 12 months

were more likely to refuse to provide partner information. Song et al. posit that MSM and IDUs may be more reluctant to share personal information because of social stigma or more negative feelings about being HIV positive. The proportion of partners that were located, notified, and counseled differed by approach used, ranging from 38% when patients agreed to notify their partners within a certain time frame or else a health care professional would notify them to 98% when patients notified their partners with a health professional present.

ETHICAL, LEGAL, AND MORAL DILEMMAS OF PARTNER NOTIFICATION. Worldwide, there is increasing emphasis on partner notification as a strategy with the potential not only to prevent HIV transmission to partners at risk but also to promote early diagnosis and prompt treatment for those found to be infected. In "Partner Notification in the Context of HIV: An Interest-Analysis" (*AIDS Research and Therapy*, vol. 12, no. 15, May 5, 2015), Amos K. Laar, Debra A. DeBruin, and Susan Craddock consider partner notification from the perspective of the individual, the state and public health, and the bioethicist (an expert in the ethical implications of biological and medical discoveries and advances).

Laar, DeBruin, and Craddock explain that state and public health interests in partner notification are based on the premise that partners are entitled to this knowledge, which can help them to avoid continuing risks, obtain early treatment, and alter their behavior to prevent transmission of infection to others. Persons infected with HIV often have opposing interests such as the desire to maintain their privacy because of the negative consequences of disclosure. Bioethicists attempt to resolve these seemingly incompatible interests. Laar, DeBruin, and Craddock conclude that "partner notification is grounded in credible evidence, and is sound in public health standings, but has multivalent ethical tensions and interests."

In *The Public Health Implications of Criminalizing HIV Non-disclosure, Exposure and Transmission: Report of an International Workshop* (January 2014, http://www.hivlawand policy.org/sites/www.hivlawandpolicy.org/files/Public%20 Health%20Implications%20of%20Criminalizing%20HIV% 20Non-Disclosure,%20Exposure%20and%20Transmission .pdf), Eric Mykhalovskiy et al. assert that criminalizing people with HIV/AIDS who do not disclose their HIV status to sexual partners or who transmit HIV to others is a global policy concern. Mykhalovskiy et al. explain that there are questions about how criminal law is used to address complex public health problems.

Some of the unresolved issues include the negative impact of criminalization on public health and community-based efforts to prevent HIV transmission and to provide treatment, care and support services to people living with HIV/AIDS. There is concern that criminalization may intensify HIV-related stigma and discrimination, discourage HIV testing and compromise access to HIV care, treatment and support services. Research reveals that criminalizing HIV nondisclosure, exposure, and transmission disproportionately affects marginalized people living with HIV/AIDS. Other studies find that criminal law has a negligible or negative impact on activities known to protect against HIV transmission. Mykhalovskiy et al. conclude that further research is needed to identify legal, ethical, and practice issues faced by public health and health care providers as a result of HIV criminalization, and provide evidence to support legally and ethically sound policy and practice.

INTERNET-BASED PARTNER NOTIFICATION. Because research indicates that a substantial number of new HIV cases and STIs are acquired by MSM who meet new sexual partners on the Internet, health professionals wondered if the same medium could be used to convey information to men, such as in e-mails or e-cards informing them that they had sex with someone with an STI and providing links about the STI and where to get tested for it. In "Evaluation of inSPOTLA.org: An Internet Partner Notification Service" (*Sexually Transmitted Diseases*, vol. 39, no. 5, May 2012), Aaron Plant et al. evaluated inSPOTLA.org, an STI partner notification website that primarily targets MSM. Between December 2005 and 2009 the site received more than 400,000 visitors and resulted in nearly 50,000 e-mail postcards sent. Users of inSPOTLA choose from six different e-cards, which vary in tone from serious to humorous. They select their STI from a pull-down menu of 10 different diseases. E-cards may be sent anonymously to as many as six partners at once or can include a personal note from the sender. E-card recipients receive an e-mail from getchecked @inspotla.org. Although the site had many visitors, Plant et al. find that community awareness and utilization of the site were low. Nonetheless, the researchers believe that sites such as inSPOTLA have the potential to enhance traditional partner notification efforts.

In "'No One's at Home and They Won't Pick Up the Phone': Using the Internet and Text Messaging to Enhance Partner Services in North Carolina" (*Sexually Transmitted Diseases*, vol. 1, no. 2, February 2014), Lisa Hightow-Weidman et al. report that in November 2011 the North Carolina Division of Public Health began using text messaging as well as e-mail for partner notification. Hightow-Weidman et al. acknowledge that text messaging is not considered a secure form of communication. However, they conclude that its use "seems to represent an acceptable and potentially more effective method for reaching previously untraceable partners and augmenting traditional partner services."

Rapid Testing

Rapid testing increases access to HIV testing because it is readily performed in a variety of settings, such as correctional facilities, military battlefield operations, and worksites where occupational exposures may occur. Several rapid HIV antibody tests have been approved by the U.S. Food and Drug Administration (FDA) for use in the United States. Table 2.4 in Chapter 2 lists the FDA-approved rapid HIV screening tests and provides their features. The tests contain test strips with HIV antigens. If the blood or sputum they come in contact with contains HIV antibodies, then the antibodies bind to the antigens and a reagent in the test kit creates a color change. The tests are interpreted visually and, like conventional HIV enzyme immunoassays, positive responses are confirmed by a Western blot or immunofluorescent assay.

Because rapid HIV testing informs clients with reactive test results that it is highly likely that they are HIV positive, compared with receiving no test result information at the conclusion of a visit where a conventional HIV test specimen is drawn, it is vitally important for health care workers to explain the meaning of preliminary positive results. Counseling for patients who receive rapid HIV testing is somewhat different from conventional testing and involves determining how prepared clients are to receive test results in the same session.

In 2012 the FDA approved the first rapid response test for home use. The OraQuick In-Home HIV Test does not require sending a sample to a laboratory for analysis. It provides a result in 20 to 40 minutes. As with other rapid tests, positive test results must be confirmed by follow-up laboratory-based testing.

Home Testing

Home HIV tests were developed during the mid-1980s but were opposed by the FDA and some HIV/AIDS organizations and health care agencies. The FDA was concerned about telephone counseling for those who tested positive, the accuracy of the tests, and confidentiality. In 1996 the FDA reversed its position, deciding that despite the limitations of home testing, the benefits outweigh the risks.

Public health officials explain that many people are afraid of obtaining testing at a physician's office or public clinic because of the associated stigma. They assert that home testing may be the only way some of these people will learn their HIV status and argue that more people will then enter treatment and take precautions to prevent spreading the infection.

Some home tests use saliva, which does not require a needle stick, and others use blood samples. When blood is tested, the patient draws a few drops of blood from a fingertip, places it on filter paper, and mails the paper to a company laboratory, which performs the standard HIV assay. If the results are positive, a confirmation test is performed. Home Access HIV-1 Test System was approved by the FDA in 1996. Individuals receive results in seven days (or sooner if express service is requested). Results and counseling are available by calling a 24-hour toll-free number and giving an identification code. Home Access claims an accuracy rate of 99.9%. The Home Access Express Test System and the OraQuick In-Home HIV Test described earlier were the only FDA-approved tests as of October 2015.

Critics of home testing suggest that news of HIV infection is not as easy to accept as the results of other in-home tests, such as those for pregnancy and cholesterol. They claim that most people cannot properly prepare themselves for the news that they have a life-threatening disease. They advocate the expansion of current testing sites to include mobile vans, sports clubs, and other places that are not exclusively associated with HIV testing, but where in-person counseling can be provided.

Military Practices

The U.S. Department of Defense (DOD) regularly screens all members of the armed services as well as those seeking to join for HIV. The DOD states in "Department of Defense: Instruction" (June 7, 2013, http://www.dtic.mil/whs/directives/corres/pdf/648501p.pdf) that its policy is to "deny eligibility for military service to persons with laboratory evidence of HIV infection for appointment, enlistment, pre-appointment, or initial entry training for military service." Biannual HIV testing is required of all personnel on active duty, as well as of all members of the reserves and National Guard. In 1995, after two months of debate in Congress, federal legislators scrapped a discharge provision that would have forced the DOD to dismiss members of the military within six months of testing positive for HIV. Along with HIV infection, a number of chronic conditions, including asthma, cancer, diabetes, heart disease, or complications of pregnancy, place troops on limited assignment, precluding them from overseas service or combat.

In "Epidemiology of HIV among US Air Force Military Personnel, 1996—2011" (*PLOS One*, May 11, 2015), Shilpa Hakre et al. look at the incidence and prevalence of HIV in the U.S. Air Force between 1996 and 2011.The researchers find the highest risk of HIV infection in the air force among young unmarried males who had not yet been deployed, especially those in higher risk occupation groups. Hakre et al. conclude that these young men "may benefit from more frequent HIV testing than the biennial compulsory force testing currently in place."

Pregnant Women and Newborns

The issue of testing newborns has placed the rights of mothers at odds with those of their newborns. States have kept HIV test results anonymous to preserve a mother's right to privacy. Civil libertarians (those that actively support the strengthening and protecting of individual rights and freedoms) and some groups that represent women, gays, and lesbians support anonymous testing, claiming that attaching names to test results would start local, state, and federal governments down the "slippery slope" of mandatory testing of adults. They also raise further privacy concerns, contending that once names are known, there is no guarantee they will not fall into the hands of employers, insurance companies, and others who might discriminate on the basis of HIV status.

The CDC recommends HIV testing of all pregnant women as a standard part of prenatal care to identify and treat HIV and to prevent transmission of HIV to infants. Testing is also advised for any newborn whose mother's HIV status is unknown. When treatment begins early in pregnancy, the risk of mother-to-child HIV transmission is reduced to 2% or less.

In May 1996 the U.S. House of Representatives and the U.S. Senate passed bills that would cut off federal money for HIV/AIDS treatment to states that failed to comply with the new disclosure requirements. In 1996 New York became the first state to mandate that health officials tell parents the results of HIV tests that the state routinely performs on all newborns. Before June 1996 parents in New York did not receive results unless they requested them, as was still the case in many states in 2015.

NEW JERSEY LEGISLATION MANDATES TESTING OF PREGNANT WOMEN AND SOME NEWBORNS. In 2007 New Jersey legislators approved a bill requiring pregnant women and some newborns—infants born to mothers who have tested positive or those whose HIV status is unknown at the time of birth—to be tested for HIV. The law requires that pregnant women be tested twice for HIV, once early and once late during the pregnancy, unless the mother specifically requests not to be tested.

Supporters of this legislation contend that the requirement for testing will save children's lives. Detractors argue that all infants of HIV-infected mothers test positive for HIV antibodies because they inherit their mother's antibodies. This initial positive result does not necessarily mean the infant is infected. Because it takes several months for the mother's antibodies to clear from the infant, it may be more prudent to test infants when they are between three and six months old to determine their HIV status. According to the Kaiser Family Foundation, in "New Jersey Legislature Approves Bill Requiring Pregnant Women, Some Infants to Receive HIV Tests" (June 25, 2007, http://www.kaiserhealthnews.org/daily-reports/2007/june/25/dr00045784.aspx?referrer=search), the American Civil Liberties Union and women's health advocacy groups assert that the legislation "deprives women of authority to make medical decisions."

Although the CDC recommends routine opt-out HIV screening of all pregnant women and newborn testing if the mother's HIV status is unknown, state policies vary. The National HIV/AIDS Clinicians' Consultation Center at the University of California, San Francisco, reports in *Compendium of State HIV Testing Laws—Perinatal Quick Reference Guide: Guide to States' Perinatal HIV Testing Laws for Clinicians* (April 2011, http://nccc.ucsf .edu/wp-content/uploads/2014/03/State_HIV_Testing _Laws_Perinatal_Quick_Reference.pdf) that as of 2011 (the most recent year for which data were available as of October 2015), 20 states, the District of Columbia, and Puerto Rico had no specific provisions regarding prenatal testing. The balance of the states had provisions for prenatal testing. Ten states had opt-out HIV testing—it is part of routine prenatal care and pregnant women are tested unless they refuse or "opt-out." The remaining 40 states had opt-in HIV testing of pregnant women—an HIV test is not part of routine prenatal care and pregnant women must specifically request or "opt-in" to receive an HIV test.

Health Care Workers

There has been a continuing debate over whether health care workers should be required to obtain HIV tests. As of 2015 there was no law requiring health care workers to submit to HIV testing, although many employers require it as a condition of employment. They cannot, however, discriminate against health care workers on the basis of their HIV status because like other employees, they are covered by the Americans with Disabilities Act of 1990, the federal law that prohibits discrimination against individuals with disabilities.

According to the CDC, in "HIV Transmission" (January 16, 2015, http://www.cdc.gov/hiv/basics/transmission .html), the risk of health care workers becoming infected with HIV on the job is very low, especially if they follow prudent safety measures known as universal precautions—gloves, goggles, and masks to prevent HIV and other blood-borne infections. The largest risk is posed by accidental needle-stick injuries, but even this risk is less than 1%.

Testing Policies in U.S. Prisons

Guidelines for the testing of inmates for HIV exist in all 50 states, in the District of Columbia, and in the regulations of the Federal Bureau of Prisons. However, the timing of testing varies. In "HIV in Correctional Settings" (June 2012, http://www.cdc.gov/hiv/resources/factsheets/ pdf/correctional.pdf), the CDC recommends that HIV screening be provided on entry into prison and before release and that voluntary HIV testing be offered periodically during incarceration.

The CDC acknowledges that some correctional systems face logistical, security, and financial constraints that hamper testing. Using rapid HIV tests within the first 24 hours after incarceration may overcome issues such as quick turnover of jail inmates. Laboratory costs associated with HIV testing and lack of familiarity with confidentiality and reporting requirements may be obstacles for some correctional systems.

PREVENTION
Critics Fault Programs' Focus and Funding

The objective of HIV-prevention programs is to reduce the number of new cases to as close to zero as possible. All prevention efforts are based on the belief that individuals can be educated in a way that will lead to changes in behavior, which will help bring an end to the spread of HIV/AIDS. However, many AIDS advocacy groups have long been critical of the ways the CDC has communicated this message. In 1987 CDC officials chose to emphasize the universality of AIDS, instead of focusing efforts on those most at risk: MSM and IDUs. According to AIDS advocates, this strategy misdirected the spending of available prevention dollars during the first decade of the epidemic. In 2015, although the number of infected people outside of these two groups was growing, HIV/AIDS was still largely a threat to MSM, IDUs, their partners, and their children. Most women with HIV/AIDS were IDUs or were sex partners of IDUs.

CDC Prevention Activities

The CDC's HIV-prevention strategy, as described in "About the Division of HIV/AIDS Prevention (DHAP)" (July 27, 2015, http://www.cdc.gov/hiv/dhap/about.html), aims to reduce the incidence and prevalence of HIV infection as well as the morbidity (illnesses) and mortality (deaths) that result from HIV infection by working with communities and other partners. The agency's efforts focus on four areas:

- Capacity building—strengthening and supporting the HIV-prevention workforce

- Program evaluation—assessing the effectiveness, costs, and impact of HIV-prevention strategies, policies, and programs

- Communication—developing and disseminating scientific and informative communications on HIV/AIDS for providers, people at risk, and the public

- Research—conducting research to design and test interventions to prevent HIV transmission

The prevention strategy capitalizes on rapid test technologies, interventions that bring people unaware of their HIV status to HIV testing, and behavioral interventions that provide prevention skills to people living with HIV/AIDS. To carry out its strategy, the CDC works in conjunction with governmental and nongovernmental partners to implement, evaluate, and further develop and strengthen effective HIV prevention efforts nationwide.

CDC health education and disease prevention efforts continue to emphasize that the most reliable ways to avoid HIV infection or virus transmission are by abstaining from sexual intercourse; maintaining a mutually monogamous, long-term relationship with a partner who is uninfected; and/or refraining from sharing needles and syringes in drug use. Although seemingly logical, critics contend that the CDC's emphasis on abstinence burdens people with an unrealistic expectation. Critics also point to the insistence on abstinence policies as a condition of U.S. government assistance for other countries' health programs to be an ill-advised foreign policy intrusion.

According to the Kaiser Family Foundation, in the fact sheet "U.S. Federal Funding for HIV/AIDS: The President's FY 2016 Budget Request" (April 2015, http://files .kff.org/attachment/fact-sheet-u-s-federal-funding-for-hivaids-the-presidents-fy-2016-budget-request), for FY 2016 just 3% of the budget allocation was for domestic HIV/AIDS-prevention activities, a 1.4% increase from FY 2015.

Prevention Efforts Aimed at Persons with HIV

In December 2014 the CDC in collaboration with a number of HIV/AIDS agencies and health care organizations released *Recommendations for HIV Prevention with Adults and Adolescents with HIV in the United States, 2014* (http://stacks.cdc.gov/view/cdc/26062). The recommendations identify challenges and offer strategies to overcome them including:

- Screening for behaviors that could transmit HIV and interventions to reduce the risk of transmission

- STI screening and treatment to the reduce the risk of HIV transmission

- Services for sex partners and drug-injection partners of people with HIV

- Individual, social, structural, ethical, legal, policy, and programmatic factors that influence HIV transmission and use of HIV-prevention and care services

- Use of antiretroviral therapy (ART) to improve health and prevent HIV transmission and approaches to

achieve ongoing adherence to ART to reduce infectiousness

- Reproductive health care to reduce the risk of HIV transmission when attempting conception or in unintended pregnancies

- Monitoring, evaluating, and improving the quality of HIV prevention and care services and programs for people with HIV

Table 8.1 identifies some prevention challenges—the factors that may affect the health and lives of adolescents with HIV and some of the recommended services to address some of these barriers to access to care.

Figure 8.1 shows strategies that reduce infectiousness of HIV and the risk of exposure, which together may act to reduce the number of people newly infected with HIV and improve the health and life spans of people with HIV.

EDUCATING YOUTH

Although most states offer prevention programs for students in public schools, as noted in Chapter 7, the prevalence of HIV education in school fell between 1992 and 2013. Further, youths who are not in school may not have ready access to such programs. Many homeless shelters and local health departments employ roving counselors who seek out these young people to offer prevention information and direct them to health and social service agencies.

Sexual Health Education

Many education programs offer students sufficient information about STIs and HIV/AIDS, but only quality education affects behavior. In "The Effectiveness of Group-Based Comprehensive Risk-Reduction and Abstinence Education Interventions to Prevent or Reduce the Risk of Adolescent Pregnancy, Human Immunodeficiency

TABLE 8.1

Factors that affect the health and access to care of adolescents with HIV

Factor(s)	Possible effect on health, quality of life, HIV transmission, and use of services	Examples of specialty services
Adolescence and legal minor status	Factors may • hinder access to HIV services because of lack of awareness about ability to access services without parental consent and concern about confidentiality of medical records • preclude having an established health care provider, having experience navigating HIV services, or having documents to confirm eligibility for HIV services (e.g., family income records needed for medical assistance programs) • hinder access to age-appropriate specialty services (youth-friendly services) • hinder HIV disclosure because of fear of parental abuse, loss of financial support or housing, or stigma about sexual or drug activity	• Youth-friendly services • Health literacy and peer education services • Psychosocial counseling and support services (e.g., group counseling, peer support) • Housing services for homeless youth • Case management and navigation assistance to assist with care coordination

SOURCE: Adapted from "Table 12-1. Factors That Can Influence Health, Quality of Life Risk of HIV Transmission, and Use of HIV Prevention, Medical, and Social Services among Persons with HIV; and Specialty Services That Address These Factors," in *Recommendations for HIV Prevention with Adults and Adolescents with HIV in the United States, 2014*, Centers for Disease Control and Prevention, Health Resources and Services Administration, National Institutes of Health, American Academy of HIV Medicine, Association of Nurses in AIDS Care, International Association of Providers of AIDS Care, the National Minority AIDS Council, and Urban Coalition for HIV/AIDS Prevention Services, December 11, 2014, http://stacks.cdc.gov/view/cdc/26062 (accessed August 6, 2015)

FIGURE 8.1

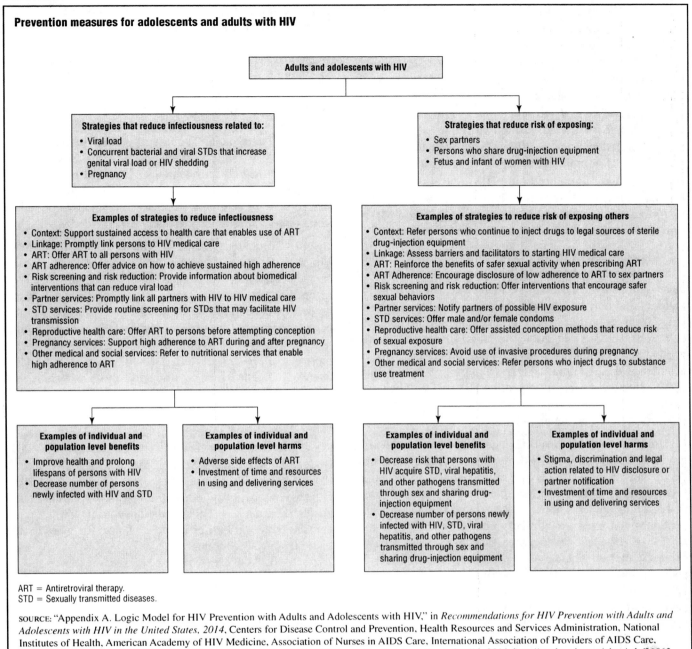

Prevention measures for adolescents and adults with HIV

ART = Antiretroviral therapy.
STD = Sexually transmitted diseases.

SOURCE: "Appendix A. Logic Model for HIV Prevention with Adults and Adolescents with HIV," in *Recommendations for HIV Prevention with Adults and Adolescents with HIV in the United States, 2014*, Centers for Disease Control and Prevention, Health Resources and Services Administration, National Institutes of Health, American Academy of HIV Medicine, Association of Nurses in AIDS Care, International Association of Providers of AIDS Care, the National Minority AIDS Council, and Urban Coalition for HIV/AIDS Prevention Services, December 11, 2014, http://stacks.cdc.gov/view/cdc/26062 (accessed August 6, 2015)

Virus, and Sexually Transmitted Infections: Two Systematic Reviews for the Guide to Community Preventive Services" (*American Journal of Preventive Medicine*, vol. 42, no. 3, March 2012), Helen B. Chin et al. examine interventions that address the sexual behavior of adolescents such as use of condoms by sexually active teenagers and aim to reduce the incidence of pregnancy, HIV, and other STIs in this group. They also look at abstinence education, which has as its exclusive purpose teaching the social, psychological, and health gains to be realized by abstaining from sexual activity.

Chin et al. find that comprehensive risk-reduction programs delayed or decreased sexual behaviors and/or increased condom and contraceptive use. Although the abstinence education interventions showed a potentially meaningful effect on sexual activity, the researchers find that these interventions did not have a significant effect on the frequency of sexual activity.

The provision of comprehensive sex education remained controversial in 2015. Some people do not agree that information about sexual health or decisions should be offered in public schools, preferring that parents instill their own values in their children. However, others point out that some parents never talk to their children about sex and drugs and that school may be the only place a child can get reliable information. According to the Guttmacher Institute, in "State Policies in Brief: Sex and STI/HIV Education" (October 1, 2015, http://www.guttmacher.org/statecenter/spibs/spib_SE.pdf), 33 states and the District of Columbia required HIV/AIDS prevention education in 2015. Twenty states and the District of Columbia required HIV education and sex education, and 13 required only HIV education. Twenty-two states and the District of Columbia required schools to notify parents that HIV education or sex education will be provided to students.

Although laws vary from state to state, and some states allow local school districts to decide on curricula, many of these states have one or more mandates determining the material that may be taught in the programs. The mandates range from requiring age-appropriate materials, to teaching comprehensive sex education programs (advocating contraceptive and condom use), to providing programs in which abstinence from premarital sex is presented as the only 100% effective means of preventing HIV/AIDS. The Guttmacher Institute notes that in 2015 only 13 states required the information that is taught be medically accurate.

Federal funding for abstinence-only educational programs was initiated in 1998. Proponents of these programs claim they change attitudes about casual sex by reducing both teen pregnancies and rates of STIs. They also maintain that teaching students about contraceptive and condom use condones, or even encourages, unsafe sexual behavior. Critics of these programs argue that there is no reliable evidence that abstinence-only programs are effective. In addition, they contend that for the five out of 10 teens aged 15 to 19 years who do choose to have sex, lack of knowledge about contraception and condom use will result only in continued teen pregnancies, STIs, and HIV infections.

The U.S. Department of Health and Human Services concludes in *Review of Comprehensive Sex Education Curricula* (May 2007) that abstinence-only education is ineffective. The review finds that students given abstinence-only education were no more likely to abstain from sex, that those who had sex did so with a similar number of partners as those who had not received abstinence-only education, and that students first had sex at the same age, independent of the type of education they had received.

In "Invited Commentary: Broadening the Evidence for Adolescent Sexual and Reproductive Health and Education in the United States" (*Journal of Youth and Adolescence*, vol. 14, no. 10, October 2014), Amy T. Schalet et al. explain that from 1998 to 2009, federal funding for was almost exclusively for ineffective and scientifically

inaccurate abstinence-only-until-marriage (AOUM) programs. During this period, the federal government spent nearly $2 billion for AOUM programs. Since 2009, funding AOUM programs has decreased but federal and state-funded AOUM programs are still offered, despite scientific and human rights concerns raised by medical and public health organizations, including "concerns about scientific accuracy, the withholding of life-saving information from young people, a lack of program efficacy, promotion of gender and racial stereotypes, insensitivity to non-heterosexual youth, and harm to traditional sexual health education." Rigorous evaluations of AOUM programs find that they do not delay initiation of sexual intercourse, reduce the number of partners, increase condom use, or reduce sexual intercourse among sexually experienced youth.

In "Community-Based Abstinence Education Project: Program Outcomes" (*Nursing Forum*, vol. 50, no. 1, January–March 2015), Denise Nagle Bailey and Zane Robinson Wolf concede that although there is little evidence that abstinence education is broadly effective, it may be useful in certain communities and with specific religious and cultural groups. Bailey and Wolf assert that the abstinence-only message offers the greatest potential benefit for children attending middle school, particularly those who may lack the knowledge to protect themselves by making choices and decisions to reduce their risk of HIV infection.

The Sexuality Information and Education Council of the United States notes in "The President's FY 2016 Budget Shows Strong Support for Effective Adolescent Sexual Health Promotion Programs" (February 3, 2015, http://www.siecus.org/index.cfm?fuseaction=feature.show Feature&FeatureID=2395&varuniqueuserid=74691326832) that the budget does not include funding for what it calls "harmful" AOUM programs.

CONDOM USE

In the fact sheet "Condoms and STDs: Fact Sheet for Public Health Personnel" (March 25, 2013, http://www.cdc.gov/condomeffectiveness/latex.htm), the CDC indicates that studies provide compelling evidence that latex condoms are highly effective in protecting against HIV infection when used properly for every act of intercourse. However, the agency warns that "the most reliable ways to avoid transmission of sexually transmitted diseases (STDs), including human immunodeficiency virus (HIV), are to abstain from sexual activity or to be in a long-term mutually monogamous relationship with an uninfected partner."

The CDC's analysis of data from the Youth Risk Behavior Surveys conducted between 1991 and 2013 finds that U.S. high school students are engaging in fewer HIV-related risk behaviors—decreasing percentages of students reported being sexually active and having had sexual intercourse with four or more people during their life. Condom use increased between 1991 and 2003, but since then has leveled off. Condom use among sexually active students rose to 59.1% in 2013 from 46.2% in 1991. (See Table 5.9 in Chapter 5.)

Other Forms of Protection

In 1993 the FDA approved Reality, a female condom that serves as a mechanical barrier to viruses. The condom is designed for women and protects against STIs, including HIV. It is made of polyurethane (a resin made of two different compounds used in elastic fibers, cushions, and various molded products) and is unlikely to rip or tear. The condom is prelubricated and is intended for use during only one sex act.

The use of female condoms is low. Margaret R. Weeks et al. cite in "Initial and Sustained Female Condom Use among Low-Income Urban U.S. Women" (*Journal of Women's Health*, vol. 22, no. 1, January 2013) the findings of a Hartford, Connecticut, study— that 29% of women had ever used female condoms before the study but after a demonstration of their use and given free samples, nearly three-quarters (73%) of never users reported sustained use. Weeks et al. assert that women will use female condoms when they are educated about them and given free trial samples and call for inclusion of this approach in standard clinical practice and public health education.

CIRCUMCISION MAY SLOW THE SPREAD OF HIV

According to the press release "WHO and UNAIDS Announce Recommendations from Expert Consultation on Male Circumcision for HIV Prevention" (March 28, 2007, http://www.who.int/hiv/mediacentre/news68/en/index.html), in 2007 the World Health Organization (WHO) and the Joint United Nations Programme on HIV/AIDS (UNAIDS) recommended circumcision as a strategy to prevent heterosexually acquired HIV infection in men. Circumcision (the surgical removal of the foreskin from the penis) has long been thought to reduce men's susceptibility to HIV infection because the skin cells in the foreskin are especially vulnerable to the virus. Kevin De Cock, the director of the WHO HIV/AIDS Department, asserted that "countries with high rates of heterosexual HIV infection and low rates of male circumcision now have an additional intervention which can reduce the risk of HIV infection in heterosexual men. Scaling up male circumcision in such countries will result in immediate benefit to individuals. However, it will be a number of years before we can expect to see an impact on the epidemic from such investment."

Three randomized clinical trials conducted in sub-Saharan Africa demonstrate that circumcision reduces HIV incidence. In "The Long Term Efficacy of Medical Male Circumcision against HIV Acquisition" (*AIDS*, July 3, 2013), Supriya D. Mehta et al. assessed 2,784 men aged 18 to 24 years who were randomly assigned to immediate circumcision in December 2006 or to a control group, which was not circumcised. The men were followed through September 2010 and circumcision was found to reduce HIV infection by 60%.

SYRINGE EXCHANGE PROGRAMS

IDUs often share the syringes they use to inject drugs into their body. When an HIV-positive IDU uses a syringe, he or she may contaminate it with HIV-positive blood that can then spread the disease to other IDUs who use that syringe. Syringe exchange programs (SEPs) attempt to prevent the spread of HIV in this manner by encouraging IDUs to bring in their used, unsafe syringes and exchange them for new, safe syringes. The reasoning behind these programs is that if people are going to use drugs, at least an effort can be made to make sure they do not contract HIV because of it. Proponents of these programs point out that the spread of HIV among IDUs threatens everyone, as people who contract HIV through drug use can then pass it on to their sexual partners and children.

Despite these arguments, SEPs are highly controversial due to their connection to drug use. Some opponents see them as helping IDUs avoid the consequences of their actions, or even providing them with the means to continue their illegal activities. In April 1998, after much debate, the administration of President Bill Clinton (1946–) decided not to lift a nine-year-old ban on federal financing for programs to distribute clean needles to drug addicts. This meant that state and local governments that received federal block grants for HIV/AIDS prevention were not permitted to use this money for SEPs. Public health experts and advocates for people with HIV/AIDS criticized the decision. The ban was lifted in 2009, and state and local health authorities sought and obtained federal funds for SEPs. However, the ban was reinstated in late 2011 and was still in full force as of October 2015.

The Foundation for AIDS Research (amfAR) details in "Syringe Exchange Program Coverage in the United States—June 2014" (2014, https://nasen.org/site_media/files/amfar-sep-map/amfar-sep-map-2014.pdf) the location of SEPs by state. In 2014 there were 194 SEPs in 33 states, the District of Columbia, Puerto Rico, and the Native American nations. Overall, 196 cities had SEPs.

SEPs Reduce Risk of HIV Transmission

In "Are Needle and Syringe Programmes Associated with a Reduction in HIV Transmission among People Who Inject Drugs: A Systematic Review and Meta-analysis" (*International Journal of Epidemiology*, vol. 43, no. 1, February 2014), Esther J. Aspinall et al. looked at 12 studies that assessed the effectiveness of needle and SEPs to reduce HIV transmission and infection. The investigators found evidence that the programs reduced HIV transmission, which supports previous study findings that these programs are important elements of HIV prevention efforts.

In "State Laws, Syringe Exchange, and HIV among Persons Who Inject Drugs in the United States: History and Effectiveness" (*Journal of Public Health Policy*, vol. 36, no. 1, May 2015), Heidi Bramson et al. confirm that public funding of SEPs is associated with lower rates of HIV infection, greater numbers of syringes distributed, and greater numbers of health and social services provided. Bramson et al. opine, "Experience in the United States may prove useful in other countries: state, provincial, and local governments may need to move ahead of central governments in addressing HIV infection among persons who inject drugs."

Trang Quynh Nguyen et al. estimated the impact on HIV transmission of increased investment in SEPs. The researchers analyzed costs associated with the supply and exchange of syringes and their impact on syringe sharing and contamination, and estimated the number of HIV infections averted and HIV treatment costs avoided. In "Syringe Exchange in the United States: A National Level Economic Evaluation of Hypothetical Increases in Investment" (*AIDS and Behavior*, vol. 18, no. 11, November 2014), Nguyen et al. find that with an annual $10 million to $50 million increase in funding increase, 194 to 816 HIV infections would be averted. The cost per infection averted ranged from $51,601 to $61,302. The researchers aver, "These analyses indicate that it would be highly cost-saving to invest additional funds to expand syringe exchange services in the U.S. Over the course of one year an additional investment of only $10 million would avert an estimated 194 HIV infections and avoid $75.8 million in lifetime HIV treatment costs."

PHYSICIANS SUPPORT ACCESS TO STERILE SYRINGES FOR IDUS. In many states syringe prescription laws effectively block access to sterile syringes for IDUs. Pharmacists may be reluctant to sell syringes to suspected IDUs, and police may take possession of syringes or arrest IDUs who cannot demonstrate a medical need, other than injection drug use of illegal drugs, for the syringes they possess. These barriers could be eliminated by physician prescription of syringes.

Grace E. Macalino et al. conducted the first national survey of physicians to determine their willingness to prescribe syringes for IDUs and reported the results in "A National Physician Survey on Prescribing Syringes as an HIV Prevention Measure" (*Substance Abuse Treatment, Prevention, and Policy*, vol. 4, June 8, 2009). The researchers find that despite the fact that physicians have, in general, never actually prescribed syringes to IDUs, most

would consider doing so. Macalino et al. conclude, "The physicians in our study were generally amenable to participating in syringe prescription programs, but physician willingness to act can be supported by better communication of what constitutes evidence-based practice, alleviation of legal concerns, and explicit validation by peers and professional organizations. Requiring substance abuse as a subject in medical training and continuing medical education would also promote better care for IDUs."

In "Threading the Needle—How to Stop the HIV Outbreak in Rural Indiana" (*New England Journal of Medicine*, vol. 37, no. 5, July 30, 2015), Steffanie A. Strathdee and Chris Beyrer assert that lifting the ban on using federal funds to support needle-exchange programs is a crucial component of HIV prevention since these programs reduce HIV incidence. Strathdee and Beyrer exhort physicians to provide IDUs with sterile syringes or refer them to places where they can obtain them and to support legislative reforms to expand Medicaid and to allow federal funds to support needle-exchange programs. They call for state action to support needle-exchange programs and legal access to over-the-counter syringe purchase without a prescription.

Legal Barriers to Federal Funding of SEPs

Despite the preponderance of evidence from myriad sources that SEPs are effective strategies for the prevention of HIV transmission, the federal government, as well as most local and state governments, have not made them legal. They argue that taxpayers should not finance illicit drug use. Since 1988 Congress has passed at least six laws that contain provisions that specifically prohibit or restrict the use of federal funds for SEPs and activities. The Comprehensive Alcohol Abuse, Drug Abuse, and Mental Health Amendments Act of 1988 requires states, as a condition for receiving block grant funds, to agree that funds will not be used "to carry out any program of distributing sterile needles for the hypodermic injection of any illegal drug or bleach for the purpose of cleansing needles for such hypodermic injection."

SEP advocates were heartened by a 2011 determination by Regina Benjamin (1956–), the U.S. surgeon general. In "Determination That a Demonstration Needle Exchange Program Would Be Effective in Reducing Drug Abuse and the Risk of Acquired Immune Deficiency Syndrome Infection among Intravenous Drug Users" (*Federal Register*, vol. 76, no. 36, February 23, 2011), Benjamin opined that SEPs "would be effective in reducing drug abuse and the risk of infection with the etiologic agent for acquired immune deficiency syndrome" and that the scientific evidence supporting the health benefits of SEPs fulfills "the statutory requirement permitting the expenditure of Substance Abuse Prevention and Treatment (SAPT) Block Grant funds."

The same year, the administration of President Barack Obama (1961–) designated needle exchanges as a drug treatment program, allowing federal money allocated to treat addictions to be used to distribute syringes and needles to IDUs. According to Scott McCabe, in "White House Moves to Fund Needle Exchanges as Drug Treatment" (WashingtonExaminer.com, March 19, 2012), Benjamin indicated "that needle exchange programs can serve as a gateway to treatment for drug addiction, HIV and other diseases" and endorsed the use of federal funds. However, later that year Congress reinstated the ban.

Austin Coleman observes in "Needle Exchange Programs" (June 25, 2015, http://knowledgecenter.csg.org/kc/content/needle-exchange-programs) that the United States has one of the lowest rates of needle-exchange availability in the developed world. The use of federal funds for needle exchange programs has been banned since 1988, with a brief period of reversal between 2009 and 2011. He reports that 16 states and the District of Columbia have provisions explicitly authorizing needle-exchange programs, but notes that "the lack of federal funding has slowed adoption."

Coleman cites ENCORE (Education, Needle Exchange, Counseling, Outreach and Referral), located in Rhode Island, as a model program in the United States. ENCORE provides services in five cities, using a combination of fixed sites and mobile exchange units. In addition to providing new syringes, alcohol swabs, antibiotic ointment, ascorbic acid, adhesive bandages, biohazard sharps containers, cookers, cotton, rubber tip covers, sterile water, and tourniquets in order to reduce harm and reduce the spread of HIV and other diseases, it provides disease testing and treatment and counseling services.

CHAPTER 9

HIV AND AIDS WORLDWIDE

Ending the AIDS epidemic as a public health threat by 2030 is ambitious, but realistic, as the history of the past 15 years has shown.

—Michel Sidibé, Joint United Nations Programme on HIV/AIDS Executive Director and Under-Secretary-General of the United Nations, *How AIDS Changed Everything* (2015)

SCOPE OF THE PROBLEM

Few factors have changed global demographics as inalterably as the HIV/AIDS pandemic (worldwide epidemic). The Joint United Nations Programme on HIV/AIDS (UNAIDS) says in *Fact Sheet 2014* (2014, http://www.unaids.org/sites/default/files/en/media/unaids/contentassets/documents/factsheet/2014/20140716_FactSheet_en.pdf) that an estimated 35 million people were living with HIV/AIDS in 2013. Nearly three-quarters of people living with HIV were in sub-Saharan Africa.

The number of new HIV infections reported each year has been in decline, from a peak of 3.2 million in 1997 to approximately 2.1 million in 2013. The decline in HIV incidence is attributable not only to the effectiveness of HIV prevention activities but also to the natural course of HIV epidemics. The prevalence of HIV in a population does not increase indefinitely, because at some point the population is saturated. Generally, after the initial spread of HIV there is likely to be a decrease in the incidence of infection, which results in a decrease in prevalence.

The global HIV/AIDS pandemic is actually many separate epidemics, each with its own distinctive origin and shaped by specific geography and populations. Each epidemic involves different risk behaviors and practices, such as unprotected sex with multiple partners or sharing injection drug equipment. According to UNAIDS, some countries have made tremendous strides in expanding and ensuring access to treatment. It also notes that there has been progress in advancing HIV prevention

programs—new HIV infections are declining in many countries that have been hardest hit by the epidemic and some of the big epidemics in sub-Saharan Africa have stabilized or are beginning to decline.

However, the epidemics are not subsiding everywhere. For example, in Indonesia, new HIV infections increased 48% between 2005 and 2013 and new infections rose 5% in eastern Europe and central Asia and 7% in the Middle East and North Africa during the same period.

UNAIDS reports that AIDS-related deaths fell 35% between their peak in 2005 and 2013. It estimated that 37% of all people living with HIV (12.9 million) had access to antiretroviral therapy (ART) in 2013. While this is a significant percentage, the Kaiser Family Foundation (KFF) reports in "The Global HIV/AIDS Epidemic" (July 31, 2015, http://kff.org/global-health-policy/fact-sheet/the-global-hivaids-epidemic) that most people living with HIV/AIDS or at risk for HIV do not have access to prevention, care, and treatment.

Global Trends

UNAIDS explains in *How AIDS Changed Everything* (2015, http://www.unaids.org/sites/default/files/media_asset/MDG6Report_en.pdf) that although fewer people are becoming HIV infected and fewer are dying from AIDS, HIV/AIDS remains a global health problem of enormous scope.

According to the KFF, in "The Global HIV/AIDS Epidemic," the global prevalence rate (the percentage of people aged 15 to 49 years who are infected) has leveled off since 2001 and was 0.8% in 2014. The KFF explains that HIV disproportionately affects people during their most productive years; 38% of all new infections occur in people under the age of 25 years. The KFF reports that there were 1.2 million AIDS deaths in 2014. This was down 42% since 2004, but clearly AIDS remains a deadly threat to many people, and in fact it was the leading cause of death in Africa in 2014.

In "A New Infectious Disease Model for Estimating and Projecting HIV/AIDS Epidemics" (*Sexually Transmitted Infections*, vol. 8, suppl. 2, December 2012), Le Bao of Pennsylvania State University observes that as the global HIV pandemic entered its fourth decade, countries have collected more surveillance data and the AIDS-related mortality has been substantially reduced by the increasing availability and use of ART. Bao presents a model that enables the HIV infection rate to change over the years in response to past prevalence and the past infection rate as the epidemic in a country stabilizes. This model also considers the impact of prevention programs and helps policy makers and planners grade their epidemics as generalized, concentrated, or low level. In generalized epidemics HIV prevalence is more than 1% in pregnant women in urban areas. By contrast, in low-level and concentrated epidemics HIV infection is not at a significant level in the general population, although in concentrated epidemics it is high in at-risk populations such as injection drug users (IDUs) and men who have sex with men (MSM).

PATTERNS OF INFECTION

Globally, HIV/AIDS is primarily a sexually transmitted infection (STI) that is spread through unprotected sexual intercourse between men and women or MSM. Like some other STIs, HIV can also be spread through blood, blood products, donated organs, semen, or vaginal fluids and perinatally from a pregnant mother to her unborn child. The majority of worldwide cumulative (over the entire time that statistics have been kept) HIV infections in adults are estimated to have been transmitted through heterosexual intercourse, although the relative proportion of infections resulting from heterosexual contact as opposed to MSM varies greatly in different parts of the world.

More than 90% of children with HIV acquired the virus perinatally, during birth, or through breast-feeding. The balance were infected by contaminated injections, transfusion with infected blood, sexual abuse, or sexual intercourse.

HIV-1 and HIV-2

Kevin Peterson et al. explain in "Antiretroviral Therapy for HIV-2 Infection: Recommendations for Management in Low-Resource Settings" (*AIDS Research and Treatment*, February 9, 2011) that two types of HIV have been recognized and identified: HIV-1, the predominant worldwide virus, and HIV-2. HIV-2 has much lower rates of progression and infectivity than does HIV-1, and the majority of people that become infected are likely to be long-term nonprogressors (people who become infected

but do not develop AIDS). HIV-2 also responds differently to antiretroviral drugs and is frequently resistant to two of the major classes of antiretroviral drugs—the fusion inhibitors and the nonnucleoside reverse transcriptase inhibitors—that are the standard treatment for HIV-1.

HIV-1 and HIV-2 also show an extraordinary difference in global distribution. In North and South America HIV-1 has reached pandemic proportions among certain risk groups, primarily through MSM and IDUs. Some African and Asian countries have also experienced extensive heterosexual transmission of HIV-1. HIV-2 is largely restricted to West Africa, where it is mostly attributable to heterosexual transmission and accounts for one-third of the HIV prevalence cases. Other countries with sizable populations infected with HIV-2 are European countries with colonial links to West Africa, such as France, Portugal, and the United Kingdom, as well as other countries with previous Portuguese ties, such as Angola, Brazil, India, and Mozambique.

In "Characteristics of HIV-2 and HIV-1/HIV-2 Dually Seropositive Adults in West Africa Presenting for Care and Antiretroviral Therapy: The IeDEA-West Africa HIV-2 Cohort Study" (*PLoS One*, vol. 8, no. 6, June 18, 2013), Didier K. Ekouevi et al. observe that HIV-2 is widespread in West Africa and many people are infected with both HIV-1 and HIV-2. The researchers also note that HIV-2 may be underreported because antibody cross-reactivity between HIV-1 and HIV-2 is common and often results in misdiagnosis of HIV-2 as HIV-1 or dual infection. Ekouevi et al. assert that clinical trials to determine optimal treatment for people with dual infection are needed.

DIFFERENCES IN EPIDEMIOLOGY, INCIDENCE, AND TRANSMISSION. The epidemiological characteristics (factors such as distribution, incidence, and prevalence that determine the presence, extent, or absence of a disease) of HIV-2 are different from those of HIV-1. Perhaps reflecting these differences, the international spread of HIV-2 is quite limited. During the early course of infection, people with HIV-2 are less infectious than those with HIV-1. This is due to the low levels of the virus found in the blood of immunodeficient people with HIV-2. Over time, as an individual's immunodeficiency progresses, HIV-2 probably becomes more infectious, but this more infectious period is relatively shorter than for HIV-1 and tends to occur in older individuals.

According to Elizabeth Pádua et al., in "Assessment of Mother-to-Child HIV-1 and HIV-2 Transmission: An AIDS Reference Laboratory Collaborative Study" (*HIV Medicine*, vol. 10, no. 3, March 2009), multiple studies demonstrate evidence that HIV-2 is not frequently transmitted from mother to child. Although the mechanics of perinatal transmission are not completely understood, advanced immunodeficiency of the mother is certainly a risk factor. Low levels of the virus are not sufficient to transmit to the baby, and higher levels of virus infection in women past childbearing years may explain why perinatal transmission is less frequent. This is the most likely explanation for the observation that HIV-2 infection is so rare in children.

In "Mortality Rates in People Dually Infected with HIV-1/2 and Those Infected with Either HIV-1 or HIV-2: A Systematic Review and Meta-analysis" (*AIDS*, vol. 4, no. 28, February 20, 2014), Puck D. Prince et al. reviewed many studies to compare disease progression and mortality in people with both HIV-1 and HIV-2 infection with those infected with either HIV-1 or HIV-2. Prince et al. find that people infected with just HIV-2 have lower mortality rates than those who are infected with HIV-1 alone or those who are infected with both types of HIV.

INTERACTION OF HIV AND OTHER SEXUALLY TRANSMITTED DISEASES

One of the major concerns of public health officials worldwide is the possible interaction between HIV and other infections. The same risky behaviors that expose individuals to potential HIV infection also expose them to other sexually transmitted diseases (STDs), such as gonorrhea, syphilis, and chancroid (a genital ulcer). Considerable data suggest that other STDs, particularly herpes simplex, chancroid, and syphilis (which all cause ulcerative lesions), promote the transmission of HIV.

In "Infectious Co-factors in HIV-1 Transmission Herpes Simplex Virus Type-2 and HIV-1: New Insights and Interventions" (*Current HIV Research*, vol. 10, no. 3, April 2012), Ruanne V. Barnabas and Connie Celum observe that there is a strong relationship between genital herpes simplex virus type 2 (HSV-2) and HIV; HSV-2 infection significantly increases the risk of HIV acquisition.

TUBERCULOSIS AND HIV/AIDS

HIV infection is recognized as the strongest known risk factor for the development of active tuberculosis (TB), because people with a latent TB infection are more apt to develop the disease once their immune system has been compromised by HIV. According to the World Health Organization (WHO), in *Guidelines for Intensified Tuberculosis Case-Finding and Isoniazid Preventive Therapy for People Living with HIV in Resource-Constrained Settings* (2011, http://whqlibdoc.who.int/publications/2011/9789241500708_eng.pdf), people with HIV have 20 to 37 times the risk of developing TB as people without HIV infection. More than one-quarter of all deaths of people with HIV are attributable to TB.

UNAIDS notes in *Fact Sheet 2014* that although TB was still a leading cause of death among people with HIV between 2004 and 2013, TB-related deaths among people living with HIV/AIDS fell 33% worldwide. TB claimed the lives of an estimated 360,000 people with HIV in 2013. However, the percentage of HIV-infected tuberculosis patients that started or continued on ART rose from 60% in 2012 to 70% in 2013.

People infected with HIV who test tuberculin-positive are not only much more likely to develop TB, they are also likely to develop TB more rapidly than people without HIV infection. An even more disastrous consequence is that half of all people infected with both will develop contagious TB, which they could then spread to susceptible people, even those not infected with HIV.

The WHO 2011 guidelines offer recommendations that are intended to reduce TB in people living with HIV/AIDS, their families, and their communities via a combination of screening for TB and preventive therapy. The guidelines advise screening all people with HIV for TB and treating those with positive test results prophylactically (to prevent the disease from becoming active). Furthermore, they advise starting all HIV-infected people who also have active TB on ART regardless of their CD4 cell counts.

ART reduces the risk of TB among HIV-infected people by 65%. UNAIDS states that tuberculosis-related AIDS deaths fell from 520,000 in 2001 to 348,000 in 2014 and that its goal is that there will be no such deaths in 2030. It reports that among 41 countries with the highest burden of HIV-TB coinfection, 17 were estimated to have met the target for reducing mortality by 50% by 2013.

Highly Drug-Resistant Tuberculosis

In *TB/HIV Facts 2012–2013* (2013, http://www.who.int/hiv/topics/tb/tbhiv_facts_2013/en), UNAIDS observes that people living with HIV/AIDS are at a greater risk from multidrug-resistant tuberculosis (MDR-TB), a type of TB that does not respond to two first-line anti-TB drugs, than people who are not HIV infected. There were an estimated 310,000 MDR-TB cases worldwide in 2011. Extensively drug-resistant tuberculosis (XDR-TB), a type of TB that does not respond to first- or second-line anti-TB drug treatments, is rarer than MDR-TB but is associated with extremely high mortality rates in people with HIV/AIDS.

To a large extent, drug-resistant TB occurs in response to inadequate TB control, poor patient or clinician adherence to TB treatment regimens, poor-quality drugs, or a lack of drug supplies. People living with HIV/AIDS are particularly vulnerable to developing drug-resistant TB because of their compromised immune system, which makes them more susceptible to infection and more likely to progress to active TB.

Disparities in access to health care and the quality of health care exacerbate the problem of drug-resistant TB in developing countries. MDR- and XDR-TB arose largely in response to inadequate care of poor and neglected populations. Inappropriate drug choices, drug doses, and duration of treatment, as well as an irregular supply of drugs, poorly trained personnel, and poor adherence to treatment, all act to increase the development and transmission of drug-resistant TB.

Promising Research

New anti-TB drugs are urgently needed to overcome drug resistance and to eliminate TB as a public health threat. Keith D. Green and Sylvie Garneau-Tsodikova explain in "Resistance in Tuberculosis: What Do We Know and Where Can We Go?" (*Frontiers in Microbiology*, vol. 4, July 23, 2013) that current strategies focus on generating compounds that will avoid or overcome the defenses of *Mycobacterium tuberculosis* (*Mtb*). Research is being carried out to find new compounds that will disrupt deoxyribonucleic acid, cell membrane biosynthesis, and general cellular metabolism. Other studies combine drugs to achieve effects greater than those achieved by either alone.

In "Antituberculosis Thiophenes Define a Requirement for Pks13 in Mycolic Acid Biosynthesis" (*Nature Chemical Biology*, vol. 9, no. 8, August 2013), Regina Wilson et al. report on a new class of compounds that kill *Mtb* by dissolving its protective fatty coating. The compounds, known as thiophenes, killed *Mtb* in the laboratory by disabling an enzyme that connects the fatty acids that coat the bacterium. More important, it appears that TB does not develop resistance to this class of compounds. Researchers hope that these compounds may be used to develop more effective TB treatments.

UNAIDS Calls for TB Testing of Every Person Living with HIV/AIDS

Since 2013 UNAIDS has called for zero parallel systems for HIV and TB. Under this ideal, "every person living with HIV/AIDS is tested for TB and . . . every person with TB is offered an HIV test, and people with TB who are HIV-positive are started on antiretroviral treatment immediately." The fact sheet *HIV/AIDS* (July 2015, http://www.who.int/mediacentre/factsheets/fs360/en) reiterates the importance of TB testing and treatment.

GEOGRAPHIC DIFFERENCES

In North America and Europe during the 1980s and early 1990s, HIV was transmitted predominantly through unprotected sexual intercourse among MSM and among IDUs who shared contaminated needles. Since that time, heterosexual contact has also become an important means of transmission in these regions.

In sub-Saharan Africa the overwhelming mode of transmission has been heterosexual intercourse. In this part of the world, transmission through MSM contact or through injection drug use is slight. Because many women have been infected, preventing perinatal transmission is very important. UNAIDS notes in *How AIDS Changed Everything* that the increasing numbers and percentages of HIV-infected pregnant women receiving antiretroviral drugs to prevent mother-to-child transmission of HIV has effectively reduced transmission.

The rates of MSM transmission in Latin America are similar to those of Europe and the United States, injection drug use transmission is less frequent, and heterosexual transmission is considerably higher. Furthermore, there are high rates of transmission among IDUs and sex workers and their clients.

The number of new HIV infections in Asia decreased in the early 21st century, but increased 3% between 2010 and 2014. China, India, and Indonesia accounted for more than three-quarters (78%) of new HIV infections in the region in 2014. The highest national HIV infection levels in Asia continued to be found in Southeast Asia, where combinations of unsafe practices with sex workers and MSM, along with injection drug use, continue to fuel and maintain the epidemics. Although the HIV infection rate had peaked and leveled off in other parts of the world, it was escalating in Bangladesh, China, Indonesia, Pakistan, and Vietnam, largely from heterosexual intercourse and through sex workers.

Unless otherwise noted, the following data and statistics, which describe the epidemics in various regions and countries, are drawn from UNAIDS reports, especially *The Gap Report* (2014, http://www.unaids.org/sites/default/files/en/media/unaids/contentassets/documents/unaidspublication/2014/UNAIDS_Gap_report_en.pdf). UNAIDS and the WHO provide the most recent and reliable estimates of HIV incidence and prevalence, generally from 2011 to 2014.

NORTH AFRICA AND THE MIDDLE EAST

Unreliable and often inadequate HIV surveillance systems complicate an accurate assessment of the patterns and trends of the epidemics in many countries in North Africa and the Middle East, especially among high-risk populations—IDUs, MSM, and sex workers and their clients. UNAIDS reports in "July 2015 Core Epidemiology Slides" (July 2015, http://www.unaids.org/sites/default/files/media_asset/20150714_epi_core_en.pdf) that there were about 22,000 new HIV infections in the region in 2014 and approximately 240,000 people in the region were living with HIV/AIDS. There were an estimated 12,000 AIDS deaths in 2014, of which about 1,200 were children. AIDS-related deaths rose 66% between 2005 and 2013 and new HIV infections rose 5% during the same period.

Improved data collection and surveillance in some countries such as Algeria, Iran, Libya, and Morocco show that HIV epidemics do exist across the region and that an epidemic continues in Sudan. In Algeria and Morocco the majority of reported HIV infections are attributable to unprotected sex, and women make up a growing proportion of people living with HIV/AIDS. Treatment levels are low in North Africa and the Middle East. Overall, just 11% of people with HIV were receiving ART in 2013.

Sudan

The largest epidemic in the region is in Sudan. The HIV epidemic in Sudan is attributable primarily to heterosexual transmission of the virus. Here, as in other countries, an increasing number of women are acquiring the virus from husbands or boyfriends who became infected from injection drug use or paid sex. UNAIDS indicates in "Sudan" (2014, http://www.unaids.org/en/regionscountries/countries/sudan) that in 2014 an estimated 53,000 people were living with HIV in that country, including 23,000 women aged 15 years and older and 2,900 children.

In *Global AIDS Response Progress Reporting 2012– 2013: Sudan National AIDS and STI Control Program* (March 2014, http://www.unaids.org/sites/default/files/ country/documents//SDN_narrative_report_2014.pdf), the government of Sudan reported on its HIV/AIDS epidemic to UNAIDS. Sudan's government notes that it has weathered sociopolitical challenges since the secession of South Sudan in 2011 and that conflicts have contributed to nearly half the population living below the poverty line. This poverty, coupled with low rates of knowledge of HIV transmission (just 6.7% of the population had comprehensive knowledge about HIV) and low availability of preventive services, contributed to the epidemic.

Some progress, however, was reported. From 2011 to the close of 2013, the number of people that had received HIV testing and counseling had increased sevenfold (from 32,329 to 233,617). The percentage of MSM and female sex workers who had received HIV prevention packages (e.g., condoms) had increased from 10% at the end of 2012 to 30% at the end of 2013. Those who had received HIV testing and counseling increased from 1% to 4% over the same period.

SUB-SAHARAN AFRICA

UNAIDS states in "July 2015 Core Epidemiology Slides" that sub-Saharan Africa remained the most severely affected region in 2014. There were an estimated 25.8 million people living with HIV in the region that year, including 2.3 million children aged 14 years and under. Of the 1.2 million worldwide AIDS-related deaths in 2014, 790,000 occurred in the region. (130,000 of these deaths were children.) Ten countries—Ethiopia, Kenya, Malawi, Mozambique, Nigeria, South Africa, Uganda, Tanzania, Zambia, and Zimbabwe—account for 81% of people living

with HIV in the region. Fully half of the HIV-infected population is in two countries: Nigeria and South Africa.

There have, however, been some gains. The annual number of new HIV infections in the region decreased between 2001 and 2014, from an estimated 2.4 million to 1.4 million, and nearly half of adults know their HIV status. More than three-quarters (86%) of people living with HIV in the region who know their status are receiving ART and 76% have achieved viral suppression.

Nonetheless, nearly one in every 20 adults is living with the virus in this region. About three-quarters of new HIV infections in 2014 were in sub-Saharan Africa, and one-in-four new HIV infections there were in adolescent girls and young women. And while the number of AIDS-related deaths decreased 39% between 2005 and 2013, the region still accounted for 74% of all the people dying from AIDS-related causes in 2013.

Since 1995 ART has prevented 4.8 million deaths in sub-Saharan Africa. But preventive measures remain in short supply. Only eight condoms per year were available for each sexually active adult, and young people had even less access to condoms.

Transmission and Gender

Heterosexual contact is the predominant mode of transmission in sub-Saharan Africa. UNAIDS reports that the majority of people living with HIV in the region (58%) are women. In fact, 80% of all women aged 15 to 24 years who are living with HIV/AIDS are in sub-Saharan Africa. Social and economic inequality limit women's access to care and their ability to take measures to prevent infection, such as by insisting on condom use.

Sex workers and their customers play a significant role in the spread of HIV in many countries. Throughout the region, about 20% of sex workers are HIV infected. However, three countries, the Comoros, the Democratic Republic of the Congo, and Madagascar, report that fewer than 6% of sex workers are living with HIV.

Mother-to-child transmission also contributes to the pandemic; ART coverage, however, for pregnant women with HIV has improved markedly. In 2009, 67% of HIV-positive women were not receiving ART during pregnancy; by 2013 this percentage had fallen to 32%. There was a similar improvement in the percentage of breast-feeding women living with HIV who were receiving ART.

Kenya

Although Kenya had experienced the ravages of AIDS for about a decade, the Kenyan parliament and cabinet did not debate the issue publicly until 1993. Physicians diagnosed the first AIDS cases in 1984, but the government did not issue national statistics until

1986, when it announced one AIDS-related death. The nation's president and vice president regularly warned the public in speeches to avoid infection, and national officials instructed district administrators, including local tribal chiefs, to encourage their people to practice safe sex and limit their partners, but there had been no official statement.

Since then, Kenya has instituted programs to address its epidemic. In its March 2014 report to UNAIDS, *Kenya AIDS Response Progress Report* (http://www.unaids.org/sites/default/files/country/documents/KEN_narrative_report_2014.pdf), Kenya's National AIDS Control Council estimates that in 2013 there were 1.6 million people in Kenya living with HIV/AIDS. The majority of those infected (57%) were women. The prevalence of HIV infection among all Kenyan adults aged 15 to 49 years was 5.3%; this represented a 40% decline from the peak of the epidemic in 1993. It was estimated that there were 100,000 new HIV infections in 2013, a 15% reduction from 2009. The 58,047 AIDS-related deaths in 2013 were significantly less than the 85,840 reported in 2009. Figure 9.1 shows the trends in HIV prevalence, new infections, and AIDS deaths in Kenya from 1990 through 2013.

Some of this decline may be attributable to changing behaviors. Kenyans are less than half as likely to have multiple sex partners than they were during the late 1990s and condom use has increased dramatically. However, it is also believed that the lower prevalence of HIV infection may reflect the saturation of the infection in the at-risk population, meaning that the peak of the epidemic

has passed and/or that deaths from AIDS have served to reduce HIV prevalence.

Gender inequality, sexual violence, and HIV stigma increase HIV risk and vulnerability, while long-standing social and cultural practices promote HIV transmission. For example, "wife inheritance," which was once a socially useful tradition, continues to contribute to the spread of HIV/AIDS. In western Kenya, when a woman is widowed, her former husband's family takes care of her and her children. For generations, a brother-in-law or male cousin took her in with his family. Initially, tradition frowned on his having sexual relations with the inherited wife. Eventually, the inheritors began to ignore this restriction and had sex with the widow. If the widow's former husband had died of AIDS, she was likely to be infected and could pass the virus on to her inheritor, who would pass it on to his wife, causing the disease to spread.

Uganda's Efforts to Reduce HIV Infection

Scientists think that during the early 1980s truck drivers first spread HIV in Uganda's Rakai District, which lies along a Lake Victoria trade route to the capital city of Kampala. Because commercial sex is widely available along the trade route, HIV quickly spread throughout Uganda and all of Africa. At one time, Uganda had the world's highest prevalence of HIV. At the turn of the 21st century, there was nationwide evidence of declining HIV prevalence in response to strong prevention programs.

Uganda was the first African country to respond powerfully to its HIV/AIDS epidemic. The government

FIGURE 9.1

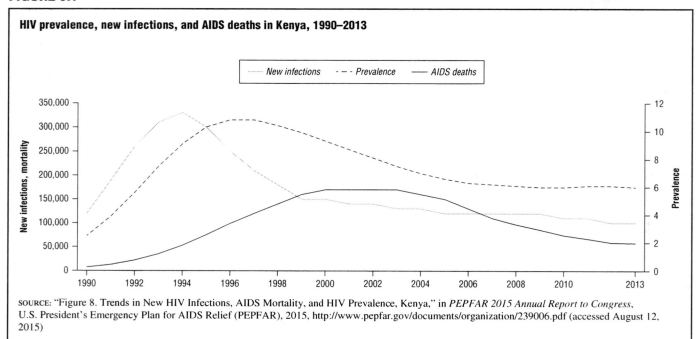

HIV prevalence, new infections, and AIDS deaths in Kenya, 1990–2013

SOURCE: "Figure 8. Trends in New HIV Infections, AIDS Mortality, and HIV Prevalence, Kenya," in *PEPFAR 2015 Annual Report to Congress,* U.S. President's Emergency Plan for AIDS Relief (PEPFAR), 2015, http://www.pepfar.gov/documents/organization/239006.pdf (accessed August 12, 2015)

began by gathering religious and traditional leaders, along with representatives of other sectors of society, in an effort to reach agreement that the problem had to be confronted. Prevention efforts targeted specific populations or communities. For example, prevention programs that focused on safe sex practices and/or delaying sex were presented in schools. Community groups were formed to counsel and support those living with the virus. Condom use was heavily promoted.

Unlike Kenya, Uganda began an aggressive campaign against the spread of HIV/AIDS during the mid-1980s, when it had the highest number of recorded HIV cases in Africa. With virtually every family touched by HIV/AIDS, much of the cultural, religious, and psychological stigma disappeared in Uganda. HIV prevalence eventually declined from a high of 18.5% in 1992 to 7.3% in 2014. Although education did prompt behavior changes that in turn resulted in lower HIV prevalence among pregnant women in Kampala and other cities from the early 1990s through the first decade of the 21st century, the decline was also due in part to increased AIDS mortality.

Despite these efforts, Uganda is still had a large HIV-positive population in 2014 and, as shown in Figure 9.2, the rate of new infections in the country increased between 2005 and 2013. However, efforts were underway to reduce new infections, and there was a decline from 2011 to 2013. (See Figure 9.3.) Uganda's government reports in *The HIV and AIDS Uganda Country Progress Report 2014* (2015, http://www.unaids.org/sites/default/files/country/documents/UGA _narrative_report_2015.pdf) that 95% of pregnant HIV positive mothers accessed ART in 2014, up from 49% in 2011, dramatically reducing the number of babies born HIV positive by end of 2014.

The populations at greatest risk of HIV infection were female sex workers and their clients, MSM, people living in fishing communities, and plantation workers. The lowest HIV prevalence was among university students, presumably in large part because they have knowledge of how to prevent infection.

In 2014 the key drivers of HIV continued to be:

- High risk sexual behavior, such as multiple sexual partners and inconsistent condom use, coupled with low levels of knowledge of HIV status

- Low levels of perceived risk and negative and stigmatizing attitudes toward people living with HIV

- High STD prevalence

- Low utilization of prenatal, delivery, and postnatal medical services

- Low prevalence of circumcision

- High numbers of HIV positive patients not on ART

- Sexual and gender based violence stemming from gender inequalities

- Alcohol consumption

- Poverty

The country continues to address the epidemic by providing psychosocial support, protection, and empowerment, especially for youth, people living with HIV and orphans and vulnerable children. Examples of these initiatives include the Support on AIDS and Life through the Telephone (SALT) program, which provides telephone counseling services, and the Y+ Beauty Pageant 2014, which was developed to combat discrimination

FIGURE 9.2

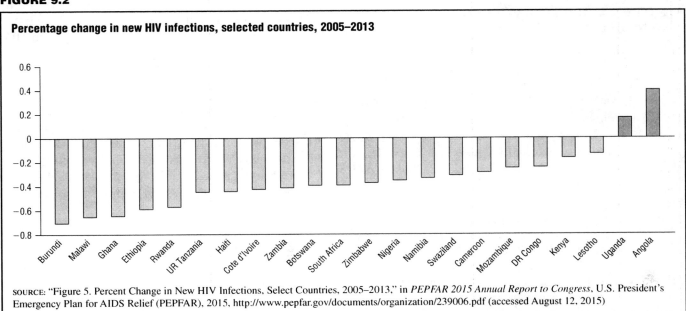

Percentage change in new HIV infections, selected countries, 2005–2013

SOURCE: "Figure 5. Percent Change in New HIV Infections, Select Countries, 2005–2013," in *PEPFAR 2015 Annual Report to Congress*, U.S. President's Emergency Plan for AIDS Relief (PEPFAR), 2015, http://www.pepfar.gov/documents/organization/239006.pdf (accessed August 12, 2015)

FIGURE 9.3

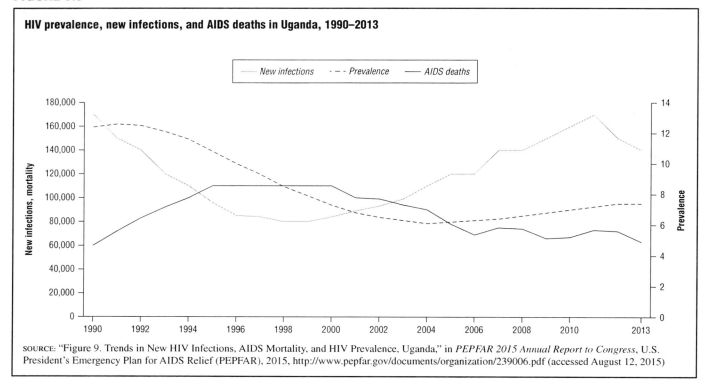

HIV prevalence, new infections, and AIDS deaths in Uganda, 1990–2013

SOURCE: "Figure 9. Trends in New HIV Infections, AIDS Mortality, and HIV Prevalence, Uganda," in *PEPFAR 2015 Annual Report to Congress*, U.S. President's Emergency Plan for AIDS Relief (PEPFAR), 2015, http://www.pepfar.gov/documents/organization/239006.pdf (accessed August 12, 2015)

against HIV positive youth and reduce HIV stigma in Uganda.

In 2014 services targeting sex work settings also intensified their efforts to test and treat sex workers. An estimated 10,000 sex workers, MSM, and members of communities they interact with received services in the target districts of Kampala, Kalangala, Gulu, Arua, Pader, Rakai, and Kiryandongo.

WESTERN AND CENTRAL EUROPE AND NORTH AMERICA

According to "July 2015 Core Epidemiology Slides," in 2014 there were an estimated 2.4 million people living with HIV in western and central Europe and North America, including 3,300 children. There were 85,000 new infections in 2014, over half of which (56%) were in the United States. Prevention coverage for mother-to-child transmission exceeded 95% in 2014. As a consequence, fewer than 500 children in this region were newly infected in 2014 and most countries in the region were close to achieving the goal of eliminating mother-to-child HIV transmission.

In western and central Europe, a median of 6.5% of people who inject drugs and 6.7% of gay men and other men who have sex with men were living with HIV. Condom use among sex workers was high across most countries in western and central Europe. Two of nine

reporting countries in 2014 found more than 80% of sex workers used a condom with their last client.

From 2000 to 2014 AIDS-related deaths fell by 12% in the region. In 2014 and there were 26,000 AIDS-related deaths, fewer than 200 of whom were children.

United Kingdom

In *HIV in the United Kingdom: 2013 Report* (November 2013, http://www.unaids.org/sites/default/files/country/documents//GBR_narrative_report_2014.pdf), the government of the United Kingdom reports that at the close of 2012 an estimated 98,400 people were living with HIV/AIDS in that country. Of this total, 21,900 (22%) were unaware of their infection status. The balance (77,610) was diagnosed and receiving care. In 2012 there were 490 HIV-related deaths.

There were 6,360 new HIV infections diagnosed in 2012. Of these, 3,250 (51%) were among MSM, the highest number ever recorded for that group. The U.K. government explains that this high number of diagnoses may be due to rising rates of transmission, increased testing, or both.

Just 120 (fewer than 2% of new infections) were acquired through injection drug use. The low number of new infections among IDUs was attributed to the institution of needle exchange programs during the 1980s. Since the mid-1990s AIDS diagnoses and deaths have declined significantly in the United Kingdom. In 2003 there were 1,030 AIDS-related deaths, compared with 390 in 2012.

Perinatal transmission of HIV has been all but eliminated in the United Kingdom. This is due in part to the fact that 98% of pregnant women received HIV testing. Between 2005 and 2011 an estimated 2% of children born to mothers living with HIV became infected themselves; less than 1% of children whose mothers had been diagnosed with HIV prior to giving birth were infected.

Netherlands

In *UNGASS Country Progress Report: The Netherlands and Parts of the Dutch Kingdom in the Caribbean* (March 31, 2014, http://www.unaids.org/sites/default/files/country/documents//NLD_narrative_report_2014.pdf), the Netherlands reports to UNAIDS about HIV/AIDS in its territory. The report observes that the Netherlands has a low prevalence of HIV infection concentrated in specific subpopulations. The principal high-risk populations are MSM and migrants from high-prevalence countries. The primary route of HIV transmission in the Netherlands is MSM. UNAIDS estimates that in 2011 there were 25,000 people living with HIV in the Netherlands.

In 2013 HIV prevalence was 0.2%, unchanged from in 2011. Of people living with HIV/AIDS, 55% were attributed to MSM, 40% to heterosexual contact and 4% to injection drug use. About 60% of people with HIV were thought to have been diagnosed. Among at-risk groups, an estimated 65% of HIV-infected MSM were diagnosed, compared with just 34% of infected sex workers. Among IDUs, the estimated proportion of diagnosed individuals varied from 57% in Rotterdam to 91% in Amsterdam.

About two-thirds (67%) of new infections occurred via MSM, while heterosexual transmission accounted for 30% of new infections (16% among men and 87% among women). Routine screening for HIV infection has been offered to all pregnant women since January 2004 and 99.8% of pregnant women are screened. Just one child was born HIV-infected in 2012.

Spain

Historically, Spain had the highest number of HIV/AIDS cases per capita in the European Union. The first case of HIV was reported in Spain in 1981; by the end of 2001, 110,000 to 150,000 people were living with HIV/AIDS. In *Informe Nacional Sobre los Progresos Realizados en la Aplicación Del UNGASS España: Enero de 2013–Diciembre de 2013* (2014, http://www.unaids.org/sites/default/files/country/documents//ESP_narrative_report_2014.pdf) the Spanish government reports to UNAIDS that there were 3,210 new cases of HIV infection in 2012 (in the 18 regions that reported these data, representing roughly 82% of Spain's population). About half (51%)

were attributed to MSM, 31% were to heterosexual transmission, and 5% were related to injection drug use.

The low percentage of cases attributed to injection drug use represents a change for Spain. In decades past IDUs were the highest risk group in the country. "Spain's War on AIDS Visits the Prado" (NYTimes.com, August 27, 1997) explains that drug use in Spain began to increase during the 1970s and 1980s, after the long Francisco Franco (1892–1975) dictatorship ended. Isabel Noguer of the Ministry of Health describes this period as a time of heavy heroin use, with addicts sharing infected needles. In 1997 IDUs still made up the highest risk group, whereas unprotected heterosexual relations was the next most common form of transmission. By 2003 HIV prevalence among IDUs declined in cities that had instituted effective long-standing harm reduction programs. In *Global Report: UNAIDS Report on the Global AIDS Epidemic, 2010* (2010, http://www.unaids.org/globalreport/documents/20101123_Global Report_full_en.pdf), UNAIDS notes that in 2006 Spain was one of just eight countries that provided comprehensive harm reduction programs, which included needle and syringe exchange and treatment programs for IDUs in prisons.

Marta Torrens et al. observe in "Methadone Maintenance Treatment in Spain: The Success of a Harm Reduction Approach" (*Bulletin of the World Health Organization*, vol. 91, no. 2, February 2013) that during the 1980s and 1990s Spain was the European country with the highest number of AIDS cases attributable to injection drug use. The researchers describe the HIV epidemic in Spanish prisons and how the implementation of comprehensive harm reduction, including needle and syringe exchange programs, significantly reduced both the incidence and prevalence of HIV/AIDS.

EASTERN EUROPE AND CENTRAL ASIA

The HIV pandemic did not reach eastern Europe until the mid-1990s. According to UNAIDS, in "July 2015 Core Epidemiology Slides," after sub-Saharan Africa and the Caribbean, eastern Europe and central Asia is the region hardest hit by the epidemic. The 1.5 million people there living with HIV/AIDS in 2014 (17,000 of whom were children) made up 0.9% of the region's population. In 2014 new infections were diagnosed in 140,000 adults and children and 62,000 people died from AIDS.

The numbers of people living with HIV/AIDS has increased throughout the region, but prevalence in eastern Europe and central Asia varies by country. Between 2001 and 2014 the most dramatic increases were in Belarus, where the number of people living with HIV rose from 4,900 to 29,000, and in Kazakhstan, where the number rose from 9,200 to 20,000.

UNAIDS indicates that although injection drug use is the "main mode of HIV transmission" in the region, there are few harm reduction programs (strategies like needle and syringe exchange that reduce the negative consequences of drug use) in place, and there is very limited access to drug rehabilitation services. Furthermore, because possession of even small amounts of narcotics is harshly punished in many countries in the region, IDUs are understandably reluctant to participate in needle exchange programs.

In a May 2014 speech at the Fourth Conference on HIV/AIDS in eastern Europe and central Asia, "The Courage to Reflect, Question and Commit" (May 12, 2014, http://www.unaids.org/sites/default/files/media_asset/20140512_SP_EXD_Moscow_en_0.pdf), Michel Sidibé, the executive director of UNAIDS, remarked on the situation in the region. He observed that despite decades of effort and financial investment, eastern Europe and central Asia still had the highest rates of new HIV infections and AIDS-related deaths, even as other regions of the world, such as Africa and Asia, had experienced declines. Sidibé noted that just 30% of infected people in the region were receiving ART and that IDUs, the most affected population in the region, continued to face barriers to treatment. He asserted that "eastern Europe and central Asia has two urgent priorities: to ensure that all injecting drug users have access to clean injection equipment; and to implement scientifically proven, evidence-based methods of drug treatment." Sidibé acknowledged that Armenia, Azerbaijan, Belarus, Georgia, Moldova, Ukraine, and several countries in central Asia were already using harm reduction to manage HIV epidemics among IDUs.

ASIA AND THE PACIFIC

The HIV/AIDS pandemic arrived in Asia much later than in the rest of the world. Until the mid-1990s HIV/AIDS was uncommon, but infections have increased considerably since that time. According to "July 2015 Core Epidemiology Slides," an estimated 5 million people in the Asia and the Pacific region, including 200,000 children, were living with the disease in 2014. This was the second-highest total for any region, but the prevalence among adults (ages 15 to 49) stood at 0.2%. This was lower than prevalence in most other regions.

UNAIDS estimates that there were 350,000 new infections in the region in 2013, a 5% decrease since 2005. UNAIDS believed that only one-third of all people living with HIV were receiving ART that year, and noted that there were only 5 countries in the region where more than 50% of infected individuals were on ART. New infections among children decreased 28% between 2001 and 2012, to 23,000.

Regionally, an estimated 250,000 people died from AIDS-related causes in 2013. This marked a 26.5% decline from 2005. However, this masked significant differences between countries in the region. Some countries saw major increases in AIDS-related mortality over the period, most notably Indonesia (427%) and Pakistan (352%).

Thailand

Thailand's commercial sex industry is notorious, and travel packages based on the availability of sex workers in Thailand are common in Asia and elsewhere. In the capital city of Bangkok, brothels are found in virtually every neighborhood. Cheewanan Lertpiriyasuwat, Tanarak Plipat, and Richard Jenkins find in "A Survey of Sexual Risk Behavior for HIV Infection in Nakhonsawan, Thailand, 2001" (*AIDS*, vol. 17, no. 13, September 5, 2003) that in 1990, 20% of all Thai men reported having paid for sex in the previous year. All of this contributed to a rapid spread of HIV/AIDS in Thailand. However, after a military coup in 1991, the transitional government instituted a comprehensive HIV/AIDS education program, which included a media campaign and condom distribution to brothels and massage parlors. Brothels that refused to use condoms were closed down. Although the anti-HIV program came too late for those infected during the mid-to-late 1980s, Thailand recorded a drop in new HIV infections until the late 1990s.

In *2015 Thailand Global AIDS Response Progress Report* (2015, http://www.unaids.org/sites/default/files/country/documents/THA_narrative_report_2015.pdf), Thailand tells UNAIDS that it has had mixed results in reaching its goals of helping HIV-positive people and preventing new transmissions. There were an estimated 445,504 people living with HIV in fiscal year (FY) 2014. During that same period, Thailand estimated that 7,816 people became newly infected and that 20,492 individuals suffered AIDS-related deaths. These were substantial improvements over the statistics from 2000. However, the most dramatic changes were years in the past. Between FY 2010 and FY 2014 these measures had changed only modestly.

One area where Thailand had achieved notable success was the effort to eliminate new HIV infections in children. In FY 2014, 121 children were newly infected with HIV, a 41% reduction since 2010. Furthermore, in 2014 the mother-to-child transmission rate was just 2.1% In addition, over the same period 70% of female sex workers received prevention services and knew their HIV status and 95% reported condom use during their most recent sexual encounter.

Cambodia

Cambodia has been the hardest hit country in Southeast Asia, but there is evidence that the epidemic is subsiding. HIV prevalence among adults dropped from a peak of 2% in 1998 to 0.6% in 2014. UNAIDS estimates that in 2014 there were 75,000 people living with HIV, and 2,600 deaths due to AIDS, in Cambodia. The number of people living with HIV/AIDS has declined steadily in response to fewer new infections, increased ART coverage, and effective HIV prevention programs. Increased ART coverage has also served to reduce the mortality rate of HIV-infected people.

In a May 2015 report to UNAIDS, *Cambodia Country Progress Report* (http://www.unaids.org/sites/default/files/country/documents/KHM_narrative_report_2015.pdf), Cambodia's National AIDS Authority explains that in 2014 sexual contact was the primary method through which HIV was being transmitted. About 48% of all new infections resulted from spousal transmission, 25% from sex workers, 11% from casual sex, and 3% from MSM transmission. An additional 13% of new infections were due to injection drug use, but the report notes that the high prevalence of the disease among IDUs was troubling. The National AIDS Authority asserts that "with continued targeted and effective interventions and by maintaining the current high level of coverage of ART among persons living with HIV, Cambodia is poised to become the first low-income country to achieve virtual elimination of HIV transmission by 2020."

India

At the International AIDS Conference held in Vancouver, Canada, in July 1996, a United Nations official reported that India had emerged as the country with the most people infected with HIV. This news came as a surprise to many of the conferees because HIV was not detected in India until 1986. According to UNAIDS, approximately 2.1 million people in India were HIV positive in 2013. This was down from 2.5 million in 2001. The 2013 total included an estimated 750,000 women and 140,000 children aged 14 years and under. In 2013, 130,000 deaths were attributable to AIDS.

In *Statement Containing Brief Activities of the Department of AIDS Control in 2013* (2014, http://www.unaids.org/sites/default/files/country/documents//IND_narrative_report_2014.pdf), India's government reports to UNAIDS that as of 2013 the epidemic was declining in most states in India. Most new HIV infections were attributable to unprotected heterosexual relationships. Researchers speculated that more than 90% of women with HIV acquired the virus from their regular partners, who had been infected during paid sex.

India has made tremendous strides in reducing new infections, improving access to prevention services for key populations and treatment services for people living with HIV, reducing AIDS related mortality, and reducing in mother-to-child transmission. India has been scaling up the availability of free ART since 2004, and it estimates that by doing so it has saved 1.5 million lives by reducing AIDS-related deaths. From 2007 to 2011 AIDS-related deaths

decreased 29%. New infections are also prevented through education, and three-quarters of HIV positive pregnant women and their babies receive ART to prevent mother-to-child transmission.

Sex trafficking and female sex workers contribute to the epidemic in many states. Jhumka Gupta et al. examine this issue in "History of Sex Trafficking, Recent Experiences of Violence, and HIV Vulnerability among Female Sex Workers in Coastal Andhra Pradesh, India" (*International Journal of Gynecology and Obstetrics*, vol. 142, no. 2, August 2011). The researchers find that one out of five female sex workers met the United Nations definition of sex trafficking (exploitation and abuse of people for revenue through sex) and that these sex workers were at increased risk for both violence and HIV.

According to Puspen Ghosh et al., in "Factors Associated with HIV Infection among Indian Women" (*International Journal of STD and AIDS*, vol. 22, no. 3, March 2011), the most common risk factor for HIV transmission for women was an exclusive sexual relationship with their husband. The researchers analyzed data from the National Family Health Survey 2005–06 to identify other risk factors. They find that women at highest risk were those aged 26 to 35 years, were impoverished, and had more than one sexual partner during their lifetime. Women with a history of a genital sore (a marker for other STIs) were also at increased risk. Because most HIV transmission in women took place within marriage, Ghosh et al. advocate targeting risk-reduction programs to this population, especially in view of their finding of a low percentage of condom use by married men with their wife and other sexual partners.

China

The first HIV case in China was identified in 1985, but the disease did not begin to spread until the early 1990s, when changes in the structure of the economy produced an increase in drug use and prostitution. The U.S. embassy in China indicates in *Flying Blind on a Growing Epidemic: AIDS in China* (2002) that the government of China estimated in 1997 that between 100,000 and 300,000 people were living with HIV/AIDS. By the beginning of 1998 this estimate had doubled.

In *2015 China AIDS Response Progress Report* (May 2015, http://www.unaids.org/sites/default/files/country/documents/CHN_narrative_report_2015.pdf), the government of China reports to UNAIDS that at the close of 2014 an estimated 501,000 people were living with HIV/AIDS in China. The prevalence of the disease was low, with 0.037% of the overall population infected. However, the number of people known to be living with HIV/AIDS was growing due to increased testing, life-prolonging ART, and new transmissions. The number of cases increased 63% between 2010 and 2014. Also, prevalence was much higher among IDUs (6%) and MSM (7.7%) than in the general population.

China's government noted that while the number of people living with AIDS grew between 2013 and 2014, the number of AIDS-related deaths fell slightly. It attributed this to better and more widely available treatments for the disease. The number of people receiving treatment increased from 227,485 in 2013 to 295,358 in 2014.

As in other countries, HIV transmission and infection in China have migrated from the typical high-risk populations—sex workers, IDUs, and the overlap of these populations—to the general population. As a result the number of HIV infections in women is growing. In 2006 and earlier, injection drug use was the primary means of HIV transmission in China, but since that time its significance has fallen. In 2014 just 6% of new cases were attributed to injection drug use. From 2007 on, heterosexual contact has been the primary means of transmission, and between 2010 and 2014 it accounted for well over half of all new cases. However, this means of transmission declined from 69.4% of new cases in 2013 to 66.4% in 2014. Meanwhile, MSM's share of transmissions has been growing rapidly, from 2.5% in 2006 to 25.8% in 2014.

Some observers, such as Jane Qiu, in "Stigma of HIV Imperils Hard-Won Strides in Saving Lives" (*Science*, vol. 332, no. 6035, June 10, 2011), Talha Khan Burki, in "Discrimination against People with HIV Persists in China" (*Lancet*, vol. 377, no. 9762, January 2011), and Laurie Abler et al., in "Affected by HIV Stigma: Interpreting Results from a Population Survey of an Urban Center in Guangxi, China" (*AIDS and Behavior*, July 27, 2013), are concerned that stigma about homosexuality and discrimination against people living with HIV/AIDS may hamper China's efforts to further reduce the size of its epidemic. People with HIV are often barred from education and employment opportunities and may be demoted or forced to resign. Hospitals and universities frequently disclose workers' HIV test results to employers and policies regarding confidentiality and consent vary from one province to the next.

LATIN AMERICA

UNAIDS indicates that approximately 1.7 million people (including 33,000 children) in Latin America were living with HIV/AIDS in 2014. This was up from 1.3 million in 2005, but the overall prevalence of the disease remained at 0.4% (among adults aged 15 to 49 years). There were 41,000 AIDS-related deaths (including 1,800 children) in 2014, down 29% from 60,000 in 2005.

Although new HIV infections decreased 17% between 2000 and 2014, there was little change in the annual number of new infections from 2009 through 2014. There were also major differences between countries. For example, new

infections declined 39% in Mexico between 2005 and 2013, but increased 11% in Brazil over the same period.

Since 2010 HIV testing efforts have been intensified. As a result, in 2013 about 70% of the HIV-positive population had been diagnosed and was aware of their status. Unfortunately, about 38% of new HIV diagnoses were late diagnoses with a CD4 count below 200, for whom treatment was less likely to be effective. In 2013 about half (48%) of people living with HIV were receiving treatment, and, of these, two-thirds (66%) were virally suppressed.

The majority of HIV/AIDS cases in Central and South America can be traced to MSM and men who have sex with both men and women. HIV prevalence in MSM was higher than 10% in 9 of 15 countries reporting in 2015. Of the estimated 1.7 million people living with HIV, 1.1 million were men. While sex workers continue to contribute to the epidemics in many countries in the region, HIV prevalence was below 10% among sex workers in all reporting countries between 2011 and 2014 except for Guyana and Uruguay. Condom use among sex workers was high throughout the region. Between 84% and 99% of sex workers reported using condoms with their last clients and nearly three-quarters (72%) had been tested for HIV in the past 12 months and knew the result.

CARIBBEAN

The first suspected AIDS cases in the Caribbean appeared in Jamaica in 1982. UNAIDS indicates in "July 2015 Core Epidemiology Slides" that in 2014 the prevalence of HIV among adults (aged 15 to 49 years) was 1.1%, the second-highest rate in the world (after sub-Saharan Africa). A total of 280,000 people (including 13,000 children) were thought to be living with HIV that year.

An estimated 13,000 people were newly infected with HIV in 2014. This was a 50% decline from 2000, the largest such drop in any region. Haiti accounted for about half of all new HIV infections in 2014 and the Dominican Republic had the second largest number of new infections. Also in 2014, the number of newly infected children fell below 500. UNAIDS credits this to the fact that 89% of HIV-positive pregnant women received ART in 2014, up more than 40% from 2010. In 2015 the agency praised Cuba for being one of the first countries to have virtually eliminated mother-to-child transmission.

The Caribbean also had a significant decrease (59%) in AIDS-related deaths between 2005 and 2014. There were a total of 8,800 such deaths in 2014. Additionally, the Caribbean was the only region in which the TB-related deaths in people living with HIV had declined more than 50%. Roughly 44% of adults and 36% of children eligible for ART were receiving it in 2014.

Since its inception, the HIV/AIDS epidemic in the region has changed from a mostly homosexual phenomenon to a largely heterosexual one. This was driven in part by people who have sex with multiple partners, such as sex workers and those who use their services. A positive sign in 2014 was that condom use among sex workers in the region ranged from 72% to 98%. That same year the percentage of sex workers who had been recently tested for HIV varied considerably by country, from a low of 7% to a high of 85%. HIV prevalence among sex workers ranged from 1% in Antigua and Barbuda to 8% in Haiti.

MSM are another group that was at heightened risk in the Caribbean. The prevalence of HIV among MSM ranged from 2% in Antigua and Barbuda to 38% in Jamaica during the span 2011 to 2014. Condom during last sex for MSM ranged from 40% to 81%. Depending on the country, 16% to 99% of MSM had been recently tested for HIV and knew the results of their tests.

TRIUMPHS AND CHALLENGES

Great strides have been made in the treatment of HIV infection and AIDS and in raising public awareness about the nature of the disease and preventing its spread; however, issues, challenges, and controversies continue to hamper the unity of purpose that is required to effectively combat HIV/AIDS worldwide.

In "UNAIDS Announces That the Goal of 15 Million People on Life-Saving HIV Treatment by 2015 Has Been Met Nine Months Ahead of Schedule" (July 14, 2015, http://www.unaids.org/en/resources/presscentre/pressrelea seandstatementarchive/2015/july/20150714_PR_MDG6report), UNAIDS reviews the progress made in combating HIV/ AIDS since 2000. In 2000 the global community established ambitious goals intended to halt and reverse the spread of HIV/AIDS, goals that UNAIDS says some "deemed impossible" when they were set. Yet the agency was able to state that the goal of having 15 million people on ART worldwide by 2015 had been met 9 months ahead of schedule. Furthermore, UNAIDS said that investment in the global AIDS response was on track, and that "concerted action over the next five years can end the AIDS epidemic by 2030."

Along with the achievement of the goal of having 15 million in treatment, UNAIDS detailed strides made in improving access to treatment and described how "the inequity of access and injustice sparked global moral outrage, which created one of the most defining achievements of the response to HIV—massive reductions in the price of life-saving antiretroviral medicines."

Cost of Drugs

The high price of HIV/AIDS drugs has been and continues to be a contentious issue. In *How AIDS Changed Everything*, UNAIDS observes that, among other strategies, the "use of generic drugs, flexibilities in the Trade-Related

Aspects of Intellectual Property Rights agreement, and tiered pricing schemes" helped to substantially reduce the cost of first-line drugs. A year's worth of treatment with drugs that would have cost $10,000 in 2000 had dropped to less than $100 by 2011. UNAIDS notes, however, that the prices of second- and third-line medications were still much too high for many in the developing world, and that there was an urgent need for negotiations to reduce their prices.

Increasing Access to HIV/AIDS Drugs in Developing Countries

The Clinton Health Access Initiative (CHAI; http://www.clintonhealthaccess.org) was founded by former U.S. president Bill Clinton (1946–) to assist countries to implement large-scale prevention and treatment programs. CHAI works with the governments of countries in Africa, the Caribbean, and Asia and provides technical assistance and human and financial resources to ensure the delivery of quality care and treatment. The initiative also provides access to reduced prices for HIV/AIDS drugs and diagnostics to countries. In total, CHAI represents over 90% of people living with HIV/AIDS in developing countries.

In "About CHAI" (2015, http://www.clintonhealth access.org/about), CHAI reports that as of 2014 it had successfully negotiated price reductions for antiretroviral drugs that have benefited millions of people in 70 countries. CHAI's efforts resulted in price reductions of 60% to 90% and have saved countries more than $1 billion. CHAI works in concert with governments to support and strengthen their capacities to care for their citizens. For example, in South Africa CHAI has assisted the government to extend ART to more than 2.3 million people and to offer HIV testing to more than 15 million individuals. CHAI also negotiated a global access price for testing to measure viral load, which will save more than $150 million over five years and will improve the quality of care people with HIV receive.

UNITAID is an international drug purchase facility that was established in 2006 by Brazil, Chile, France, Norway, and the United Kingdom. UNITAID is an innovative funding mechanism that focuses on speeding access to quality drugs and diagnostics for HIV/AIDS, malaria, and TB in countries where these diseases pose serious threats to the health of their residents. In "Increasing Access to Better and Cheaper Medicines and Diagnostics for HIV/AIDS" (2015, http://www.unitaid.eu/en/what/hiv), UNITAID describes its role as closing "gaps in global public health funding for HIV/AIDS treatment" and discusses its work with CHAI, the WHO, and the United Nations Children's Fund.

UNITAID notes that besides expanding access to, availability, and affordability of antiretroviral drugs, its accomplishments include price reductions of up to 60% for the more-potent ART drugs many patients need when first-line drugs no longer keep the virus in check and enabling more than 100,000 patients per year to obtain these lifesaving drugs.

President's Emergency Plan for AIDS Relief

The President's Emergency Plan for AIDS Relief (PEPFAR) is a U.S. government initiative to help people suffering from HIV/AIDS worldwide. Launched by President George W. Bush (1946–) in 2003, PEPFAR is responsible for saving millions of lives. In "Bush Signs Bill to Triple AIDS Funding" (Associated Press, July 30, 2008), Katharine Euphrat describes the program as "one of the major achievements of the Bush presidency." In 2008 the program was renewed for five years and the controversial requirement that 33% of prevention funds be used for abstinence-until-marriage programs was eliminated.

Abstaining from sexual intercourse does prevent the sexual transmission of HIV. Nonetheless, most experts, who agree that it is not realistic to expect sexual abstinence from many segments of the population, stress that condom use is essential to stop the spread of the disease. Abstinence education remains a key component of PEPFAR, although in 2007 the program's prevention strategy was broadened to include "ABC—Abstain, Be faithful, and correct and consistent Condom use," the prevention of mother-to-child transmission, activities that focus on blood safety, and interventions aimed at IDUs.

PEPFAR was reauthorized by the Tom Lantos and Henry J. Hyde United States Global Leadership against HIV/AIDS, Tuberculosis, and Malaria Reauthorization Act in July 2008. The reauthorization act stipulates that "in countries with generalized HIV epidemics, at least half of all money directed towards preventing sexual HIV transmission should be for activities promoting abstinence, delay of sexual debut, monogamy, fidelity, and partner reduction," but it does not mandate abstinence-only education and prevention programs as a requirement for receiving funds.

PEPFAR helped provide ART to 7.7 million people in FY 2014 and PEPFAR aimed to serve 9.4 million in 2015. (See Figure 9.4.) It also supported HIV testing and counseling for more than 14.2 million pregnant women. The launch of PEPFAR significantly boosted U.S. spending to support the fight against the global HIV/AIDS pandemic. Spending increased from $2.3 billion in FY 2004 to $6.8 billion in FY 2015. (See Table 9.1.) For FY 2016 President Barack Obama (1961–) requested $6.5 billion in funding for PEPFAR.

FIGURE 9.4

PEPFAR treatment results and fiscal year 2015 target

[Fiscal year 2015 ART target 9.4 million*; APR fiscal year 2014 ART result: 7.7 million*]

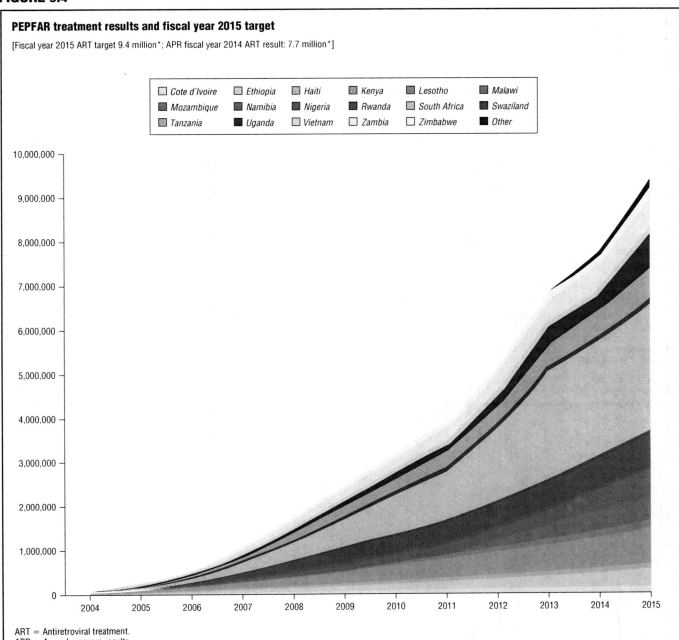

ART = Antiretroviral treatment.
APR = Annual program results.
PEPFAR = President's Emergency Plan for AIDS Relief.
*These figures represent both those receiving direct PEPFAR support and those benefiting from essential PEPFAR technical support to partner countries.

SOURCE: "Figure 15. PEPFAR Treatment Results and FY 2015 Target," in *PEPFAR 2015 Annual Report to Congress*, U.S. President's Emergency Plan for AIDS Relief (PEPFAR), 2015, http://www.pepfar.gov/documents/organization/239006.pdf (accessed August 12, 2015)

TABLE 9.1

President's Emergency Plan for AIDS Relief funding, fiscal years 2004–16

[U.S. dollars in millions]

	Programs			
Fiscal year	Bilateral HIV/AIDS programs[a]	Global fund	Bilateral tuberculosis programs	Total PEPFAR (without malaria)
2004 enacted	1,643	547	87	2,277
2005 enacted	2,263	347	94	2,704
2006 enacted	2,654	545	91	3,290
2007 enacted	3,699	724	95	4,518
2008 enacted	5,028	840	163	6,031
2009 enacted	5,503	1,000	177	6,680
2010 enacted	5,574	1,050	243	6,867
2011[b] enacted	5,440	5,440	239	6,725
2012[c] enacted	5,083	1,300	256	6,639
2013[d] enacted	4,726	1,569	233	6,527
2014 enacted	4,940	1,650	243	6,833
2015 enacted	5,238	1,350	242	6,830
Total enacted[e]	**51,791**	**11,968**	**2,163**	**65,921**
2016[f] request	5,240	1,107	195	6,542

PEPFAR = President's Emergency Plan for AIDS Relief.

[a]Bilateral HIV/AIDS Programs includes funding for bilateral country/regional programs, UNAIDS, International AIDS Vaccine Initiative, Microbicides and National Institutes of Health HIV/AIDS research.

[b]Fiscal year 2011 enacted level includes across the board and Department of Health and Human Services (HHS) agency-wide rescissions.

[c]Fiscal year 2012 enacted Global Fund contribution reflects an increase of $250M over original congressional allocation.

[d]Fiscal year 2013 enacted level reflects full-year continuing resolution reduced by rescission and sequestration.

[e]Includes enacted funding for fiscal year 2004-fiscal year 2015.

[f]Fiscal year 2016 allocations are initial estimates only.

SOURCE: "Fiscal Year 2014–2016 PEPFAR Funding (U.S. Dollars in Millions)," in *PEPFAR Funding*, PEPFAR, July 2015, http://www.pepfar.gov/documents/organization/189671.pdf (accessed August 12, 2015)

CHAPTER 10
KNOWLEDGE, AWARENESS, BEHAVIOR, AND OPINION

CONCERN ABOUT HIV/AIDS

During the first decades of the 21st century the U.S. public appeared less concerned about HIV/AIDS and its impact on health care than at any time since it first became known during the 1980s. According to the Gallup Organization, the number of Americans who named AIDS as the most urgent health problem facing the country had declined steadily when compared with 68% of Americans in 1988. It declined to 41% in 1992 and to 29% in 1997. By late 2014 just 1% of Americans considered AIDS the most urgent health problem. (See Table 10.1.)

Access to health care and health care costs overshadowed diseases as the most pressing health problems facing the country. (See Table 10.1.) Interestingly, Ebola and obesity were the most frequently named health problems, outpacing cancer, heart disease, diabetes, AIDS, and flu.

Knowledge Is Necessary but Not Sufficient to Halt the HIV/AIDS Epidemic

Although raising awareness and improving knowledge about HIV/AIDS and how to prevent transmission are necessary prerequisites to combating the epidemic, researchers have sought to determine whether knowledge alone was sufficient to alter risk-taking behavior and maintain behavioral change.

In "Knowing Is Not Enough: A Qualitative Report on HIV Testing among Heterosexual African-American Men" (*AIDS Care*, vol. 27, no. 2, 2015), Keosha T. Bond et al. interviewed heterosexual African American men aged 18 to 45 years in New York City to find out if HIV knowledge was related to rates of HIV testing and perceived risk of HIV infection. The researchers find that while HIV testing was frequent, the study subjects had low levels of HIV knowledge, perceived little risk of HIV, and misused HIV testing as a prevention method. For example, subjects who perceived themselves as having low HIV risk after receiving negative HIV test results were not motivated to use condoms. Bond et al. report, "When asked how it felt to receive negative HIV test results, one participant stated that it was acceptable to have unprotected sex because he was HIV-negative."

Bond et al. find that among study subjects the primary motivators for HIV testing were recent exposure risk, having a new sexual partner, and gaining knowledge of their status. Barriers to testing not only included low perceived risk of infection but also fear of being HIV-positive and stigma. Many of the subjects opined, "their peers avoided testing because of the stigma that they would be subjected to [in] the community if they test positive."

In "Is Knowledge Enough? Considering HIV/AIDS Risk Behaviors and HIV/AIDS Knowledge with African American Women" (*International Journal of High Risk Behavior and Addiction*, vol. 3, no. 3, September 2014), Emory L. Perkins et al. questioned two groups of African American women aged 24 to 44 years to determine whether knowledge alone was sufficient to alter African American women's risk-taking behaviors in terms of HIV/AIDS. The first group included 53 women who were HIV positive; the second group included 62 women who were HIV negative. The study specifically looked at knowledge of risk-taking behavior including heterosexual transmission, low and sporadic condom use, illicit drug use, and multiple sex partners.

Although the investigators anticipated that knowledge of HIV would be higher in the HIV negative group, this was not the case. Both groups were equally knowledgeable. Perkins et al. conclude, "this study reveals that knowledge about HIV/AIDS is not enough to impact practice behaviors associated with contracting HIV/AIDS. While the study does not negate the importance of knowledge, it simply confirms that knowledge alone does not have a significant relationship with HIV/AIDS related risk-behaviors."

TABLE 10.1

Percentage of people naming AIDS as the most urgent health problem, November 2013 and November 2014

WHAT WOULD YOU SAY IS THE MOST URGENT HEALTH PROBLEM FACING THIS COUNTRY AT THE PRESENT TIME?

	Nov 7–10, 2013	Nov 6–9, 2014
	%	%
Affordable healthcare/health insurance; costs	23	19
Access to healthcare/universal health coverage	16	18
Ebola virus	—	17
Obesity	13	10
Cancer	10	10
Finding cures for diseases	1	3
Diabetes	2	2
Heart diseases	2	2
Government interference	9	2
Drug/alcohol abuse	1	1
Flu	—	1
Mental illness	2	1
AIDS	1	1
Other	6	3
No opinion	13	10

SOURCE: Lydia Saad, "What Would You Say Is the Most Urgent Health Problem Facing This Country at the Present Time?" in *Ebola Ranks among Americans' Top Three Healthcare Concerns*, The Gallup Organization, November 17, 2014, http://www.gallup.com/poll/179429/ebola-ranks-among-americans-top-three-healthcare-concerns.aspx?utm_source=most%20urgent%20health%20problem&utm_medium=search&utm_campaign=tiles (accessed August 13, 2015). Copyright © 2015 Gallup, Inc. All rights reserved. The content is used with permission; however, Gallup retains all rights of republication.

Knowledge about the HIV/AIDS Epidemic among Men Who Have Sex with Men

Although Americans may no longer view HIV/AIDS as a key health problem facing the nation, a 2014 Kaiser Family Foundation survey of 431 men who have sex with men (MSM) focusing on their attitudes, knowledge, and experiences with HIV/AIDS and new HIV therapies finds that MSM "see HIV/AIDS as the number one health issue, and as a top priority among overall issues facing their community today."

In "HIV/AIDS in the Lives of Gay and Bisexual Men in the United States" (September 25, 2014, http://kff.org/hivaids/report/hivaids-in-the-lives-of-gay-and-bisexual-men-in-the-united-states), Liz Hamel et al. of the Kaiser Family Foundation report the survey findings. About half of the MSM surveyed (49%) responded that HIV/AIDS is a "very" or "somewhat" important issue for them personally. The other half (52%) viewed it as "not too significant" or "not a significant issue" in their lives. About one-third (35%) were personally concerned about becoming infected, but more than half (56%) said they are not personally concerned about it.

Even this community, which names HIV/AIDS as the most pressing health issue, is not well informed about the epidemic or current treatment guidelines. Only one-third (32%) of MSM in the survey were aware that new infections

are on the rise among gay men. Nearly one-quarter (22%) mistakenly responded that new infections are decreasing, and the balance stated the situation is staying the same or admitted that they do not know.

Most MSM in the survey were unaware of current treatment recommendations for people who are HIV positive or of the current guidelines about how to reduce new infections. Just one-quarter (26%) reported knowing about pre-exposure prophylaxis (PrEP), daily prescription medication that people who are HIV negative can use to reduce their risk of becoming infected. Just 10% said they knew someone who used PrEP, and the majority of survey respondents (80%) claimed they had heard only a little or nothing at all about PrEP. Fewer than half (46%) of the men surveyed knew that antiretroviral treatment (ART) should begin immediately upon diagnosis of HIV infection, and just one-quarter (25%) knew that using ART significantly reduces the risk of HIV transmission to sexual partners.

Three-quarters (75%) of survey respondents stated that the reason it has been challenging to control the epidemic among MSM is that too many MSM do not know their HIV status. Nearly two-thirds (65%) believe the gay community has become too complacent about the epidemic, and more than half (56%) responded that HIV stigma hampers efforts to reduce the spread of HIV.

About 70% of MSM said they had been tested for HIV at some point in their lives, but few are tested as often as is recommended. Thirty percent reported that they had been tested in the year prior to the survey, and the same proportion said they had never been tested. Surprisingly, more than half (56%) said their physicians had never advised them to get tested, and 61% said they never or only rarely discussed HIV with their doctors. One of the reasons physicians have not advised testing may be that about half of MSM surveyed admitted that they had never discussed their sexual orientation with their doctors.

The survey found that the knowledge and behavior of MSM varied by race/ethnicity. MSM of color (64%) were more likely than white MSM (42%) say that HIV/AIDS was a significant issue for them personally, and more were worried about becoming infected—53% compared with 28%. MSM of color were more likely that white MSM to report consistent condom use (61% versus 39%) and were more likely to say that they wanted additional information about HIV/AIDS.

Personal experience with the epidemic varies by age, and it shapes the opinions and behaviors of MSM. About half (47%) of MSM aged 35 years and older said they had lost someone close to them from the disease compared with 8% of MSM aged 18 to 34 years. Older MSM also were more likely to know a person living with HIV

(54%) than were younger men (39%). MSM younger than age 35 (44%) were more likely than older men (21%) to report having never had an HIV test. These findings may explain why more younger than older MSM said they would be uncomfortable having sexual or nonsexual relationships with someone who is HIV positive.

Older MSM were more inclined to express support for PrEP (64% endorsed its widespread use, and 35% said it should be used on a more limited basis), while younger MSM were less enthusiastic about its use (56% thought it should be used on a limited basis, and 43% supported widespread use).

DIFFERING OPINIONS: AIDS DISSIDENTS AND DENIALISTS

In 1987 Peter Duesberg (1936–) of the University of California, Berkeley, published "Retroviruses as Carcinogens and Pathogens: Expectations and Reality" (*Cancer Research*, vol. 47, no. 5, March 1, 1987), in which he asserts that HIV does not cause AIDS. Duesberg believes that HIV is a harmless virus and one of many organisms that may reside in humans but will not harm them. One of his arguments is that most viruses make people ill very quickly before they can mount an immune response. People infected with HIV may not become ill for more than a decade. Duesberg posits that it is the use of illicit drugs that compromises the immune system, not infection with HIV. He feels that maintaining a healthy diet and abstaining from harmful drug use is sufficient to prevent and even cure AIDS. Duesberg is considered by many to be at the forefront of a small but vocal minority of people who do not accept the direct connection between HIV infection and AIDS.

In a highly controversial article published in a peer-reviewed journal, "AIDS since 1984: No Evidence for a New, Viral Epidemic–Not Even in Africa" (*Italian Journal of Anatomy and Embryology*, vol. 116, no. 2, 2011), Duesberg et al. contend, "there is as yet no proof that HIV causes AIDS" and refute the effectiveness of ART. Two years prior, an earlier version of the article, "HIV-AIDS Hypothesis out of Touch with South African AIDS–A New Perspective" was published online in the July 2009 issue of the journal *Medical Hypotheses* but was withdrawn. The publisher issued a statement about the withdrawal, which read in part, "The editorial policy of *Medical Hypotheses* makes it clear that the journal considers 'radical, speculative, and non-mainstream scientific ideas' . . . we received serious expressions of concern about the quality of this article, which contains highly controversial opinions about the causes of AIDS, opinions that could potentially be damaging to global public health."

Christine Maggiore (1956–2008) was another vocal critic of the generally accepted premise that HIV causes AIDS. Diagnosed as HIV positive in 1999, Maggiore was a positive activist who believed that flu shots and other common viral infections could cause a person to test positive for HIV. In "Christine Maggiore, Vocal Skeptic of AIDS Research, Dies at 52" (LATimes.com, December 30, 2008), Anna Gorman and Alexandra Zavis report that Maggiore refused treatment and gave birth to two children, one of whom died in 2005 of what an autopsy determined was AIDS-related pneumonia at age three. Maggiore self-published a book, *What If Everything You Thought You Knew about AIDS Was Wrong?* and founded Alive & Well AIDS Alternatives, a nonprofit group that challenged conventional understanding of HIV/AIDS. At its website (http://www.aliveandwell.org), the group describes its mission as offering "information that raises questions about the accuracy of HIV tests, the safety and effectiveness of AIDS drug treatments, and the validity of most common assumptions about HIV and AIDS." Maggiore also broadcast a podcast about the topic and served on the board of Rethinking AIDS, another nonprofit group.

Besides rejecting HIV as the cause of AIDS, others argue that the risks of antiretroviral drugs far outweigh the benefits. Some even assert that ART is poison and is promoted to generate profits for pharmaceutical companies. Other dissidents aver that there is no AIDS epidemic in sub-Saharan Africa. They maintain that the deaths attributed to AIDS resulted from malnutrition and the lack of clean, safe water supplies—circumstances that most observers believe have hindered efforts to stem the epidemic but did not cause it.

Critics of Duesberg and other AIDS denialists contend that the adoption of their beliefs has led to the premature death of hundreds of thousands of people affected by HIV. In "Death by Denial: The Campaigners Who Continue to Deny HIV Causes AIDS" (Guardian .com, February 12, 2012), Brian Deer reports that the denialist beliefs of Thabo Mbeki (1942–), who as president of South Africa from June 1999 to September 2008 delayed widespread use of ART, resulted in more than 300,000 deaths and 35,000 preventable infections.

Other denialists seek to promote alternative treatment to ART. For example, Matthias Rath (1955–), a German physician, urges people living with HIV/AIDS to abandon prescribed treatment in favor of high doses of vitamins and other nutrients. Rath claims that his vitamin regimens will prevent or even cure AIDS as well as other chronic diseases. Michael Specter notes in "The Denialists" (NewYorker.com, March 12, 2007) that Rath has been criticized by many organizations, including the Joint United Nations Programme on HIV/AIDS and the South African Medical Association, and that the U.S. Food and Drug Administration deems material on Rath's website to be misleading.

AIDS denialism persists in the 21st century. In "'There Is No Proof That HIV Causes AIDS': AIDS Denialism Beliefs among People Living with HIV/AIDS" (*Journal of Behavioral Medicine*, vol. 33, no. 6, December 2010), Seth C. Kalichman, Lisa Eaton, and Chauncey Cherry report the results of their study of the prevalence of AIDS denialism beliefs and their association to health-related outcomes among people living with HIV/AIDS. The researchers surveyed African American men and women living with HIV/AIDS. One out of five survey participants expressed the belief that there is no proof that HIV causes AIDS and that treatment does more harm than good. The respondents who held these beliefs were less likely to be on ART and as a result were in poorer health. Kalichman, Eaton, and Cherry conclude, "Openly discussing the baseless views of AIDS denialists and exposing the pseudoscience behind AIDS denialism is key to diluting its impact.... Ignoring AIDS denialism undermines our best efforts to test, engage, and care for people living with HIV/AIDS."

In September 2014 Patricia Goodson, a professor of health education at Texas A&M University, published "Questioning the HIV-AIDS Hypothesis: 30 Years of Dissent" in *Frontiers in Public Health*, a peer-reviewed journal. Publication of the paper was immediately questioned, and the journal opted to call the paper an opinion piece and publish an argument against it.

HIV/AIDS AWARENESS EFFORTS

Many national and global initiatives and observances are conducted in an effort to inform the public, heighten awareness, and improve understanding of the HIV/AIDS pandemic. This section describes some of the activities, individuals, and groups that are involved in the ongoing effort to educate, motivate, and mobilize people to prevent the spread of HIV and to assist those who are living with HIV/AIDS.

The U.S. Department of Health and Human Services (2015, http://www.aids.gov/news-and-events/awareness-days) designates the annual observation of HIV/AIDS Awareness Days. These include:

- February 7, National Black HIV/AIDS Awareness Day—this annual awareness day was created by a community-based coalition to raise awareness among African Americans about HIV/AIDS and its disproportionate and devastating impact on African American communities.

- March 10, National Women and Girls HIV/AIDS Awareness Day—this day aims to raise awareness of the increasing impact of HIV/AIDS on the lives of women and girls.

- March 20, National Native HIV/AIDS Awareness Day—this day was created to increase awareness of the impact of HIV/AIDS on Native Americans, Alaskan Natives, and Hawaiians.

- April 10, National Youth HIV & AIDS Awareness Day—this day was created to educate the public about the impact of HIV and AIDS on young people as well as highlight the work young people are doing to combat the HIV/AIDS epidemic.

- May 18, HIV Vaccine Awareness Day—this day recognizes and acknowledges the people who are working to help find an HIV preventive vaccine, such as the clinical trial volunteers, the nurses, the community educators/recruiters, and the researchers.

- May 19, National Asian and Pacific Islander HIV/AIDS Awareness Day—this awareness day intends to increase awareness among Asians and Pacific Islanders about the ruinous impact of HIV/AIDS.

- June 8, Caribbean American HIV/AIDS Awareness Day—this day is a national mobilization effort that is designed to encourage Caribbean American and Caribbean-born individuals across the United States and its territories to become better informed and educated, obtain testing, and seek treatment.

- June 27, National HIV Testing Day—this day aims to provide opportunities for testing, especially for those who have never been tested or who have engaged in high-risk behavior since their last test, and to help dispel the myths and stigmas that are associated with HIV.

- September 18, National HIV/AIDS and Aging Awareness Day—this day aims to heighten awareness of the impact of HIV/AIDS on older adults. It intends to focus on HIV prevention, care, and treatment of people aged 50 years and older.

- September 27, National Gay Men's HIV/AIDS Awareness Day—this day aims to regain and refocus the attention of a community that has been disproportionately affected by the HIV/AIDS epidemic at a time when the United States confronts the simultaneous challenges of a resurgence of new HIV infections among gay men and growing complacency about HIV/AIDS among gay men.

- October 15, National Latino AIDS Awareness Day—this awareness day marks an opportunity to communicate the devastating and disproportionate effects AIDS is having on the Hispanic community.

- December 1, World AIDS Day—started by the World Health Organization in 1988, this day serves to focus global attention on the HIV/AIDS pandemic. Observance of this day provides an opportunity for governments, national AIDS programs, churches, community organizations, and individuals to demonstrate the importance of the fight against HIV/AIDS.

The AIDS Memorial Quilt

The AIDS Memorial Quilt is not only an ongoing community art project that pays tribute to and commemorates the lives claimed by AIDS but also serves as a powerful visual way to inform, educate, and heighten awareness of the lives lost in this epidemic. The AIDS Memorial Quilt notes in "History of the Quilt" (2015, http://www.aidsquilt.org/about/the-aids-memorial-quilt) that the quilt consists of cloth panels that have been designed and made by friends and families of people who died from AIDS-related illnesses. Cleve Jones (1954–), a San Francisco, California, gay rights activist, had the idea for the quilt in November 1985, and the quilt was started in June 1987, when Jones and a group of his friends in San Francisco decided to memorialize people who had died from AIDS-related illnesses.

The first public display of the quilt was at the National Mall in Washington, D.C., in October 1987. It contained 1,920 panels and was larger than a football field. The quilt, and enthusiasm for it, grew quickly. One year later the quilt had grown to 8,288 panels. Each time the quilt was displayed the names of those honored by it were read aloud by celebrities, politicians, family members, and friends.

As reported in "History of the Quilt," by 2015 more than 14 million people had seen the 1.3-million-square-foot (121,000-square-m) quilt. The quilt has traveled around the world, raising awareness and money (more than $4 million) for AIDS-related research and programs. It has been the subject of stories, papers, articles, and books and was nominated for a Nobel Peace Prize in 1989. That same year a feature-length documentary about it, *Common Threads: Stories from the Quilt*, won an Academy Award.

In "The AIDS Quilt, and Hoping for 'The Last One'" (CNN.com, July 24, 2012), Julie Rhoad of the NAMES Project Foundation, an international nonprofit organization that is the caretaker of the AIDS Memorial Quilt, states: "Throughout its 25-year history, [it] has been used to fight prejudice, and to raise awareness and funding for direct service and advocacy groups. The Quilt is a catalyst and conduit, a tool for healing and grief therapy, a springboard for frank dialogue.... It gives voice to far too many lives lost, telling us that never again should we ever leave a community in need and dying, ignored and uncared for. It is a stark reminder that we can never forget that we are all inextricably linked in life."

AIDS Activists

AIDS activists have been credited with raising awareness and attracting money and media attention to the pandemic. Many groups, individuals, and celebrities have taken on the cause and become champions of HIV/AIDS research, prevention, and treatment. Others have agitated to change the course of national and government policy and to improve access to and availability of quality care, especially affordable drug treatment. Still others have defended the rights of people living with HIV/AIDS in an effort to counter stigmatization and discrimination. Using a variety of approaches—from fund-raising campaigns and political lobbying to protests and guerrilla theater (dramatization of a social issue, often performed outdoors in a park or on the street)—AIDS activists have raised their voices and the consciousness of people around the world.

Although there are many groups and organizations engaged in AIDS activism, the most effective and vibrant organization is probably the AIDS Coalition to Unleash Power (ACT UP). ACT UP (2015, http://www.actupny.org) describes itself as "a diverse, non-partisan group of individuals united in anger and committed to direct action to end the AIDS crisis." It states, "We advise and inform. We demonstrate. We are not silent. Silence = Death." ACT UP has thousands of members in more than 70 chapters in the United States and worldwide. The organization advocates nonviolent direct action through vocal demonstrations and acts of civil disobedience that are intended to make the public aware of the crucial issues of the AIDS crisis. During a span of more than 25 years, ACT UP members have staged scores of protests and demonstrations and have often been arrested, usually for civil disobedience.

AIDS United (2015, http://www.aidsunited.org/About.aspx), another national organization, describes its mission as "strategic grantmaking, capacity building, and advocacy." AIDS United has played a key role in the development and implementation of public health policies to improve the quality of life for Americans who are HIV positive. It also works with the public health community to enhance HIV-prevention programs and care and treatment services.

The AIDS Treatment Activists Coalition is also a national coalition of AIDS activists who work together to end the AIDS epidemic by advancing research on HIV/AIDS. The coalition's mission statement (2015, http://www.thebody.com/content/art53683.html) has as its goals:

- To encourage greater and more effective involvement of people with HIV/AIDS in the decisions that affect their lives by identifying, mentoring and empowering treatment activists in all communities affected by the epidemic

- To develop within all communities affected by HIV/AIDS and related coinfections the leadership to provide the knowledge and skills needed to advocate for improved research, treatment and access to care

- To enable treatment activists to speak with a united, powerful voice to provide meaningful input into issues concerning HIV disease and related complications and coinfections

- To facilitate communications and set agenda items...between HIV/AIDS treatment activists and government, industry and academia in matters affecting research, treatment and access [and] among HIV/AIDS treatment activists and the larger HIV community in keeping up to date with the latest developments in research, treatment and access

CELEBRITIES SHINE A SPOTLIGHT ON HIV/AIDS. When celebrities endorse or lend their name to charitable causes, the causes often benefit from increased media attention and visibility. When celebrities actively work to promote their chosen causes, the results can be even more dramatic. For example, Tyler Curry lists in "10 Celebrity Icons of HIV Activism" (Advocate.com, April 5, 2015) Madonna (1958–), Elizabeth Taylor (1932–2011), Bono (1960–), Alicia Keys (1981–), Rihanna (1988–), former President Bill Clinton (1946–), Annie Lenox (1954–), Elton John (1947–), Joan Rivers (1923–2014), and Miley Cyrus (1992–).

The Irish musician Bono uses his celebrity to champion the fight against HIV/AIDS. In 2002 he formed the organization Debt AIDS Trade Africa (DATA), an advocacy organization that was dedicated to eradicating extreme poverty and AIDS in Africa. In 2005 Bono was named *Time*'s Person of the Year along with Bill Gates (1955–) and Melinda Gates (1964–). The following year he was nominated for a Nobel Peace Prize.

In 2008 DATA merged with ONE (http://www.one.org/us), a global antipoverty organization that pursues high-level global advocacy in concert with grassroots mobilization efforts. Like DATA, ONE's (2015, http://www.one.org/international/about/faqs/what-is-ones-mission) mission is to "fight extreme poverty and preventable disease in the poorest places on the planet, particularly in Africa." ONE partners with other global relief and HIV/AIDS initiatives, including the Bill and Melinda Gates Foundation, Bread for Life, CARE, Islamic Relief, Malaria No More, Oxfam America, Physicians for Peace, (RED), Save the

Children, and the White Ribbon Alliance for Safe Motherhood.

(RED) (2015, http://www.red.org) involves the private and public sectors in a fund-raising initiative. Companies whose products carry the (RED) insignia pledge to contribute a significant percentage of their sales or a portion of their profits from those products to the Global Fund to finance AIDS programs in Africa, with an emphasis on the health of women and children. The Global Fund (2015, http://www.red.org/en/learn/the-global-fund), which is supported by the funds that (RED) generates, is the world's leading financer of programs to fight AIDS, tuberculosis, and malaria. The Global Fund invests $4 billion per year for programs in 140 countries. Since 2003 PEPFAR and the Global Fund have provided funding for free antiretroviral drugs to countries where they are urgently needed.

Other celebrities including George Clooney (1961–), Matt Damon (1970–), Richard Gere (1949–), Whoopi Goldberg (1955–), Lady Gaga (1986–), and Sharon Stone (1958–) contribute their time, energy, and money to combat the HIV/AIDS pandemic.

Many young celebrities have also taken up the cause. The article "Celebrities Changing the World for HIV-Positive People" (HIVPlusMag.com, July 21, 2013) indicates that Vinny Guadagnino (1988–), Khloe Kardashian (1984–), and Snoop Dog (1971–) have promoted HIV prevention. The music industry has also taken up the cause. Educational material about HIV and free condoms were offered by Lifebeat's Tour Outreach program (2015, http://lifebeat.org/programs/outreach) at concerts by A$AP Ferg (1988–), Fools Gold Day Off , Wiz Khalifa (1987–), Kendrick Lamar (1987–), Lil' Kim (1975–), Mad Decent Block Party, Madonna, Mac Miller (1992–), and Sam Smith (1992–). Lifebeat's Hearts & Voices Program (2015, http://lifebeat.org/programs/hearts-voices) brings concerts to hospitals, residential facilities, and day-treatment programs. Among the musicians and groups that have participated are Destiny's Child, Jewel (1974–), LL Cool J (1968–), Maroon 5, Jon Secada (1962–), and Kanye West (1977–).

IMPORTANT NAMES
AND ADDRESSES

ACT UP/New York
332 Bleecker St., PMB G5
New York, NY 10014
URL: http://www.actupny.org/

AIDS United
1424 K St. NW, Ste. 200
Washington, DC 20005
(202) 408-4848
FAX: (202) 408-1818
URL: http://www.aidsunited.org/

American Foundation for AIDS Research
120 Wall St., 13th Floor
New York, NY 10005-3908
(212) 806-1600
FAX: (212) 806-1601
URL: http://www.amfar.org/

America's Essential Hospitals
1301 Pennsylvania Ave. NW, Ste. 950
Washington, DC 20004-1712
(202) 585-0100
FAX: (202) 585-0101
E-mail: info@essentialhospitals.org
URL: http://essentialhospitals.org/

Center for Women Policy Studies
1776 Massachusetts Ave. NW, Ste. 450
Washington, DC 20036
(202) 872-1770
FAX: (202) 296-8962
E-mail: cwps@centerwomenpolicy.org
URL: http://www.centerwomenpolicy.org/

Centers for Disease Control and Prevention
1600 Clifton Rd.
Atlanta, GA 30329-4027
1-800-232-4636
URL: http://www.cdc.gov/

Human Rights Campaign
1640 Rhode Island Ave. NW
Washington, DC 20036-3278
(202) 628-4160

1-800-777-4723
FAX: (202) 347-5323
URL: http://www.hrc.org/

Joint United Nations Programme on HIV/AIDS
20 Ave. Appia
CH-1211 Geneva 27
Switzerland
(011-41-22) 791-3666
FAX: (011-41-22) 791-4187
URL: http://www.unaids.org/

Kaiser Family Foundation
2400 Sand Hill Rd.
Menlo Park, CA 94025
(650) 854-9400
FAX: (650) 854-4800
URL: http://www.kff.org/

National Hemophilia Foundation
7 Penn Plaza, Ste. 1204
New York, NY 10001
(212) 328-3700
1-800-424-2634
FAX: (212) 328-3777
E-mail: handi@hemophilia.org
URL: http://www.hemophilia.org/

National Institute of Allergy and Infectious Diseases
6610 Rockledge Dr., MSC 6612
Bethesda, MD 20892-6612
(301) 496-5717
1-866-284-4107
FAX: (301) 402-3573
URL: http://www.niaid.nih.gov/

National Minority AIDS Council
1931 13th St. NW
Washington, DC 20009-4432
(202) 483-6622
FAX: (202) 483-1135
E-mail: communications@nmac.org
URL: http://www.nmac.org/

National Prevention Information Network
PO Box 6003
Rockville, MD 20849-6003
(404) 679-3860
1-800-458-5231
FAX: 1-888-282-7681
E-mail: NPIN-info@cdc.gov
URL: https://npin.cdc.gov/

National Women's Health Network
1413 K St. NW, Fourth Floor
Washington, DC 20005
(202) 682-2640
FAX: (202) 682-2648
E-mail: nwhn@nwhn.org
URL: http://www.nwhn.org/

ONE
1400 Eye St. NW, Ste. 600
Washington, DC 20005
(202) 495-2700
URL: http://www.one.org/us/

TeenAIDS-PeerCorps
PO Box 8460
Norfolk, VA 23503
(757) 352-2055
E-mail: teenaids@gmail.com
URL: http://www.teenaids.org

U.S. Department of Health and Human Services
AIDSinfo
PO Box 4780
Rockville, MD 20849-6303
1-800-448-0440
FAX: (301) 315-2818
E-mail: contactus@aidsinfo.nih.gov
URL: http://aidsinfo.nih.gov/

U.S. Food and Drug Administration
10903 New Hampshire Ave.
Silver Spring, MD 20993
1-888-463-6332
URL: http://www.fda.gov/cder

RESOURCES

The Centers for Disease Control and Prevention (CDC) provides the most current accounting of the HIV/AIDS epidemic in the United States. Publications cited in this text include "1993 Revised Classification System for HIV Infection and Expanded Surveillance Case Definition for AIDS among Adolescents and Adults" (Kenneth G. Castro et al., December 1992), "Revised Surveillance Case Definitions for HIV Infection—United States, 2014" (Richard M. Selik et al., April 2014), "Basic Statistics" (May 2015), "Current Trends Update: Impact of the Expanded AIDS Surveillance Case Definition for Adolescents and Adults on Case Reporting—United States, 1993" (*Morbidity and Mortality Weekly Report*, March 1994), "Populations at Higher Risk for HIV: Route of Transmission" (September 2014), "STDs and HIV—CDC Fact Sheet" (April 2015), "HIV in Correctional Settings" (June 2012), "Updated U.S. Public Health Service Guidelines for the Management of Occupational Exposures to HIV and Recommendations for Postexposure Prophylaxis" (Adelisa L. Panlilio et al., September 2005), "Surveillance of Occupationally Acquired HIV/AIDS in Healthcare Personnel, as of December 2010" (May 2011), "Updated U.S. Public Health Service Guidelines for the Management of Occupational Exposures to HIV and Recommendations for Postexposure Prophylaxis" (September 2013), and "Integrated Prevention Services for HIV Infection, Viral Hepatitis, Sexually Transmitted Diseases, and Tuberculosis for Persons Who Use Drugs Illicitly: Summary Guidance from CDC and the U.S. Department of Health and Human Services" (Hrishikesh Belani et al., November 2012).

HIV Surveillance Reports are prepared by the CDC and describe and quantify transmission categories, risk factor combinations, demographics, and people living with HIV/ AIDS. Other CDC publications that were used to prepare this book include *Epidemiology of HIV Infection through 2012* (2015), *HIV Surveillance Report: Diagnoses of HIV Infection and AIDS in the United States and Dependent Areas, 2013* (February 2015), "HIV among African Americans" (July 2015), *HIV Surveillance in Women* (June 2015), *HIV Surveillance Report: Diagnoses of HIV Infection in the United States and Dependent Areas, 2013,* (February 2015), "HIV among Pregnant Women, Infants, and Children" (June 2015), and "HIV among People Aged 50 and Over" (May 2015).

The National Institutes of Health's Panel on Antiretroviral Therapy and Medical Management of HIV-Infected Children published *Guidelines for the Use of Antiretroviral Agents in Pediatric HIV Infection* (March 2015). The CDC National Center for Health Statistics publishes findings from the Youth Risk Behavior Surveys, the National HIV Behavioral Surveillance System, and the *National Vital Statistics Reports*.

Information about the worldwide effects of HIV/AIDS, as well as global projections, were provided by the World Health Organization reports, including *How AIDS Changed Everything* (July 2015), *HIV/AIDS Data and Statistics* (2015), "Blood Safety and Availability" (June 2015), *Consolidated Guidelines on HIV Prevention, Diagnosis, Treatment and Care for Key Populations* (July 2014), *Guidelines for Intensified Tuberculosis Case-Finding and Isoniazid Preventive Therapy for People Living with HIV in Resource-Constrained Settings* (2011), and *Guidelines on HIV and Infant Feeding 2010: Principles and Recommendations for Infant Feeding in the Context of HIV and a Summary of Evidence* (2010). Furthermore, the Joint United Nations Programme on HIV/AIDS published *2014 China AIDS Response Progress Report* (June 2014) and *Fact Sheet 2014* (2014), and the United Nations Children's Fund released *HIV/AIDS and Children: Analysis of Achievements and Challenges* (September 2014).

Medical and scientific journals provide a wealth of information about the HIV/AIDS pandemic. Articles cited in this publication were published in *AIDS and Behavior, AIDS Care, AIDS Care: Psychological and Socio-medical*

Aspects of AIDS/HIV, AIDS Research and Human Retroviruses, AIDS Research and Therapy, AIDS Research and Treatment, American Journal of Preventive Medicine, Annals of Internal Medicine, Archives of Oral Biology, BMC Public Health, British Medical Journal, Cancer Research, Clinical Infectious Diseases, Clinical Microbiology and Infection, Clinics in Chest Medicine, Clinics in Perinatology, Current HIV Research, European Heart Journal, Frontiers in Microbiology, Frontiers in Public Health, HIV Clinician, HIV Medicine, Indian Journal of Experimental Biology, Infectious Disease Clinics, International Journal of Epidemiology, International Journal of High Risk Behavior and Addiction, Issues in Mental Health Nursing, Journal of AIDS & Clinical Research, Journal of Behavioral Medicine, Journal of Experimental Medicine, Journal of the International AIDS Society, Journal of the National Cancer Institute, Journal of Public Health Policy, Journal of Women's Health, Journal of Youth and Adolescence, Lancet, Lancet Infectious Diseases, Maternal and Child Health Journal, Medical Care, Modern Healthcare, Molecular Therapy, Nature, Nature Chemical Biology, Nature Immunology, Nature Medicine, New England Journal of Medicine, Nursing Forum, Open AIDS Journal, PLoS Medicine, PLoS One, Proceedings of the American Thoracic Society, Retrovirology, Science, Science & Society, Science Translational Medicine, Sexually Transmitted Diseases, Sexually Transmitted Infections, Social Science and Medicine, and Substance Abuse Treatment, Prevention, and Policy.

Timely information about many facets of HIV/AIDS may be found at the website TheBody.com and the American Foundation for AIDS Research (http://www.amfar.org/). The National AIDS Housing Coalition provided information on housing opportunities for people with HIV/AIDS.

The Kaiser Family Foundation publications "HIV/AIDS in the Lives of Gay and Bisexual Men in the United States" (Liz Hamel et al., September 2014), *Health Insurance Coverage for People with HIV under the Affordable Care Act: Experiences in Five States* (Jennifer Kates et al., December 2014), the fact sheet "U.S. Federal Funding for HIV/AIDS: The President's FY 2016 Budget Request" (April 2015), and "The Global HIV/AIDS Epidemic" (July 2015) were used to prepare this publication. The Kaiser Family Foundation also provides daily updates about a variety of issues that are related to HIV/AIDS on its website (http://www.kff.org/).

We are grateful to the Gallup Organization for permitting us to present the results of its renowned opinion polls and graphics depicting Americans' feelings about HIV/AIDS.

INDEX

PEPFAR treatment results, 125*f*
scope of problem, 111–112
sub-Saharan Africa, 115–118
triumphs/challenges, 123–124
tuberculosis, HIV/AIDS and, 113–114
Uganda, HIV prevalence/new infections/
AIDS deaths in, 118*f*
western/central Europe, 118–119
young people, global HIV infection
among, 67–68

X

XDR-TB. *See* Extensively drug-resistant
TB

Y

Yanik, Elizabeth L., 20
Young adults
adults ever tested for HIV by age group/
sex, 94*f*
as AIDS activists, 70–71
HIV diagnoses in persons aged
13–24, by transmission category,
95*f*
with HIV/AIDS, 93–94
patterns of infection among,
68–70
See also Adolescents
Young, Saundra, 13

"The Youth Risk Behavior
Surveillance—United States, 2013"
(Kann et al.), 69
Youth Risk Behavior Surveys (CDC),
106–107

Z

Zavis, Alexandra, 129
Zeidler, Sari, 27
Zidovudine
ADAPs established to help pay
for, 74
for early intervention, 99
effects of, 83